MW00568928

The University of Rochester Medical Center

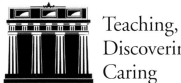

Teaching,
Discovering,
Caring

With thanks for
all you've done
and best wishes
[signature]

The University of Rochester Medical Center

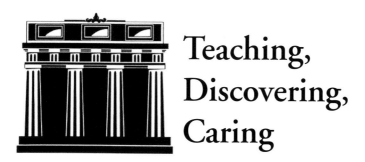

Teaching,
Discovering,
Caring

Seventy-Five Years of Achievement

1925–2000

EDITED BY
JULES COHEN AND ROBERT J. JOYNT
WITH THE EDITORIAL ASSISTANCE OF
NANCY W. BOLGER

University of Rochester Press
Rochester, New York

First published 2000
by the University of Rochester Press

The University of Rochester Press is an imprint of Boydell & Brewer, Inc.
668 Mount Hope Avenue, Rochester, NY 14620, USA
and of Boydell & Brewer, Ltd.
P.O. Box 9, Woodbridge, Suffolk, 1P12 3DF, UK

ISBN 1580460836 (cl)
ISBN 1580460917 (pb)

Library of Congress Cataloging-in-Publication Data

Teaching, discovering, caring : the University of Rochester Medical Center : seventy-five years of achievement, 1925–2000 / edited Jules Cohen and Robert J. Joynt ;
        p. ; cm.
    ISBN 1-58046-083-6 (cloth : alk. paper)—ISBN 1-58046-091-7 (pbk. : alk. paper)
    1. Academic medical centers—New York (State)—Rochester—History, 20th entury.
2. Medical colleges—New York (State)—Rochester—History—20th century.
I. Cohen, Jules, 1931– II. Joynt, Robert J., 1925– III. Bolger, Nancy W.
[DNLM: 1. University of Rochester. Medical Center. 2. Academic Medical Centers—history—New York. 3. Education, Medical—history—New York. WX 28 AN6 T253 2000]
RA975.T43 .T43 2000
610'.71'174789—dc21   00-064787

British Library Cataloging-in-Publication Data
A catalogue record for this item is available from the British Library.

Designed and typeset by JM Book Packaging
Printed in the United States of America
This publication is printed on acid-free paper.

This volume is dedicated to
the faculty, staff, students, and alumni
of the School of Medicine and Dentistry,
the School of Nursing, Strong Memorial
Hospital, and our affiliated hospitals,
who have inspired and brought about the
achievements described in this book—and
have made the University of Rochester
Medical Center a beloved and respected
institution.

CONTENTS

FOREWORD

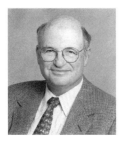

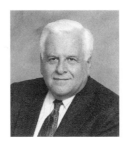

JAY H.
STEIN, M.D.

LOWELL A.
GOLDSMITH, M.D.

Early in 1923, a tough young construction crew began tearing up the sod in a field not far from the Genesee River in Rochester, New York. A steam shovel arrived and chugged into action, shattering the quiet of a peaceful rural morning on the Crittenden Tract. Hour after hour, day after day, a parade of horse-drawn wagons wheeled away mountains of displaced soil. Before long the steam shovel was joined by a monster pile driver, requisitioned to pound steel supports through layers of rock.

By September 1925, the foundations, both physical and intellectual, of a brave and innovative medical enterprise were firmly in place and the doors of the nation's newest medical school opened to its first class of twenty-two students.

The dream that was brought to reality that day had been several years in the making. Five years earlier, in 1920, the cream of the country's medical reformers, brought together by the Rockefeller Foundation and represented by its general secretary, Abraham Flexner, turned to the University of Rochester, and to its benefactor George Eastman, to create a new model of medical education. The question was set before them: Would Rochester become one of five or six new centers dedicated to transforming the nation's medical education from its haphazard Victorian state—often characterized by medical "diploma mills," unlicensed practitioners, and rowdy, undisciplined medical students—into a medical education system worthy of the 20th century? Eastman and the University of Rochester accepted the challenge.

Within the simple, spare medical school building that rose on that lot, and in the spartan hospital that grew almost simultaneously as its twin, an exceptionally gifted group of faculty gathered to meet the challenge sounded by the Rockefeller Foundation. Led by their redoubtable dean and faculty colleague George Hoyt Whipple, this small number of visionary professors— brilliant and dedicated to their work and to their students—set a standard of intellectual excellence, whose brilliance remains untarnished seventy-five years later.

In the mid-1940s, some twenty years after those first bricks were laid, another transforming event began to unfold. John Romano arrived in Rochester to become the medical school's first chair of Psychiatry; his partner in revolutionizing medical education, George Engel, was soon to follow. Together, Romano and Engel infused the curriculum with a radical idea: doctors need to be taught how to listen to their patients and they need to understand that health and illness are influenced by a multitude of forces—familial, societal, economic, cultural, and spiritual, as well as biological. Learning the art of physician-patient dialogue and understanding its importance are at the heart of what has come to be called (to use Engel's term) the biopsychosocial model. This model is still the hallmark of a University of Rochester-educated physician.

In the year 2000, we stand poised on the edge of a new medical revolution. As the mysteries of genetic makeup are rapidly being decoded, the University of Rochester Medical Center is transforming to meet the challenges of a new millenium. On the site where men with horse-drawn wagons once toiled to build a small, hopeful medical school, there now stands a major medical center ready to meet the challenges of a dramatic future.

Three years ago the most dramatic undertaking in the history of the University of Rochester began as the University of Rochester Medical Center implemented a ten-year, $400 million strategic plan which will place the Medical Center in the top echelon of medical research centers worldwide. Last year, the Arthur Kornberg Medical Research Building (named for one of our Nobel laureate alumni) and the Aab Institute of Biomedical Sciences were inaugurated. The first of the seventy new researchers and four hundred technicians and support personnel to be added to our ranks have been recruited. Research-focused centers have been created in subspecialties that include Vaccine Biology and Immunology, Cancer Biology, Human Genetics and Molecular Pediatric Disease, Aging and Developmental Biology, Cardiovascular Research, and Oral Biology, and internationally known scientists have been brought to Rochester to direct these programs.

Research is essential, but at the heart of any medical center is informed, compassionate patient care. In developing Strong Health, the University's comprehensive healthcare delivery system, we have brought together a cohort of care-giving professionals from Strong Memorial Hospital, Children's Hospital at Strong, Highland Hospital, the Eastman Dental Center, the Highlands at Pittsford and the Highlands at Brighton (both residential, long-term care facilities), the Visiting Nurse Service, and the University of Rochester Medical Faculty Group. Thanks to these professionals, we are able to respond quickly, proactively, and effectively to the needs of the more than half-million patients who turn to us each year for their health-care needs.

At the School of Nursing, other dramatic transformations are underway. As our nurse-scientists continue their research in the laboratory and in the community, their findings infuse and improve patient care, both here and around the country. A new generation of men and women are turning to the School of Nursing for a nursing education that can be combined with an MBA degree to open careers in health-care systems management and administration. At the same time, Rochester's nurse-educators have created a new curriculum that better meets the needs of today's adult learners, many of whom are practicing nurses refining and expanding their skills to meet the scientific and social challenges of the 21st century.

And at the School of Medicine and Dentistry, the Double Helix Curriculum was introduced this fall. This revolutionary program—the most dramatic shift in American medical education in more than half a century—has captured the attention of medical educators across the nation. In addition, the recent restructuring of our graduate programs around subspecialty research clusters promises to prepare a new generation of research scientists who will have a major impact on the understanding and treatment of cancer, heart disease, Alzheimer's disease, and other conditions.

Over the past 75 years, our world has been transformed in ways that our founders could not have imagined. They built, however, beyond their vision. They and their successors taught, mentored, and inspired thousands of alumni whose work, in a multitude of fields, has made the transformation possible.

This publication, prepared with love, to celebrate the University of Rochester Medical Center's 75th anniversary, is a rich chronicle of achievements. We congratulate the authors and editors, and all those whose work is honored within these pages. Their legacy will sustain us, as we step confidently into a bright new future.

Jay H. Stein, M.D.
Senior Vice President
and Vice Provost for Health Affairs

Lowell A. Goldsmith, M.D.
Dean, School of Medicine and Dentistry

ACKNOWLEDGMENTS

The editors and authors acknowledge with gratitude those who have contributed to the preparation of this book by providing ideas and historical memory. Some have contributed written material, others have met with one or more of the authors to provide insights and information. We are grateful to them all. These valuable contributors include:

Allan Anderson	Eleanor Hall	Sandra Morgan
William Barker	William Hall	John Morton
Robert Berg	J. Peter Harris	Gerald Murphy
Robert Betts	Diane Hartmann	J. Lowell Orbison
Donald Bordley	Arthur Hengerer	Daniel Ornt
Leo Brideau	Christopher Hoolihan	Pradyumna Phatak
Bernard Brody	Laurence Jacobs	Arvin Robinson
Andy Brooks	Jean Johnson	Philip Rubin
Richard Burton	Ralph Jozefowicz	Jacob Schlesinger
Lee Caldwell	James Kendig	Seymour Schwartz
Grace Centola	Kathleen King	Stephen Silver
Steven Ching	Christine Kurland	Jenny Smith
Frank Colgan	Robert Lawrence	Richard Sterns
James DeWees	John Leddy	David Stewart
John Dickinson	Marshal Lichtman	James Stewart
Nancy Dimmick	Arthur Liebert	Andrew Swinburne
Frank Disney	John Looney	Henry Thiede
John Frazer	Robert McCormack	Alvin Ureles
Donna Greenberg	Susan McDaniel	Mark Utell
Robert Griggs	Patricia McLane	Elizabeth White
Paul Griner	Joyce Morgan	Lyman Wynne

75th Anniversary Planning and Publication Committee

Nancy Baldwin	Gilbert Forbes	Paul Lambiase
Jacqueline Beckerman	Karin Gaffney	Ruth Lawrence

Nancy Bolger   Eleanor Hall   Harriet Kitzman
Jules Cohen   John Hansen   Leon Miller
Richard Collins   Carolyn Hunt   Christopher Raimy
Mary Jo Ferr   Robert Joynt   Elizabeth White

A special note of heartfelt thanks goes to Amy Gregory and Rebecca DiNatale who served as staff to the publication project. Without their patience, dedication to the project, and high quality efforts, this book would never have been possible. We are deeply indebted to them.

INTRODUCTION
Beginnings and Medical Center Leadership

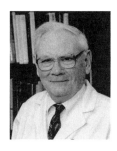

ROBERT J. JOYNT, M.D., PH.D.

PART 1: BEGINNINGS

There is an account, probably apocryphal, of a conversation between George Eastman and George Whipple. After the completion of the medical school and hospital in 1925, they took a stroll around the structure. Mr. Eastman turned to Dr. Whipple and said, "George, I don't think you will have to add another brick to that building." Their eyesight regarding the future expansion was faulty, but their vision was perfect. Although literally thousands of bricks have been added to the original structure—for the atomic energy project, Wing R, the education wing, the new Strong Memorial Hospital (now twenty-five years old), the outpatient facility, and the new Kornberg Research wing, among others—their idea of an institution where teaching, patient care, and research would progress in an integrated manner was sound and their vision of the future is as fresh today as it was 75 years ago.

While our institution is said to be a product of the Flexner Report of 1910, this is only partly true. The report, supported by the Carnegie Foundation for the Advancement of Teaching, is entitled *Medical Education in the United States and Canada*. There is no doubt that the report played a significant role in medical education, the most immediate impact being the closing of several inadequate schools; the number of schools in this country dropped from over 150 in 1910 to less than 100 in 1925. Certainly, it was the project proposal suggested by Abraham Flexner to George Eastman in 1920 that led to the construction of the medical school. However, it is equally true that George Whipple, the driving force behind this school, had very definite views on medical education prior to the Flexner Report. From his autobiographical sketch, biographies, and personal interviews, it is clear that he had formed, very early, his own views on medical education. These are likely to have been the result of his education at Johns Hopkins where he was in the last class taught by the great clinical teacher William Osler.

The Johns Hopkins model was mentioned as the paragon of medical education in the introduction to the Flexner Report by Henry S. Pritchett, the president of the foundation, and Whipple's early views mirrored the conclusions of the Flexner Report. Early on, Whipple saw the importance of good basic science teaching, done in well-equipped laboratories, by instructors in the forefront of research. He also knew the value of research for students and had participated in research as part of his medical education. He knew the importance of a unified medical school, as opposed to what he called "a split medical school" where the basic science, the clinical teaching, and the practice were done in different locales. It was also important to him

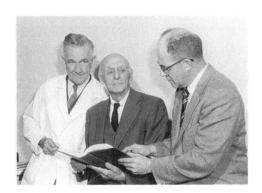

Left to right: George Whipple, Abraham Flexner, Donald Anderson

that the medical school be within a university so that a rigorous academic environment would prevail. He expressed his concern about clinical teachers who were distracted from their main role as educators by a heavy practice schedule, often removed from the medical school setting.

The events leading up to the construction of the school and hospital are described in detail by George Corner, M.D., in his biography of Whipple. Flexner convinced George Eastman to give a very generous amount for the school. Afterward, Mr. Eastman laughingly referred to Mr. Flexner as "the greatest highwayman west of the Hudson River." Nonetheless, George Eastman's vision of what could happen, when a great medical center was located in his beloved Rochester, was a necessary key. Indeed, without the initial gift of Mr. Eastman, Dr. Whipple, then forty-two years old, would not have considered coming here. The fact that $10 million, half from Eastman and half from the General Education Board of the Rockefeller Foundation, had already been received in gifts by the time of his recruitment was the major factor in his decision to move from San Francisco to Rochester. Dr. Whipple pointed out that Eastman's intense interest did not stop after his generosity; he also participated in the planning and construction of the Medical Center and supplied many useful suggestions. Much of the austerity of the construction has been attributed to Eastman; he said he was paying for "brains, not bricks."

Dr. Whipple, who disdained the idea of a "split medical school," had definite ideas about the building's construction. He felt strongly about the need to integrate teaching, research, and clinical practice. Therefore, the clinical departments, which were housed in the hospital, were juxtaposed to the basic science departments. The library was placed in the center so that it was easily accessible from all sides. The dining room was for faculty, students, and staff in order to promote collegiality. There was also horizontal integration; basic science departments were on the same floor as their related specific clinical departments. Thus, the operating room suites were next to the gross anatomy laboratories, the surgical offices were next to the surgical pathology laboratories, the medical floors were near Biochemistry, and the pediatric floors were near the bacteriology laboratories.

The final construction principle put forward was that each person was to be, as it is said, within "bare-headed distance" of one another. Thus, everything was under one roof. This theme continues today. The roof has grown very large, and occasionally leaky, but one can visit one's colleagues in any department, or in any area of the hospital, without leaving the building. This construction principle is a philosophical statement, and in the harsh upstate winters, it is also a meteorological blessing. To find out how important this idea is, one need only visit medical schools where the hospital is miles away or, as with some European universities, where each medical school department occupies a separate building.

The plans for the hospital were largely left to Nathaniel Faxon, M.D., who had been appointed hospital director by Dr. Whipple. While austerity was key to the construction

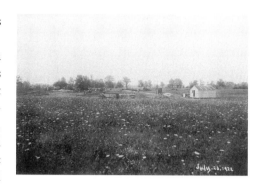

The site for the future Medical Center

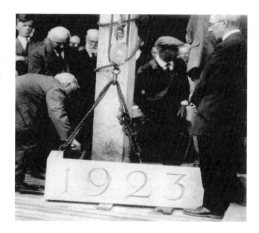

Laying the cornerstone, 1923

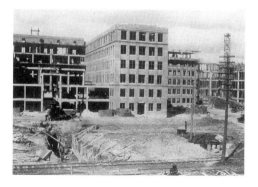

The Medical Center under construction, 1924

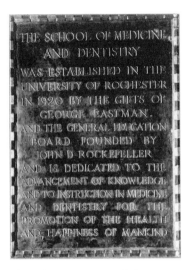

Plaque hanging in Miner Library

THE MEDICAL SCHOOL OF THE UNIVER-
SITY OF ROCHESTER

It is planned to open the new medical school of the
University of Rochester in September, 1925, and the
Strong Memorial Hospital, with its 240 beds, will
open a few weeks in advance, and the nurses' home
four months earlier, in order that its training school
may complete the training of an adequate staff of
undergraduate nurses before the hospital first opens
its doors to the public.

Considering 1925 as the year for the completion of
the building program of the school, it is estimated
that there will be available, from accumulated interest
and the Strong Memorial gift, approximately $3,-
000,000 for building expenses, without encroaching
upon the $9,000,000 capital originally donated. This
fund will be left intact, therefore, as an endowment
to provide for the running expenses of both school
and hospital. As far as is known, this is one of the
few instances on record where a large educational institution will have been built without encroaching
upon its original endowments. It is announced that
those entrusted with the destinies of the Rochester
institution have chosen deliberately to build modestly
and simply and to place the future reputation of the
school in its scholastic attainments rather than in its
outer appearance.

A final addition to the medical school and hospital
group, as at present planned, will be the new municipal hospital to contain 240 beds to be built by the
city of Rochester at some time in the near future
close by the Strong Memorial Hospital, and coordinated with it both physically and in its operation.
Piling already has been driven for the foundations
of this structure.

It will be remembered that the General Education
Board and George Eastman, of the Eastman Kodak
Company, provided the sum of $9,000,000 for the
foundation of a medical school for the University of
Rochester. To this amount was added a donation of
$1,000,000 from the two daughters of the late Henry
A. Strong for a hospital to be built in conjunction
with the school in order to enable it to carry out its
work under the most favorable conditions.

A note in Science *magazine announced
the opening of the medical school*

plan, Dr. Whipple agreed with Faxon that the entrance to the hospital should be warm and inviting. The young Rochester architect Carl Schmidt was assigned to draw up the plans for the entrance and lobby. In a taped inter-view, he recalled some of the issues surround-ing the design and construction, such as the importance of classical architectural features. Schmidt submitted the initial plans to Faxon, taking pains to detail all of the design fea-tures. Faxon indicated that in his experience, drawings with a lot of lines usually meant that construction would be expensive. Schmidt said that he erased most of the lines and Faxon approved the plans. The architect said that later he included all of the design features he had submitted in the early plans.

The building was ready for students a few years after construction began, and the first class, twenty men and two women, entered on September 17, 1925. At that time there were sixty-five faculty, handpicked by Dr. Whipple. His choices were excellent. Many faculty came from Johns Hopkins; George Corner, one of the founding faculty, said in an interview that they were known as the "Johns Hopkins Country Club of Roch-ester." While Dr. Whipple closely monitored the budget, he allowed for great scope in the faculty's teaching methods. Faculty engaged in their own research and were encouraged to include students in their programs. Stu-dent laboratories were well equipped for that time, they were not locked at night, and they were juxtaposed to faculty research laborato-ries. Dr. Edward Adolph believed this pro-vided an excellent model for the students. Re-search opportunities for students included summer and year-out fellowships, among oth-ers. An easy collegiality was set up between students and faculty and, although numbers have changed the character, much of this re-mains today.

Mr. Eastman, interested in dentistry,

ROBERT J. JOYNT

initiated a plan by which dental students would study with the medical students in basic science courses and then continue their clinical training at the dental infirmary, also started by Eastman. This plan determined the official name of the school, the School of Medicine and Dentistry. As there were no applicants for the program, the scheme was dropped after a few years but it did lead to a very successful post-graduate program in dental research. This program continues to train many international leaders. When the school is referred to as the School of Medicine, dental-faculty dentists cry: "dental extraction."

Helen Wood was appointed superintendent of nursing in 1922. Wood also designed a nursing degree program. The School of Nursing, originally a department of Strong Memorial Hospital, became a department of the medical school in 1960 and the eighth college of the university in 1972.

By 1926, all of the components of the Medical Center were in place—faculty, students, nurses, and staff. The hospital took in its first patient January 4, 1926; the first operation was performed January 7, 1926; and the first baby was delivered January 14, 1926.

There is no doubt that the success of the medical school is due to the early influence of its excellent faculty and to the first dean, Dr. George Whipple. My successor in the deanship, Marshall Lichtman, M.D., once said, "You can be a dean at Rochester, but you can never be *the* dean at Rochester." And that is as it should be.

Expenses

The tuition fee is $300 per annum, payable in equal installments at the beginning of each semester. A deposit of $25 will be required on *acceptance* of the candidate, which will apply on the first semester's fee but will be forfeited if the candidate does not enter and continue with the class for which he has enrolled.

Students will provide their own books, dissecting instruments, laboratory gowns and other equipment at a minimum cost of about $30 per year. These articles can be purchased in Rochester, and information as to the required books and equipment will be given at the beginning of the respective courses of instruction.

Each student must provide his own microscope, which will be constantly in use throughout the course and will be needed at once at the beginning of instruction. The microscope must be a compound instrument of the modern type, with 2 oculars (approximately x5 and x10) and with 3 objectives of about 16 mm., 4 mm., and 2 mm. oil immersion, and an Abbe condenser, all in good condition and yielding clear images. Arrangements can be made through the treasurer's office to purchase such an instrument on a partial payment plan.

From the first student handbook

This year we are celebrating the Medical Center's 75th year. Other publications have marked the Center's landmarks throughout the years. In 1936, a small paperbound book was published entitled *The First Decade: 1926–1936*. The anniversary committee was composed of five people, chaired by Dr. Whipple, and the book contains chapters on the beginning of the school, research, teaching programs, and clinical activities of the hospital. Although the book had no dedication, the frontispiece photograph was of George Eastman. There was also a tenth anniversary faculty lecture program, highlighted by an Eastman Lecture on diabetes given by Elliot Joslin, M.D., of Harvard University.

The quarter century was noted by a hardcover volume, *The First Quarter Century: 1925-1950*. There were eight members on this publication committee and it was chaired by Wallace Fenn, M.D. This publication expanded on the history given in the first publication and was organized in a similar manner.

The half century was marked with the publication of *To Each His Farthest Star,* which had a large editorial committee headed by John Romano, M.D. This volume is a series of essays by members of the faculty, former students, and others. Many of the essays are personal reminiscences of the school's early days. This volume is fortunate to have contributions by people who were here from the beginning. Particularly noteworthy is the inclusion of remarks by Dr. Fenn, given in 1950 at the dedication of the Whipple Auditorium, as well as an essay on the first medical school class by J. D. Goldstein, M.D. *To Each His Farthest Star* continues to be a valuable and entertaining source of information about the development of the Medical Center.

The 75th Anniversary Committee, appointed by Dean Lowell Goldsmith, was to design a program celebrating the 75th anniversary and to create a publication marking the event. The committee decided not to use the format used for *To Each His Farthest Star,* as that volume is still available. Unfortunately, we no longer have the benefit of the contributors who were present at the beginning of the institution.

We organized this publication as a historical account of the three major activities of the Medical Center—teaching, research, and clinical practice—with sections on nursing, dentistry, the library, and Strong Memorial Hospital. The authors are members of both the Anniversary Committee and the faculty and have many years of experience at the Medical Center, sharing a long perspective on its activities. In addition, we are fortunate to have a large repository of photographs, particularly depicting the first fifty years. We believe these photographs will bring back many memories.

This publication will not cover all of the history and accomplishments of the institution. While we would like it to be comprehensive, we have, necessarily, emphasized the later days that are more familiar to the contributors.

Further references are available for those who wish to learn more about the rich history of the institution. The following list includes publications available at the Edward G. Miner Library:

The First Decade: 1926-1936.

The First Quarter Century: 1925-1950.

To Each His Farthest Star, published 1975.

George Hoyt Whipple and His Friends, by George Corner.

Autobiographical Sketch, "George H. Whipple," *Perspectives in Biology and Medicine,* volume 2, spring 1959.

"George Hoyt Whipple, 1878–1976," a biographical memoir, by Leon Miller, in *Biographical Memoirs,* volume 66, 1995. National Academy Press, Washington.

Taped interviews, arranged by Edward Atwater, M.D.: George H. Whipple, Edward F. Adolph, Carl Schmidt, George Corner, Larry Kohn, William McCann, Karl Wilson.

ROBERT J. JOYNT

PART 2: MEDICAL SCHOOL AND MEDICAL CENTER LEADERSHIP

The academic and administrative titles held by the head of the School and Medical Center have changed throughout the years. The title Dean of the School of Medicine and Dentistry and Director of the University of Rochester Medical Center was held by Drs. Whipple, Anderson, Orbison, and Young. In 1981, during Young's tenure, the title of Director was dropped and was replaced by Vice President for Health Affairs. In 1984, when Dr. Joynt assumed the position, the Vice President title was dropped and he was designated Dean of the School of Medicine and Dentistry and Vice Provost for Health Affairs. In 1989 the title Vice President for Health Affairs was again activated. For a short time, while a search was underway for a new dean, Joynt was Dean and Vice President and Vice Provost for Health Affairs. In 1990 Marshall Lichtman became Dean and Joynt continued as Vice President and Vice Provost for Health Affairs. When Joynt retired from the position in 1994, Jay H. Stein, M.D., was named Vice President and Vice Provost for Health Affairs. In 1996 this title was changed to Senior Vice President and Vice Provost for Health Affairs; the following year the title Strong Health Chief Executive Officer was added. Lowell Goldsmith, M.D., became Dean of the School of Medicine and Dentistry in 1996.

The evolution of the title came about as the size and complexity of the Medical Center grew. The changes reflect a national trend in the designation of administrative and academic officers.

George H. Whipple, M.D.

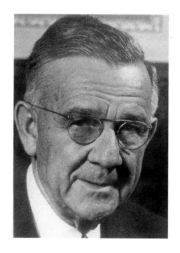

George Whipple was the first and founding dean of the medical school and hospital. Born and raised in New Hampshire, he graduated from Yale University with honors. At Johns Hopkins Medical School he became interested in pathology, which he chose as his career work.

In 1914 he went to the Hooper Institute at the University of California in Berkeley. Here he began his work on hemoglobin production, which led to his Nobel Prize in 1934.

In 1921 he was recruited by Rush Rhees, president of the University of Rochester, to form a new medical school. Whipple planned the school and the hospital and the first class entered in 1925.

As dean he set a tone for the medical school that continues today. He recruited the first faculty, who proved to be remarkable teachers, researchers, and clinicians. He encouraged collegiality between the students and the faculty and fostered research as part of the medical school education. He personally supervised the selection of medical students and counseled them while in school.

During Whipple's tenure there was great expansion in the institution's physical structure, including the wing for the atomic energy project, Wing-R for Psychiatry, and Q-wing for private patients.

During his time as dean he continued with active research. In addition to the Nobel Prize, he was awarded numerous honorary degrees, awards, and distinctions. He was also a member of the National Academy of Sciences.

After he retired as dean in 1953, Whipple remained active on the faculty. He died in 1976 at the age of ninety-seven.

Donald G. Anderson, M.D.

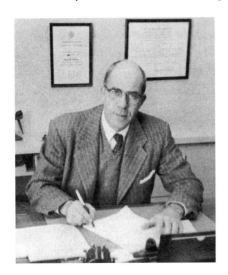

Donald Anderson succeeded Dr. Whipple as the second dean of the medical school in 1953. After graduating with honors from Harvard College in 1935, he received his medical degree from the College of Physicians and Surgeons, Columbia University, in 1939. He interned at Boston City Hospital and trained in pathology, and later in internal medicine, in New York and Boston. Anderson joined the faculty of the Boston University School of Medicine and served as dean at that institution from 1945 until 1947. While there, he collaborated in several research projects on the use of penicillin. He served as secretary for the Council on Medical Education of the American Medical Association from 1947 until 1953, when he was appointed dean at Rochester.

Several initiatives in medical education began during Anderson's deanship. Major changes in the medical curriculum were proposed by the Committee of Six, the general clerkship was started, as well as the innovative two-year internship. Medical school facilities for offices and research laboratories expanded with the construction of the GG-Wing. Anderson was also active in obtaining funds to increase faculty salaries.

While dean, Anderson was very active in national and international organizations related to medical education. He served as president of the Association of American Medical Colleges and was on the board of directors of several educational and certifying bodies.

Although Anderson left the deanship in 1965, he continued to work in the Department of Internal Medicine as an active teacher and clinician. He retired in 1978 and died in 1995.

J. Lowell Orbison, M.D.

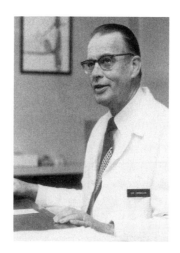

Lowell Orbison became dean in 1967 after serving one year as acting dean. He earned his undergraduate degree at Ottawa University in Ottawa, Kansas, a master's degree at Michigan State University, and his doctor of medicine degree at Northwestern University. After training in pathology in Cleveland, he joined the faculty of the medical school at Western Reserve University, where he was very active in designing a new curriculum for the medical school. He came to Rochester in 1955 as the George H. Whipple Professor of Pathology and Chair of the Department of Pathology.

While chair of Pathology, he actively combined teaching and research with his administrative duties. He served as president of the International Academy of Pathology and of the American Association of Pathologists and Bacteriologists.

Orbison's tenure as dean coincided with a time when the government was expanding health-care facilities and healthcare personnel education. The medical school class size grew from seventy-four to ninety-six students. The education wing, the cancer center, and the expansion of the R-Wing were built and, in 1975, the new Strong Memorial Hospital and the new outpatient area were finished. Other educational innovations marked his tenure, including expanded research facilities and programs and the independent study program. It was a transforming time for the Medical Center.

Dr. Orbison retired in 1979 and moved to North Carolina where he pursues his lifelong interest in nature.

Frank E. Young, M.D., Ph.D.

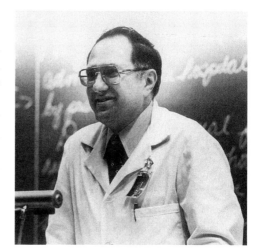

Frank Young became the fourth dean of the School of Medicine and Dentistry in 1979. He received his M.D. degree at the Upstate Medical Center in Syracuse in 1956, completed his internship at the University Hospitals in Cleveland, and then trained in pathology at Western Reserve University. Young completed his Ph.D. in the Department of Microbiology in 1962 at Western Reserve, where he served as a faculty member in Pathology until he moved to the Scripps Clinic and Research Foundation in 1965.

In 1970 Young came to the University of Rochester as Professor and Chair of Microbiology; in addition, he was Professor of Pathology and of Radiation Biology and Biophysics. He continued his active research program centering on molecular genetics, was active in many professional organizations, and consulted widely on scientific and educational matters. He is a member of the Institute of Medicine of the National Academy of Sciences.

Young became Dean and Director in 1979. In 1981 he was named Vice President for Health Affairs and took more direct responsibility for the hospital, which had attained a sound financial basis. A new curriculum was planned and put into place. Renovation of the Miner Library was initiated and extensive renovations were made to unused hospital space, providing new offices and research laboratories. Molecular biology and biotechnology initiatives were undertaken.

Young left the deanship in 1984 to become Commissioner of the Food and Drug Administration, a post he held until 1989. He then became Deputy Assistant Secretary for Science and Environment in the Department of Health and Human Services, and later he held various posts in the Public Health Service. Throughout his career he has been active in church work. In 1996 Young was ordained as a minister and currently is pastor of the Fourth Presbyterian Church and Executive Director of the Reformed Theological Seminary in Bethesda, Maryland.

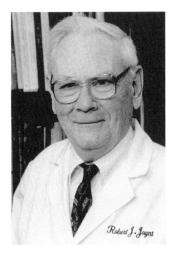

Robert J. Joynt, M.D., Ph.D.
(by Jules Cohen)

Robert Joynt was appointed Acting Dean on July 1, 1984 and Dean and Vice Provost in January, 1985. A native of Iowa, he received his M.D. at the University of Iowa in 1952 and interned at the Royal Victoria Hospital in Montreal, Canada. As a Fulbright Scholar, he did research for a year at the University of Cambridge, England. His training in neurology was at the University Hospital in Iowa City, where he remained on the staff, continuing clinical and research work, and obtaining a Ph.D. in 1963.

In 1966 Joynt came to Rochester as the first chair of the Department of Neurology. Active in neurological circles, he served as president of the American Academy of Neurology, the American Neurological Association, and the American Board of Psychiatry and Neurology. He is a member of the Institute of Medicine of the National Academy of Sciences.

During Joynt's deanship, several student programs were initiated or expanded, including the student outreach program and the foreign student study programs. The renovation of the medical library was completed and several thousand square feet of research space were added by renovating old hospital space. He appointed the first woman to chair a medical school department. Joynt served as chair to the Rochester Area Hospital Corporation, which granted a prospective payment to hospitals, dependent on the share of patient care that they contributed.

In July of 1989, Joynt became Vice President for Health Affairs and continued in this position until July of 1994. Although Marshall Lichtman, M.D., became dean in January 1990, many services of the Medical Center were reorganized to report to the Vice President's office and Joynt retained a very active role. The new outpatient facility and parking garage were constructed during this time.

Joynt retired as Vice President in July 1994 and continues as an active teacher and clinician in the Department of Neurology. In 1997, the Board of Trustees of the University designated him as a Distinguished University Professor.

Marshall A. Lichtman, M.D.

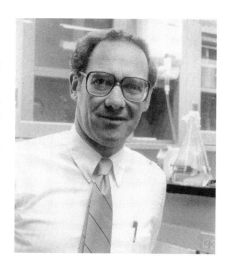

Marshall Lichtman became Dean of the School of Medicine and Dentistry in 1990. He received his undergraduate degree from Cornell University and graduated from the University of Buffalo School of Medicine in 1960. He completed his Internal Medicine training at Strong Memorial Hospital and was Chief Resident in Medicine in 1965–1966. His research training at the School of Public Health at the University of North Carolina was followed by two years of post-doctoral research training at the University of Rochester. He remained on the faculty of the Department of Internal Medicine at Rochester, where he was active in clinical work, teaching, and an extensive research program in hematology.

In 1979 Lichtman was appointed Associate Dean for Academic Affairs and Research, becoming Senior Associate Dean a year later, and Academic Dean in 1988. During his tenure in the dean's office, he initiated and organized many of the school's research programs. Additionally, he modified the faculty tracking system for promotions, giving much more weight to clinical and teaching accomplishments.

Along with his responsibilities at the University of Rochester, Lichtman was active in national and international organizations in his specialty, served as president of the American Society of Hematology, and as chair of the Board of Scientific Advisors to the American Red Cross. A Master of the American

College of Physicians, he has written and edited many books on hematology. He stepped down from the deanship in 1995 and became executive vice president of the American Leukemia Society while retaining clinical and teaching duties at the University of Rochester.

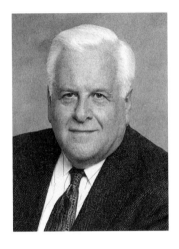

Lowell A. Goldsmith, M.D.

Lowell Goldsmith succeeded to the deanship in 1996. His undergraduate degree is from Columbia University, and his M.D. degree is from the State University of New York at Brooklyn was awarded in 1963. After interning at the UCLA Medical Center in Los Angeles, he completed further training at UCLA, the National Institutes of Health, Massachusetts General Hospital, Brandeis University, and Oxford University in England. He is certified in dermatology and has a special interest in genetic disorders.

In 1981 Goldsmith was named the James H. Sterner Professor of Dermatology and Chair of the Division (later the Department) of Dermatology at Rochester. He has published extensively on genetic diseases of the skin and served as president of the Society for Investigative Dermatology, which awarded him its highest award for investigative work.

During his deanship a major change in the medical school curriculum was introduced. The Double Helix curriculum blends basic science and clinical medicine and relies heavily on problem-based learning.

Goldsmith has initiated a county-wide program, Health Action, a consortium of individuals and agencies whose aim is to make greater Rochester the healthiest city in the country by 2020.

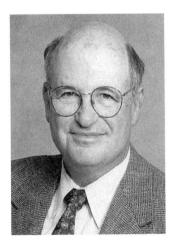

Jay H. Stein, M.D.

Jay Stein became Vice President and Vice Provost for Health Affairs in 1995. He later became Senior Vice President and Vice Provost for Health Affairs, and now carries the additional title of Chief Executive Officer of Strong Health (the university's health maintenance organization).

Stein was born in Chicago and received his undergraduate and medical degrees from the University of Tennessee. He interned and trained in internal medicine at the University of Iowa and completed special training in nephrology at Iowa and at the University of Texas, Southwestern. After serving on the faculty at Ohio State University, he went to the University of Texas at San Antonio in 1975 and in 1977 became chair of the Department of Medicine. He was appointed Senior Vice President and Provost of the Health Science Center at the University of Oklahoma.

One of the leading figures in the field of nephrology and former president of the American Society of Nephrology, Stein has done fundamental work on sodium and potassium transport, renal hemodynamics, and the pathophysiology of renal failure. He received the coveted Williams Distinguished Chair of Medicine Award from the American Association of Professors of Medicine and was made a Master of the American College of Physicians.

During his tenure as Senior Vice President at the University of Rochester, he has overseen extensive changes in healthcare delivery. The Eastman Dental Center and Highland Hospital have merged with Strong Memorial Hospital. An extensive health maintenance organization has been established, utilizing these clinical facilities as well as numerous medical practices in the community, including cooperative arrangements with other hospitals.

The research capabilities of the medical school have been greatly expanded with the construction of the Kornberg Medical Research Building, which houses the Aab Institute for Biomedical Research. An additional building to provide space for clinical departments is underway, and a new emergency care facility is being added to Strong Memorial Hospital.

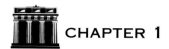 CHAPTER 1

Medical Education: Tradition to Innovation

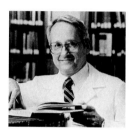

JULES COHEN, M.D.

THE UNDERGRADUATE PROGRAM: THE EARLY YEARS (1925–1940)

From its earliest days the educational program at the University of Rochester medical school was designed to express the principles embodied in the Flexner Report on medical education reform:

- Medical schools should be tied to universities.
- Clinical education should take place in teaching hospitals.
- The faculty in clinical departments, as well as in basic sciences, should have full-time university appointments.

Largely anticipated by George Whipple, as Robert Joynt points out in his introduction to this volume, these principles had three objectives: to ensure that medical education, including clinical education, would occur in a scholarly environment; that faculty would have protected time to devote to teaching and research; and that the intel-

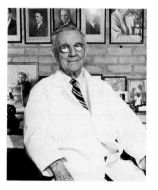

George Hoyt Whipple, 1878–1976

"I would be remembered as a teacher."

"Few people in the history of American medicine have accomplished as much as Dr. Whipple. Of all his achievements, however, perhaps the most significant was to project to his students his concern for patients as human beings."—J. Lowell Orbison

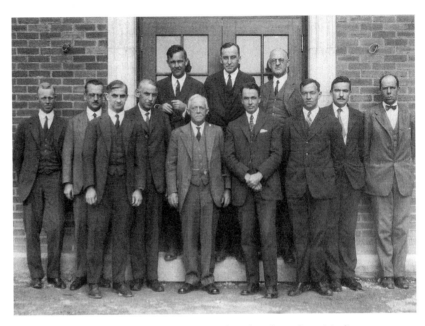

Original department chairs: back row, left to right: Whipple, Wilson, Murlin
Front row, left to right: Bayne-Jones, Clausen, Morton, Bloor, President Rhees,
McCann, Fenn, Corner, Faxon
Photo circa 1926

lectual environment would be enriched by having basic science and clinical faculty working in close physical proximity, encouraging collaboration.

It was important to Dean George H. Whipple and the energetic young faculty he recruited that the not-much-younger medical students would be treated as graduate-level learners, that they would be—to the extent possible and appropriate—colleagues in both learning and research. Department chairs and faculty were selected not only for their academic and clinical accomplishments and promise, but for their belief in these values, their capacity for collegiality, and their willingness to work together on behalf of the institution, its students, and its programs.

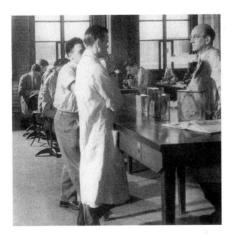

Early student laboratory

To encourage this close relationship between students and faculty, the new medical school and teaching hospital were built under one roof, with construction finished in 1925. Faculty offices, research laboratories, student-teaching laboratories, classrooms, and patient-care wards and clinics were located in close proximity to one another. The medical library and the main dining room were situated at the center of the complex,

JULES COHEN

where they would become intellectual and social gathering places. Within this carefully structured physical environment, basic science and clinical faculty, medical students, graduate students in the biomedical sciences, residents, and nurses all learned and worked "within bare-headed distance" (as the saying went) of one-another.

The facilities were designed to be functional rather than elegant. In fact, one member of the University Board of Trustees, James Cutler (of Cutler Mail Chute fame) coined the phrase "Early Penitentiary Style" to characterize the new school's physical plant—the lecture rooms, laboratories, and hallways. The hospital was more comfortable, and its memorable main lobby, now beautifully restored as part of the Miner Medical Library, was indeed elegant. But the school's physical character reflected Whipple's determination to put scarce resources "where they belonged," invested in people, programs, and equipment, rather than appearances. The environment was said to be characterized by asperity, austerity, and authenticity, terms used by many to describe Whipple himself. The absolutely essential ingredient was an insistence on *quality*—in the student body, the faculty, the school's programs, and its spaces.

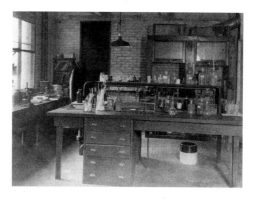

Early research laboratory

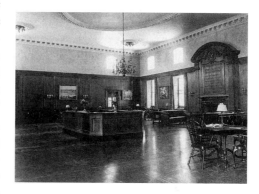

Main lobby of SMH circa 1926

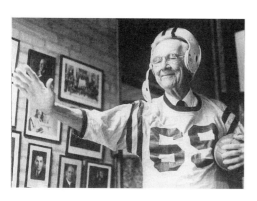

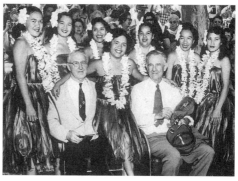

George Whipple *in moments of lesser asperity and austerity. Although he was well-known for his seriousness in all aspects of his professional life, Whipple also had a capacity for lightheartedness, reflected in these charming photographs.*

Rochester's first medical education program was designed to reflect the philosophy that medical students were to be graduate learners. At first, lectures were few or non-existent. All learning took place in laboratories, at the bedside, with students and faculty working closely together, or through independent study. Small classes encouraged easy contact between students and faculty. Over the years, when alumni have been asked to reflect on their student experiences, time and again they recall these close, collegial student/faculty interactions. This experience, built into the curriculum, was strengthened by the many opportunities students had to work in the research laboratories of their faculty mentors.

It is extraordinary to go back and look at descriptions of the curriculum from those early years. Many topics, once considered important, disappeared years ago; some of these are now reappearing. For example, the teaching of nutrition was an important ingredient of the first pre-clinical curriculum; over time, this emphasis eroded and the study of nutrition was replaced with topics presumed to have a more substantive scientific base. Now, in medical schools across the country, nutrition is a "hot topic," its scientific base re-legitimatized, making it once again important for inclusion.

The opportunity for students to engage in research, working alongside members of the faculty, was a key element in the school's programs from the beginning. The Student Summer Research Fellowship program and the "Year-Out" program attracted a high proportion of the student body; both have retained their importance over the years. The chance to pursue productive and satisfying research experiences, together with the modeling provided by faculty mentors, has inspired many of our graduates to pursue research-oriented careers. Many have become highly distinguished scientists, bringing honor to their alma mater.

The number of faculty in these early years was very small. Full-time

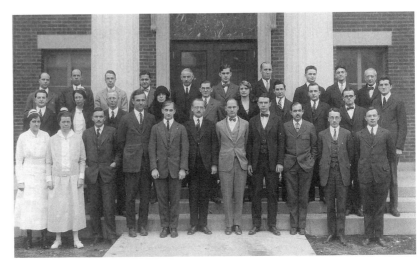

Early photo of full-time faculty, circa late 1920s

JULES COHEN

faculty in the basic biomedical sciences and in the clinical departments, in addition to their research and/or patient care responsibilities, were deeply involved in teaching medical students, graduate students, residents, and post-residency and post-doctoral fellows. High-quality part-time clinical faculty who brought their patients to Strong Memorial Hospital also made substantial contributions to teaching during the clinical years, a practice that continues to this day. While pressures on the early faculty to conduct research and to see patients were sub-

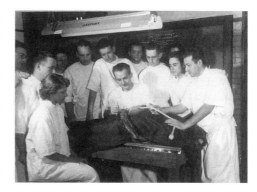

Charles Tobin *instructing first-year students in anatomy, early 1950s*

stantial, especially since resources were so limited, teaching was a high-priority from the beginning. This strong commitment to teaching, which flowed from the priorities set by Whipple and other early senior faculty, became a hallmark of our institutional culture. Rochester, then, has been a distinctively collegial, humane, student- and learning-centered school from the beginning. This character has shaped the educational experience of Rochester students, no matter what the formal curriculum has been.

ADMISSION TO MEDICAL STUDY: A COMMITMENT TO QUALITY

From the beginning the admissions process at Rochester has reflected the institution's character and has featured careful, individualized attention to each and every applicant.

This was an especially important ingredient in the work of the small admissions committee gathered together by Dean Whipple. The senior faculty who comprised the committee were searching for top-quality candidates with special personal characteristics. They wanted "young men" (a few

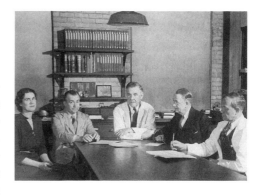

Early admission committee members
Left to right: H. DeBrine *(Administrative Assistant to Dr. Whipple),* W. Bradford, G. H. Whipple, W. S. McCann, and W. O. Fenn

women *were* successful in gaining admission, in spite of this published criterion) who would function with a high level of independence, working at graduate student level and assuming responsibility for their own education.

The admissions committee was interested in attracting candidates who would serve as colleagues for the faculty; young people capable of intellectual interchange, with a demonstrated capacity for learning and excellent performance. Each candidate's credentials were individually reviewed and each

It is enlightening to compare admission requirements as listed in the school's first bulletin in 1925 (at right) and those in the most recent bulletin from 1999 (at far right, on facing page). The emphasis on recruiting first-rate, broadly prepared students has not changed. While German or French is no longer required and Latin no longer encouraged, other requirements remain basically the same. Absent from the first bulletin, and present now, is a reference to personal attributes important to "success in medicine." (Perhaps these were assumed to be present in those who applied to medical school 75 years ago!)

Entrance Requirements

The minimum requirements for admission to the School of Medicine and Dentistry will be as follows:

1. Three full years of study in an approved university or college.

2. One year (6 semester hours) of college English. This course must be largely devoted to training in written and spoken English.

3. Three years of college chemistry, including
    (a) Inorganic chemistry (8 semester hours).
    (b) Qualitative and quantitative analysis (8 semester hours).
    (c) Organic chemistry (6 semester hours).
    N. B. A course in physical chemistry is desirable though not essential.

4. One year of college biology (8 semester hours).

5. One year of college physics (8 semester hours).

6. A reading knowledge of German or French.

It is understood that the requirements listed above indicate the *minimum* academic training necessary for admission. In general candidates who have had a more extensive training will be given preference.

In the science courses approximately one-half of the credit should be for laboratory work.

A knowledge of Latin such as is acquired in two years of a high school course is highly desirable.

The medical sciences have now become so diversified, and the opportunities for contribution to medical knowledge are so varied, that an extensive acquaintance with almost any field of scholarship may be turned to good account in the study of medicine. For this reason the Committee on Admissions will be favorably influenced by evidence of unusual attainment in any branch of learning which a candidate may appear to possess in addition to the prescribed and suggested subjects.

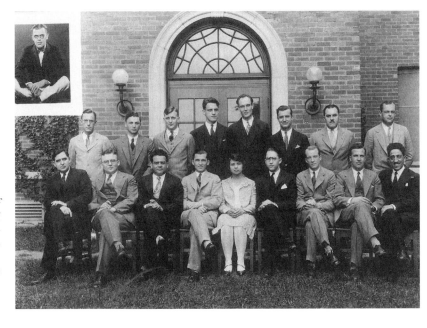

First class of the medical school, at their graduation, 1929

JULES COHEN

Admission to Medical Study

The study and practice of medicine require integrity, compassion, scholarship, responsibility, devotion, and intellectual curiosity. The individual's educational and other life experiences prior to medical school should demonstrate and strengthen these qualities.

Qualifications for Acceptance

Students should choose and pursue in depth a major field of study in an area they find most interesting and rewarding. We are particularly interested in broadly educated people who have taken advantage of intellectual opportunities. Competence in the natural sciences should be demonstrated through work done for the major or for elective courses.

Students should not attempt to anticipate the work given in medical school without considering the limitation which this places on the opportunity to explore other areas of knowledge.

Although applicants are given consideration with three years of undergraduate study, students are advised to obtain a bachelor's degree unless there are compelling reasons for seeking admission to medical school at an earlier date. All premedical requirements ordinarily must have been taken at a U.S. or Canadian college or university.

English. The ability to communicate effectively both orally and in writing is a necessary prerequisite to success in medical practice, research, or teaching. Evidence of proficiency in the use of the language is a primary criterion in the selection of candidates. *One year of expository writing—may be met with writing, English, or nonscience courses that involve expository writing.*

Chemistry. The application of chemistry to medicine is fundamental to an understanding of cellular and organ function. *Two years of college chemistry, including one year of organic chemistry or one semester of organic chemistry and one semester of biochemistry, are required. Within the two-year chemistry sequence, one year of laboratory is required.*

Biology. The study of medicine requires a sound understanding of the evolution and development of living organisms. It is strongly recommended that students' preparation include exposure to both the structure and function of organisms as well as cellular and molecular biology. *A minimum of one full year of biology, with laboratory, is required.*

Physics. The application of the principles of physics to biological systems is important. The student should have knowledge of atomic and nuclear physics. *One year of college physics, with laboratory, is required.*

Other Required Courses. In addition to the English requirement noted above, the School expects that students will enter with other undergraduate work that gives evidence of a broad, liberal, and diversified educational experience. *Two years (12–16 credit hours) of courses in the humanities and/or the social or behavioral sciences are required.*

A knowledge of mathematics is important in all phases of medicine. Although not specifically required, mathematics, including statistics and calculus, is strongly recommended.

Although not a requirement, experience in clinical practice, research, public health, or health policy issues also is recommended.

While the medical school recognizes that many able students are admitted to college with advanced placement, the School favors this practice as an aid to the student in broadening and enriching preparation for the study of medicine. With regard to the premedical requirements discussed in the preceding paragraphs, however, advanced placement courses may be used to meet only one semester of the chemistry and/or one semester of the physics requirements. Advanced placement courses will *not* satisfy the English, biology, or non-science requirements.

Success in medicine depends on many attributes. Scholastic accomplishment is only one. The Medical Admissions Committee gives careful consideration to many other factors, including integrity, judgment, maturity, general knowledge, and special aptitudes. Selection is based upon the most thorough assessment of the applicant that can be achieved during the application process.

The Medical Admissions Committee considers applicants with diverse educational backgrounds and is influenced favorably by evidence of outstanding scholarship in any field of learning.

---

applicant was personally interviewed. "One of the best parts [of the interview process]," an alumnus recalls, "was being interviewed by department chairs and other senior faculty. I was interviewed by Corner, Bradford, and Hodge." Another recalls being interviewed by Dean Whipple, who was soaking his sore feet in a basin of hot water, having just come in from pheasant hunting. An early alumnus recalls the rumor among Rochester applicants and matriculants: "If you were six feet tall and liked to fish, you were in."

But even the tall fishermen had to rise to meet the school's high standards. High quality was the *sine qua non*, but the committee was equally inter-

Harriet F. Purdy,
an institutional legend,
known to generations of Rochester
students as Dr. Whipple's secretary,
then as Secretary to the Committee on
Admissions and Director of the
Admissions Office.

ested in candidates who had already made distinctive achievements. The initial bulletin of the school, published before the first class entered, specifies: "… the Committee will be favorably influenced by unusual attainment in any branch of learning which a candidate appears to possess in addition to the prescribed and suggested subjects."

These early standards set the pattern for consideration of candidates over the years. Even as the numbers of applicants skyrocketed in the 1970s, and again in recent years, every candidate's credentials were carefully reviewed. The process currently followed, which has been in place for some time, makes clear this highly individualized attention. The admissions record of every applicant is reviewed first by two members of the Committee on Admissions so that informed judgments can be made on whom to invite for interviews. Since it is no longer possible to personally interview every applicant (5,866 applications were received in 1999 for a class limited to 100 students), preliminary review is essential. Rochester has avoided, however, what some schools have descended to: making interview decisions based on a computerized screening of undergraduate grade-point averages and scores on the Medical College Admissions Test (MCAT, or "med boards"). Indeed, for many years, until joined by Johns Hopkins, Rochester was the *only* medical school that did not require the MCAT. While we now do require it (since candidates apply from widely diverse undergraduate colleges, some little known), factors other than MCAT scores play a much larger role in admissions decisions. We look for candidates with special achievements, unusual backgrounds, special preparation, or en-

Size of applicant pool vs. class size

Entering Year	No. Applicants	Class size
1930	290	47
1940	606	53
1950	2046	70
1960	920	70
1970	1648	79
1980	3453	97
1990	1813	96
1999	4717	100

JULES COHEN

riching life experiences—all of which may remain unrevealed if one relies on grades or test scores alone.

After the decision to interview is made, the process remains highly personalized. Often, visiting applicants are hosted by medical students, whenever possible by an alum of the candidate's own alma mater. Each applicant has at least two, and usually three, interviews. One interview is always with a faculty member of the Admissions Committee; another is often with a student member of the committee. Interviews are structured to help committee members get to know students personally and to hear about their special achievements. Most important, interviewees' questions about the school are taken very seriously and fully answered. Here again, personal attention serves the interests of the applicant as well as the school.

Many applicants have told us that the application and interview experience at Rochester was special and that the way that they were treated would play an important role as they decided where to matriculate. When, at last, the full Admissions Committee reviews the qualifications of the finalists, special attention is given to the candidates' personal qualities; these are a featured part of the discussions that take place before acceptance/rejection decisions are made.

This highly personalized approach, informed by the original standards set when the school began, has characterized the medical school admissions process over the years. Insistence on quality, attention to candidates' personal strengths and achievements, and considerate treatment of applicants throughout the admissions process are important factors in bringing unusually talented students to this school.

Special Early Selection Programs

To support the school's long-standing interest in attracting candidates who have demonstrated outstanding achievement and diversity of preparation for medicine, we introduced two innovative admissions approaches, the first in the mid-1970s and another, more recently, in the early 1990s.

The Rochester Plan

In the early 1970s, the Commonwealth Foundation, under the leadership of Dr. Carleton Chapman, conceived of a plan to integrate baccalaureate and medical education. The plan involved the creation of eight-year programs that would allow students, after two baccalaureate years, to weave first- and second-year basic science medical school courses into their undergraduate programs. At the same time, students accepted into the program were encouraged to weave baccalaureate courses into their first two years of medical school.

The ultimate goal of the Commonwealth Foundation plan was to graduate a core of physicians with scholarly and personal breadth. The plan enabled students to avoid redundancies in their scientific preparation for medicine, while enriching and broadening their educational experience during both the baccalaureate and medical school years. Students were encouraged to craft distinctive, highly enriched, and innovative programs of study in the eight-year continuum. Those accepted into the program had early assurance of admission to medical studies at the institution in which they were enrolled for baccalaureate studies. No longer would they have to worry about taking the MCAT exam or compiling a highly competitive grade-point average by taking less demanding courses. Instead, they had the flexibility to create programs tailored to their own interests.

The Commonwealth Foundation issued a request to medical schools for proposals to design such programs. Along with a number of other prestigious schools, Rochester's application to the Foundation was successful. A committee of accomplished senior faculty from both the College of Arts and Science and the Medical School oversaw the Rochester Plan's development and operation. Students were interested and over the next twenty years a number of applicants were accepted. Students used the opportunity to take advanced-level courses in the sciences and humanities, which they might not have done otherwise; to pursue research with faculty; to spend time abroad in educational programs; or to study topics of special interest.

Beyond decompressing students' premedical experience and enriching their educational experience, a number of other major institutional achievements relate to the development of the Rochester Plan. Over fifty new courses were introduced; many were joint enterprises of the undergraduate college and medical school faculty. A majority of the courses were interdisciplinary and involved the medical sciences, the humanities, and the social sciences as they related to medicine and health. All were open to college undergraduates. Among the new offerings were cross-campus programs in microbiology and neurobiology, a seminar entitled "Interdisciplinary Topics in Human Aging," a course on "Religious Studies/Sociology and Preventive Medicine—Dilemmas in Healing," new courses on the history of science and medicine. In addition, a number of new degree programs were developed, including a master's degree in public policy analysis related to Community Health, and bachelor's degrees in Microbiology and in Neuroscience. These new degree programs complemented, and in some cases flowed from, the creation of new interdepartmental majors in the broad field of Health and Society.

One of the distinctive achievements of the Rochester Plan was the enhanced opportunity for faculty collaboration and the creation of new interdisciplinary programs which were offered to faculty. For example, the Faculty Bridging Fellowship supported faculty who wished to broaden their education and expertise by studying in a university department other than their own. Thus, medical school faculty working in the Department of Political Science gained greater understanding of how public policy is developed, while others working in the Department of History broadened their knowledge of how historical events shaped developments in science and medicine. In addition to the Bridging Program, faculty education was enriched through the creation of a number of interdisciplinary Faculty Clusters. The clusters addressed aging, genetics, behavioral studies, applied mathematics, women's studies, and cognitive science.

Many of these curricular offerings—for students and faculty—still enrich the institution, even though the formal Rochester Plan has been dissolved.

For philosophical, political, fiscal, and operational reasons, other universities that sponsored these programs abandoned them soon after Commonwealth Foundation funding ended. At Rochester, however, the eight-year program for undergraduates was continued, without interruption, for twenty years. Two developments in the late 1980s and early 1990s resulted in its gradual erosion. In 1985, the medical school introduced a new, more highly integrated curriculum that made it much more difficult for undergraduate students to interweave medical school and baccalaureate level courses. As a result, the Rochester Plan became more of an early acceptance/early assurance program, and student interest declined. In addition, medical school faculty no longer perceived Rochester Plan students as "special"; they seemed little different, in terms of intellectual breadth or capacity for achievement, than their peers. The central objectives of the program were not being achieved.

The Rochester Early Medical Scholars Program (REMS)

At the time that the Rochester Plan was being phased out, an increasing number of integrated baccalaureate–MD programs were being developed across the country. Some of eight years duration, others six, these programs were becoming increasingly attractive to high school seniors planning careers in medicine. At the University of Rochester, undergraduate admissions officers were looking for creative ways to attract top-quality high school seniors, and this, coupled with a declining interest in the Rochester Plan, has resulted in the creation of the Rochester Early Medical Scholars (REMS) Program. Through this program, extraordinarily talented high school seniors with a convincing commitment to the study of medicine are accepted into an eight-year continuum program of undergraduate and medical studies. Special paracurricular enrichment programs and mentoring/advising support have been created to ensure that these students feel that they are part of both the college and medical school communities. While the students have an implicit commitment to remain at Rochester for their medical studies, they are, of course, free to apply elsewhere. One of the values of the program is that the advisory system helps to redirect those students, originally committed to medicine, who realize that another career path is more appropriate to their abilities and interests.

While it is too early to draw conclusions about the success of the REMS undertaking, one thing is clear: it has brought truly gifted young people into

Rochester's undergraduate colleges and to the medical school. We are hopeful that many will continue to demonstrate that high level of ability and achievement as they pursue their medical studies and careers.

ROCHESTER'S DISTINCTIVE CONTRIBUTIONS TO MEDICAL EDUCATION

Innovations in the Formal Curriculum

For the first 25 years, the undergraduate medical education curriculum at the University of Rochester was traditional. It was departmentally based, and the content of programs and teaching methods were determined largely by departmental leaders. As the basic and clinical science of medicine evolved, changes in content were, of course, introduced to keep programs current but little in the way of paradigmatic or focused substantial change occurred in the medical student program.

When the school opened, Dean Whipple's plan was to have few, if any, lectures. Over time, fewer laboratory experiences were offered and more and more lectures were introduced. In this respect Rochester's curriculum became like that of most other medical schools. Some curricular features, however, distinguished Rochester's program from the beginning. Among these were: (1) an emphasis on keeping the student body and faculty relatively *small*, in order to insure collegiality; (2) an emphasis on preparing the *undifferentiated* physician; and (3) *balanced exposure* to generalist fields and to the specialties, to patient care and to advances in research.

Over the years, as a result of four major reviews and modifications to the curriculum—in the early 1960s, early 1970s, early 1980s, and now, in the year 2000—a number of innovative programs have been introduced. Some have lasted; others have had their time in the sun and been superceded. Progressively, there has been a move away from a heavy emphasis on laboratory instruction and/or lectures and toward a more interdepartmental/interdisciplinary education, with students being tutored in small groups and having greater responsibility for their own learning.

During each period of change key aspects of our institutional culture have facilitated the transformation. First has been the belief that change, if it is to be sustained, should be evolutionary rather than revolutionary. That is, change should be informed by past experience and introduced gradually and progressively, with results being continuously evaluated. Second, the pervasiveness of Rochester's collegiality has made possible the development of interdepartmental, as well as other forms of interdisciplinary programs that embrace the biomedical, behavioral, and social sciences. Third is the deep commitment of the administration and faculty to education and to teaching. Without this commitment, the leadership needed to initiate and promote change, and the resources required to underwrite the planning, implementation, and maintenance of new programs, would not have been available. Nor would it have been possible for faculty to devote the time and effort required to plan and implement new programs, some more labor-intensive than those offered in the past. Also critically important to the change process has been the support of major national foundations, especially the Josiah Macy, Jr. Foundation and the Robert Wood Johnson Foundation.

The diagrams below and on the following pages illustrate the evolution of curricular changes over the years. Note the gradual movement towards the development of more interdisciplinary programs, the expanded attention to behavioral and social sciences and to the humanities. Not shown, but equally important, has been the progressive introduction of more active modes of learning and self-instruction, through case and classical problem-based learning, as well as information-systems-based instruction. Through each period of significant change, the basic commitments to quality, to student-centeredness, and to the furtherance of biopsychosocial medicine (vide infra) have been sustained.

The charts below and on the following pages reflect three periods of major curricular change that led up to the introduction in 1999 of the Double Helix Curriculum. Note the progressive development of interdisciplinary programs and the gradually increasing emphasis on Biopsychosocial Medicine. Note, too, that each change was consistent with the school's overall educational philosophy and value system. Success depended on a clear statement of philosophy and objectives, committed leadership, the resources needed to support change, and a planning process that engaged all faculty and students.

1928–1929 and 1940–1941

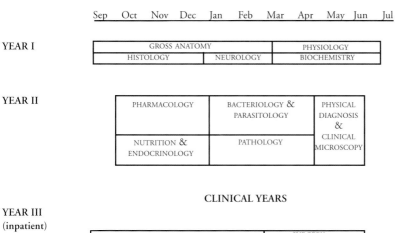

1960

Sep Oct Nov Dec Jan Feb Mar Apr May Jun Jul

YEAR I

GROSS ANATOMY	PHYSIOLOGY
HISTOLOGY / NEUROLOGY	BIOCHEMISTRY
PSYCHIATRY—WEEKLY LECTURES & CONFERENCES	
	ROLE OF THE PHYSICIAN—WEEKLY

YEAR II

PHARMACOLOGY	BACTERIOLOGY, IMMUNOLOGY, VIROLOGY, MYCOLOGY, & PARASITOLOGY	PHYSICAL DIAGNOSIS, INTERVIEWING, & CLINICAL LAB
NUTRITION & ENDO-CRINOLOGY	PATHOLOGY	
MEDICAL PSYCHOLOGY & PSYCHOPATHOLOGY—TWICE WEEKLY		

CLINICAL YEARS

YEAR III

INTRO CLERK-SHIP	INPATIENT CLERKSHIP ROTATIONS IN MEDICINE, OB/GYN, PEDIATRICS, PSYCHIATRY, & SURGERY

YEAR IV

INPATIENT & OUTPATIENT ROTATIONS THROUGH CLINICAL DEPTS. INCLUDING SURGEON SUBSPECIALTIES & ED SURGERY
COMBINED STAFF CLINIC—DAY PER WEEK

1970

Sep Oct Nov Dec Jan Feb Mar Apr May Jun Jul

YEAR I

GROSS ANATOMY/ EMBRYOLOGY	MECHANISMS IN MAMMALIAN PHYSIOLOGY
HISTOLOGY	HUMAN GENETICS
	PREVENTIVE MEDICINE—WEEKLY
BIOCHEMISTRY	ELECTIVES
PATIENT, PHYSICIAN, & SOCIETY	
HUMAN BIOLOGY—THE PSYCHOLOGICAL LEVEL OF ORGANIZATION	

YEAR II

NEURAL SCIENCES	STATISTICS—WEEKLY
	EPIDEMIOLOGY—WEEKLY
	CONCEPTS & MECHANISMS OF DISEASE—WEEKLY
MICROBIOLOGY, IMMUNOLOGY, & PARASITOLOGY	PHARMACOLOGY
PATHOLOGY	
GROWTH & DEVELOPMENT	MEDICAL PSYCHOLOGY & PSYCHOPATHOLOGY

YEAR III

GENERAL CLERKSHIP	FIVE IN-HOSPITAL ROTATIONS IN MEDICINE, OB/GYN, PEDIATRICS, PSYCHIATRY, & SURGERY
	GENERAL CLASS EXERCISES
	MATERNAL & CHILD HEALTH CONTINUITY EXPERIENCE

YEAR IV

RE-HAB	SURG SPEC	EMER-GENCY	ELECTIVES—18 WEEKS
AMBULATORY & GENERAL CLASS EXERCISES			

1980

	Sep	Oct	Nov	Dec	Jan	Feb	Mar	Apr	May	Jun	Jul

YEAR I

GROSS ANATOMY	PHYSIOLOGY	
CELL BIOLOGY (HISTOLOGY)	GENETICS	
CELL BIOLOGY (BIOCHEMISTRY)	CELL BIOLOGY (ENDOCRINOLOGY)	CELL BIOLOGY (NUTRITION)
PSYCHOSOCIAL AND COMMUNITY MEDICINE (PSYCHOSOCIAL MED, PREVENTIVE/COMMUNITY MED, PATIENT, PHYSICIAN, & SOCIETY)		

YEAR II

MICROBIOLOGY & PARASITOLOGY	
	APPLIED PATHOPHYSIOLOGY
NEURAL SCIENCES	PHARMACOLOGY
PATHOLOGY	
PSYCHOSOCIAL AND COMMUNITY MEDICINE	

INDEPENDENT STUDIES PROGRAM

CLINICAL YEARS

YEAR III

GENERAL CLERKSHIP	ROTATIONS THROUGH MEDICINE, OB/GYN, PEDIATRICS, PSYCHIATRY, & SURGERY (EACH 6 WEEKS)
	GENERAL CLASS EXERCISES

YEAR IV

SURGICAL SPECIALTIES 4 WEEKS	EMERGENCY CLERKSHIP 4 WEEKS	(2 OF 3 FROM NEUROLOGY, REHAB, MUSCULO-SKELETAL)
GENERAL CLASS EXERCISES		
AMBULATORY CARE		

1990

	Sep	Oct	Nov	Dec	Jan	Feb	Mar	Apr	May	Jun	Jul

YEAR I

Human Anatomy: Gross Structure & Function	Cell Structure & Function: Histology, Biochemistry	Adaptive & Regulatory Mechanisms: Physiology, Neural Sciences
Psychosocial & Community Medicine: Psychosocial Medicine 1; The Physician, the Patient, and Society; Community Medicine		
Introduction to Human Health and Illness 1		

YEAR II

MECHANISMS OF HUMAN DISEASE	
GENERAL SECTION: Pathology, Microbiology & Immunology, Pharmacology, Genetics	SYSTEMS SECTION: Cardiovascular; Respiratory; Gastrointestinal; Female Reproductive; Renal, Urinary, and Male Genital; Endocrine; Lymphoreticular; Musculoskeletal and Skin; Nervous
	Biostatistics, Epidemiology, Introduction to Physical Diagnosis
Psychosocial Medicine II	
Introduction to Human Health and Illness II	

YEAR III

General Clerkship 8 weeks	DEPARTMENT CLERKSHIPS (sequence varies)				
	Medicine 11 weeks	Obstetrics & Gynecology 6 weeks	Pediatrics 6 weeks	Psychiatry 6 weeks	Surgery 6 weeks
	General Class Exercises				

YEAR IV

Externship 4 or 6 weeks	Emergency Clrkshp 4 weeks	Surgical Specialties 4 weeks	Choice of 2 or 3			Electives 12–14 weeks
			Rehab 4 weeks	Neurology 4 weeks	Musculoskltl 4 weeks	
General Class Exercises						
Ambulatory Care						

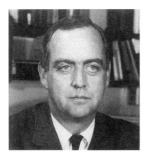

The Associate/Senior Deans who oversaw planning for the curricular changes diagrammed on the preceding pages

1960s:
Leonard Fenninger
(left)

1970s:
Sanford Meyerowitz
(right)

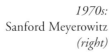

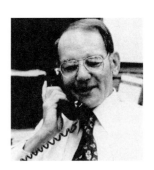

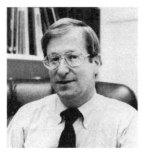

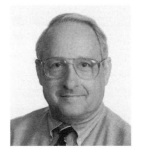

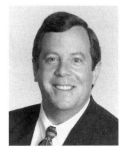

1980s:
Gordon Douglas *(left) and* Jules Cohen *(center)*

late 1990s:
Edward Hundert

Five developments which are "quintessentially Rochester" merit more detailed description. These five curricular programs are distinctive in concept and almost certainly have influenced similar efforts elsewhere. As such, they represent Rochester's special contributions to national medical education pedagogy. These are (1) The Program in Biopsychosocial Medicine, (2) The General Clerkship, (3) The Independent Studies Program, (4) Introduction to Human Health and Illness, and most recently, (5) The Double Helix Curriculum.

The Program in Psychosocial/Biopsychosocial Medicine

The first transforming change in Rochester's undergraduate curriculum followed the arrival of John Romano in 1946. As the first chair of the new Department of Psychiatry, Romano, a psychiatrist, along with his colleague George Engel, an internist, helped medical students appreciate the essential interrelationship between biological, behavioral/psychological, and social forces in human health and illness.[1] Romano and Engel came to Rochester because they perceived that the environment would support their educational philosophy. They felt that the "freely permeable departmental barriers" (Romano's words)—collegiality of the faculty, commitment to interdisciplinary research collaboration, and openness to new ideas—provided an ideal atmosphere for their work. Romano, Engel, and their colleagues saw as their primary mission not the education of psychiatrists, but the development of broadly prepared humanistic physicians, sensitive to the interactions of biological and personal forces in patient well-being and disease.

Although the reception of the new team was generally warm, it wasn't so hospitable that other departments and faculty were willing to give up that precious commodity, "curricular time." Romano relished recalling that initially they were only allowed to schedule their classes at midday on Saturday! Undeterred, students came—and were soon very interested. As word spread about the quality of the teaching and the value of this new biopsychosocial approach, upper-level students "crashed the party" and came to learn in spite of the hour. Gradually, classes offered by Romano, Engel, and their colleagues were accommodated within the regular hours of the curriculum. Very quickly thereafter, Rochester became distinctive for the number of hours and the amount of systematic attention given to the teaching of psychosocial medicine.

A key component of the Romano-Engel method was instruction in patient-centered interviewing. In small groups and under the guidance of faculty mentors, second-year students interviewed real patients. During these formal sessions, and informally on the wards of Strong Memorial Hospital, students were mentored by post-residency fellows who had come to work with Engel in the Medical-Psychiatric Liaison Unit. These fellows were top-quality graduates of residency programs in Internal Medicine, Pediatrics, and Obstetrics/Gynecology. In addition to their role in second-year teaching, the fellows were ever present on the wards as students rotated through clerkships, overseeing and guiding students in their work-ups and providing general support.

The faculty in psychiatry and the Medical-Psychiatric Liaison fellows were usually *welcomed* as teachers, reflecting the receptiveness of most department chairs and other teaching faculty to the new paradigm. The Liaison Unit became a formal unit of the Department of Medicine, and a comparable Behavioral Pediatrics Unit was later established in the Department of Pediatrics. Through the extensive teaching and interdepartmental research activities of these units, the influence of Romano, Engel, and their colleagues became a presence throughout the institution. As leaders in articulating the educational agenda, they had a profound influence in shaping institutional culture.

Through the work of the many talented heirs of the Romano/Engel

Reprinted from
8 April 1977, Volume 196, pp. 129–136

SCIENCE

Replica of the heading from Engel's paper on the Biopsychosocial model, 1977

The Need for a New Medical Model:
A Challenge for Biomedicine

George L. Engel

An Innovative Team

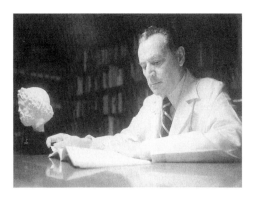

John Romano, *first Chair of Psychiatry,*
circa mid-1970s
"What I have done has been done con amore.*"*

The late John Romano (1908–1994), first chair of the Department of Psychiatry, remains a legendary figure for four generations of medical students and one of the most influential voices in American psychiatry and medicine in general. His spirit continues to animate and challenge all aspects of medical education and patient treatment, not only in Rochester but in every far-flung region where his students pass on his message of patient-centered care.

A founding father of American psychiatry, Dr. Romano is recognized worldwide as a revolutionary reformer in medical education. His bedrock belief—that a successful dialogue between patient and physician is at the heart of working scientifically with and healing patients—is the cornerstone of the Biopsychosocial model, widely recognized as a hallmark of Rochester-educated physicians in all fields and specialties.

The patient-physician dialogue, Dr. Romano taught, must move beyond immediate medical symptoms to explore a patient's concerns about self and family, addressing issues such as economic concerns, loss of personal independence, and fear of dying. Respect for the individual's cultural and spiritual beliefs must enlighten the dialogue, even when those beliefs conflict with those of the physician.

Born in Milwaukee, the son of poor Italian immigrants (his grandfather a stone cutter, his father a music teacher), the young Romano worked his way through college and medical school at Marquette University, followed by residencies at Yale, the University of Colorado, and Harvard. He was invited by Soma Weiss to become a founding member—and the first psychiatrist—of the Department of Medicine at Peter Bent Brigham Hospital. It was there that his interest in sensitizing doctors to psychological problems grew.

When he was thirty-three years old, in 1942, he was named chair of the Department of Psychiatry at the University of Cincinnati, four years later he was tapped by Dr. Whipple to found the Department of Psychiatry at Rochester. Attracted by the fact that, at Rochester, departmental boundaries were "permeable," he convinced both the dean and William McCann, M.D., founding chair of the Department of Medicine, that what was then called psychosomatic teaching must be integrated through all of the medical school years. To work with him in pursuing this agenda, he brought to Rochester his colleague from Harvard and Cincinnati, George Engel, M.D. Together the psychiatrist and internist developed an innovative partnership; with the recruitment of like-minded colleagues they infused medical education at Rochester with what became known as "the Biopsychosocial model."

Dr. Romano supervised the building in 1946 of Strong Memorial Hospital's Wing R. As one of the first psychiatric facilities in the nation to function as an integral part of a university hospital, it became a national model. At the same time, he began a decade-long battle (eventually successful) to win insurance coverage for New York State's mental health patients and to develop community-wide mental health services in Rochester.

A founding member of what later became the National Institute of Mental Health, Dr. Romano received countless awards and honors. Among the most satisfying, he said, were the founding of the John Romano Community Residence, an outpatient facility in Rochester for the care and treatment of mentally ill patients; his appointment as a Distinguished University Professor at the University of Rochester; and the establishment in 1992 of the John Romano Professorship, an honor held by the chair of the Department of Psychiatry.

In 1994, he was honored by the American Psychiatric Association at its 150th anniversary

Jules Cohen

meeting for "over a half-century of inspirational leadership for the profession of medicine as an educator, clinician, and role-model par excellence, and as the most influential voice in American psychiatric education in this century."

"Someone once said, 'A man has but one song to sing in his life,'" Dr. Romano recalled for an interviewer. "I'm not sure I agree, but I do know a major theme of my professional life has been and remains the education of the medical student." Thousands of those mentored by John Romano will attest to the success of their charismatic teacher, whose intellect, vision, and humanism was for nearly half a century the animating spirit of the Medical Center.

Few of us in medicine have the creativity, vision, or persuasiveness to have a transforming influence on the fundamental ways in which we think about health and illness and frame our approach to the care of patients. George Libman Engel *was such a person.*

Engel's early life experience undoubtedly influenced his professional career interests significantly. He, his parents, and his brothers grew up in the home of his uncle, Emanuel Libman (of Libman-Sacks endocarditis), distinguished pathologist and internist at Mt. Sinai Hospital in New York City. A superb clinician and keen

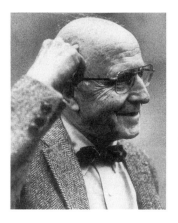

George Engel, *formulator of the Biopsychosocial model*

observer of patients, Uncle Manny, of whom Engel often spoke and wrote, surely had a profound effect on George, his twin brother Frank, and their older brother Lewis. Frank went on to become a distinguished internist/endocrinologist at Duke, and Lewis a distinguished biochemist at Harvard.

George Engel attended Dartmouth College and graduated from the Johns Hopkins Medical School in 1938. He then served a two and one half year rotating internship at Mt. Sinai before going on to the Peter Bent Brigham Hospital in Boston for fellowship training.

Engel's first paper, published in 1935 when he was a medical student at Hopkins, dealt with organic phosphorous compounds in muscle. Many of his other early papers also were principally biomedical in their orientation. One suspects, however, that the early influence of Libman, and Engel's own growing interest in the science of clinical observation, led him quite naturally to come under the influence, in his later training years, of several master clinicians and patient-centered mentors who had a broad view of human biology. Special among these were Soma Weiss and John Romano, with whom Engel worked when he was a post-residency fellow at Brigham. Both of these mentors were centrally important to Engel's growing concern with the interaction of psychological and biological forces in health and illness.

Engel accompanied Romano when the latter was recruited to become chair of Psychiatry at Cincinnati. Only a few years later, in 1946, Romano was recruited to the chair of Psychiatry at Rochester; he asked Engel to accompany him so that they could pursue their cross-disciplinary objectives for medical education and patient care. They decided to come to Rochester because of the collegiality of the faculty and because they perceived it to be a school with "freely permeable" departmental barriers— as Romano put it. Both characteristics, they felt, would make the institution hospitable to their interdisciplinary way of thinking. The support of Dean Whipple, Wallace Fenn (chair of Physiology), and William McCann (chair of Medicine) were key to their decision to come to Rochester, as well as to their ultimate success in achieving their goals.

Rather than educating psychiatrists, their objective was to focus on the education of medical students, introducing them to what Engel termed the Biopsychosocial model in his seminal paper published in Science *in 1977. It took time, but ultimately the model became accepted at Rochester, and then widely in this country and abroad. Engel was increasingly given a national and international platform to talk about his ideas, as an invited speaker and visiting professor at many institutions. His more than three hundred publications embraced the fields of psychosomatic medicine, internal medicine, neurology, and psychiatry, as well as biopsychosocial medicine and medical education, an expression of his capacity to bridge multiple disciplines. This is exemplified by his work on decompression sickness, syncope, the electroencephalogram, psychogenic pain, ulcerative colitis, delirium, and the unique psychologic long-term studies (with Reichsman et. al.) of an infant with a gastric fistula. But what he became distinctively recognized for were his many papers on biopsychosocial medicine and medical education. In many respects his studies of the relationship between behavioral and psychologic processes in changing biological systems provided the intellectual basis for the field of psychoneuroimmunology.*

Engel's leadership role in professional societies, and the many awards and honors he received, are too numerous to mention. One that he especially treasured was his selection in 1997, by the Association of American Medical Colleges, for the AOA Distinguished Teacher Award. Engel has had an enormous impact worldwide on our understanding of human disease, on the education of health professionals, and on humane patient care. [The Engel sidebar is published with permission from the American Medical Association JAMA 2000; 288:2857.]

---

legacy, the impact of Biopsychosocial Medicine continues to be felt throughout the school's educational programs. John Donovan, William Greene, Walter Hamburger, Robert Klein, Sanford Meyerowitz, Franz Reichsman, Arthur Schmale, and Otto Thaler and, in more recent years, Stan Friedman, Lawrence Guttmacher, Anthony Labrum, Jeffrey Lyness, Elizabeth McAnarney, Mary Lou Meyers, Timothy Quill, David Reiser, David Rosen, O. J. Sahler, Roger Sider, and many others are remembered by alumni. Their trainees, too nu-

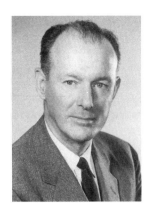

William A. Greene, M.D.

Franz Reichsman, M.D., *and*
John Donovan, M.D.

Many members of the Medical-Psychiatric Liaison Unit (now called the Behavioral and Psychosocial Medicine Unit) contributed significantly to medical education over the years. Six stand out for their many years of service in both education and research, evaluating the impact of psychological factors on the onset and course of human illness: William A. Greene, M.D., Franz Reichsman, M.D., John Donovan, M.D., Arthur Schmale, M.D., Anthony Labrum, M.D., and Otto Thaler, M.D.

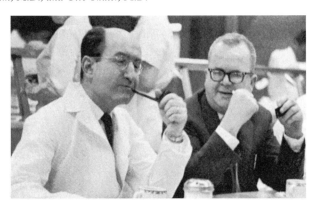

JULES COHEN

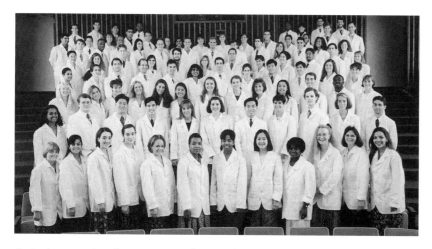

Beginning a number of years ago, at Rochester and a number of other medical schools, the White Coat Ceremony became part of the orientation program for entering medical students. The ceremony is designed to bring students at the very beginning of their training into the fellowship of the profession. Even more important, the ceremony emphasizes that their ultimate educational objective is to learn how to provide compassionate and humane care to their patients, throughout their professional lives.

merous to mention, in Medicine, Family Medicine, Obstetrics/Gynecology, Pediatrics, and Psychiatry, have been important in carrying on the legacy.

The impact of the Psychosocial/Biopsychosocial Program has influenced many other courses, clerkships, and programs. Three examples will suffice. For about twenty years a *funeral* has been held for the cadavers used in the Gross Anatomy course. Why? To teach students that the cadaver is not only their first patient, but that this first basic science course also has a human dimension. Second, Rochester was one of the first medical schools to hold a White Coat Ceremony. With support provided by the Arnold Gold Foundation, entering first-year students are presented with white coats in a ceremony

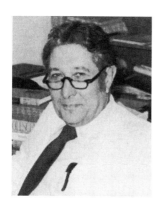

Arthur Schmale, M.D.

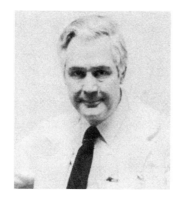

Anthony Labrum, M.D.

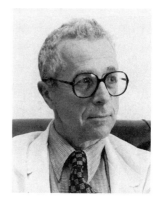

Otto Thaler, M.D.

which draws close attention to the human dimension of medicine as emphasized by the program in Biopsychosocial medicine. In a different arena, several of Rochester's most distinguished basic neuroscientists, immunologists, and psychologists have been engaged over the years in studying the effect of psychological forces on the functions of the autonomic and immune systems. The results of their work have been incorporated into the teaching of our students.

Attention to the Biopsychosocial model of patient care is now part of many student clerkship experiences and has influenced the decision to incorporate into our curriculum such programs as the Medical Humanities Seminars, Ethics and Law in Medicine, and an enriched Community Medicine Program. Similarly, the introduction of a community volunteer outreach program and a program in international health can be linked to the influence of the Biopsychosocial model.

One graduate, speaking at a recent commencement about the pervasiveness of Rochester's Romano-Engel legacy, put it this way: "The Biopsychosocial Model—it's like God. It's everywhere!"

The General Clerkship

In the late 1950s, advances in medical science, accompanied by advances in and increasing reliance on medical technology for diagnosis and treatment, produced a wave of concern. A perception arose that physicians' clinical skills might be eroding and that the human dimension of patient care was being neglected. F. W. Peabody, in his classic 1925 paper "The Care of the Patient," had warned of this possibility.[2] Regarding medical education he wrote, "And while they have been absorbed in the difficult task of digesting and correlating new knowledge, it has been easy to overlook the fact that the application of the principles of science to the diagnosis and treatment of disease is only one limited aspect of medical practice. The practice of medicine in its broadest sense includes the whole relationship of the physician with his patient." Thirty years later Peabody's concerns were becoming a reality in both clinical practice and medical education. As Romano, Engel, and their colleagues became more influential in the educational dialogue at Rochester, concerns about basic skills and patient-centeredness became central to discussions regarding the curriculum.

With the support and encouragement of Dean Donald Anderson, a major review of the undergraduate curriculum was undertaken in the late 1950s, spearheaded by "The Committee of Six," distinguished and influential department chairs, all of whom had a strong commitment to medical education. The group was chaired by J. Lowell Orbison (Pathology, and later Dean), and it included Robert L. Berg (Community and Preventive Medicine); Herbert R. Morgan (Microbiology); Charles G. Rob (Surgery); John Romano (Psychiatry); and Elmer H. Stotz (Biochemistry). Their review of the undergradu-

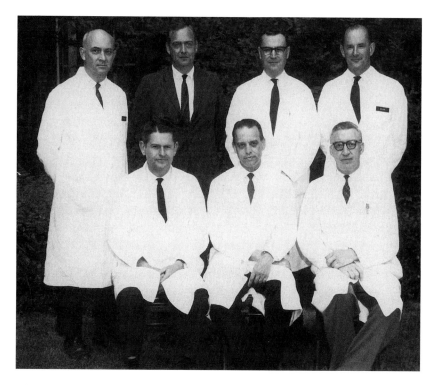

The Committee of Six: back row, left to right: R. L. Berg, L. Fenninger *(Associate Dean and Staff to the committee),* J. Romano, C. Rob; *front row, left to right:* H.R. Morgan, J. L. Orbison, E.H. Stotz

ate curriculum, conducted with the assistance of a number of subcommittees, resulted in a report accepted in 1961 by the medical school's Advisory Board. A set of broad objectives for the educational program was presented, as well as a series of very specific programmatic recommendations for both the pre-clinical and clinical years. This report had a transforming impact on medical student education at Rochester.

A central recommendation of the Committee of Six was to create an interdepartmentally taught General Clerkship of sixteen weeks duration. Elements of the recommendation are fascinating to read even now, almost forty years later. The course was designed to build on the strength of students' experiences in the second-year Psychosocial (later Biopsychosocial) Medicine program and on the second-year emphasis placed on mechanisms of disease. The Clerkship was "to be concerned with basic methods of perception of data … fundamental will be mastery of the techniques of interviewing and history taking … acquisition of skills in the examination of patients … [and] learning the use of instruments as extensions of their senses."

The revolutionary program would occupy the first sixteen weeks of the third year for all students. For the first time—anywhere in the country— medical students would be able to concentrate all their energies on developing

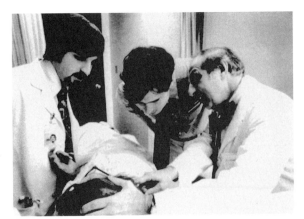

M. N. Luria
demonstrating the
evaluation of the jugular
venous pulse and
pressure, 1970s

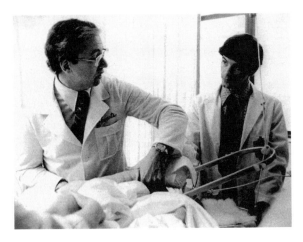

C. M. Evarts
demonstrating an
orthopedic examination

their clinical skills. Gone were the "distractions" demanded by second-year basic science courses, which had run concurrently. The program was to be offered as a continuum, featuring progressive acquisition of skills under the direct observation of carefully selected, senior, and experienced clinicians.

Once the basic concept of the General Clerkship was formally approved, detailed planning proceeded, and the clerkship took the following shape. Teams of instructors were assigned to work with groups of students. In the first section of the course students learned physical diagnosis by examining one another under close faculty supervision. These exercises were integrated with small-group instruction in interviewing and examining patients, which gave way progressively to supervision by a single instructor working with two or three students, then to one-on-one teaching of the full work-up of a patient, including a detailed, carefully reviewed write-up of the case. During the second and third periods of the course, students were assigned to work on various clinical services with teams of residents, supervised by a single senior preceptor. Through in-depth study of small numbers of patients, and as members of ward teams, students became directly engaged in evaluating and caring for "their own patients." Although lectures on basic skills were a part of the initial clerkship format, these were gradually eliminated. A formal section in basic clinical laboratory methods became part of the first section of the course. Here students learned to perform and interpret blood smears and other simple bedside laboratory investigations.

Program organization and logistics were crucially important to the program's success. First, the director of the clerkship was to be a senior highly respected clinician-teacher of professorial rank. This criterion spoke to the importance that the school placed on teaching basic skills and clinical reasoning. The first director, William L. Morgan, Jr., epitomized these skills and the school's commitment to them. Each director was advised by a com-

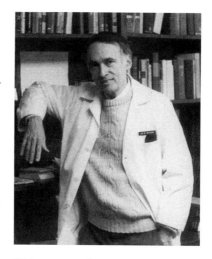

W. L. Morgan, *first Director of the General Clerkship and Associate Chair of Medicine for Educational Programs*

mittee whose members represented each of the clinical departments involved and each affiliated hospital. The course had its own budget, administered by the director, from which key faculty participants received compensation; token contributions to affiliated hospitals recognized their participation in the

program. A highly detailed and structured course guide and syllabus were created. The guide evolved to become *The Clinical Approach to the Patient*, a textbook by Morgan and Engel, which received national and international recognition and was translated into a number of languages.[3] Faculty teams met regularly during the course to discuss progress, address problems, and consider special opportunities to improve the program. Each of these organizational elements was crucial to emphasizing the importance of the program in the overall curriculum, recognizing the special efforts of participating faculty, and achieving clerkship objectives. Based on its objectives, content, structure, and organization, the General Clerkship served as a model of interdisciplinary clinical education. By the end of their clinical training, most students recognized what a valuable experience the General Clerkship had been.[4]

Within just a few years of its begin-

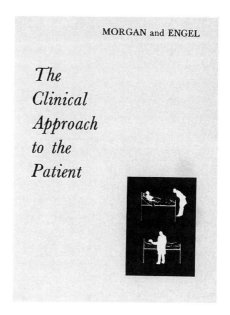

Cover of the text for the General Clerkship, The Clinical Approach to the Patient, *by* W. L. Morgan *and* G. L. Engel

nings, the clerkship was shortened to twelve, then to eleven, then to eight, six, and finally four weeks. Pressure from students eager to get on with their specialty clerkships was a contributing factor, as was pressure from department heads concerned about the erosion of time allotted to their own clerkships. All of this occurred at a time when clinical science and technology, in all specialties, were expanding rapidly. A third pressure on time allotted to the Clerkship came from the need to introduce new student experiences during the clinical years, a requirement that became apparent through subsequent curricular reviews. As a result of the progressive shortening of the General Clerkship, some of its original purposes became eroded. Although the luster of this "jewel in the crown" of clinical education at Rochester has dimmed, the basic beliefs that led to its formation are alive and well among the faculty.

There is every reason to be optimistic that the traditional Rochester emphasis on basic clinical skills and patient-centeredness—the same values that led to the development of the General Clerkship back in the 1960s—will be preserved and enhanced as Rochester's new "Double Helix" curriculum is further developed.

The Independent Studies Program

As early as the 1930s, medical education leaders around the nation began to express concerns about "curricular oppression" and "passive learning." At issue were the increasing number of lecture hours, program fragmentation resulting from increasing specialization in both basic and clinical sciences, isolation of basic science from clinical education, and marginal problem-solving skills among students as they reached their clinical training years.

In the early 1970s, responding to these concerns, a subcommittee of the medical school's Curriculum Committee, encouraged by Dean Orbison, was asked to develop a program of independent study through which students

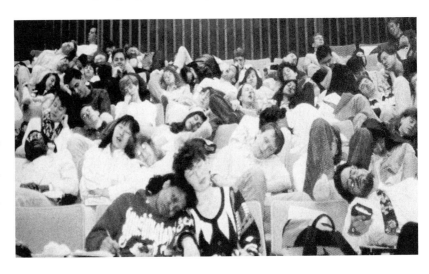

Posed photo (1994) of a class demonstrating that the lecture format for medical education does not always engage their active participation

JULES COHEN

could complete a portion or all of the first two years of medical school on a "self-motivated" basis. They would be guided by a small group of faculty who would provide appropriate instructional materials and references. The subcommittee completed its deliberations in time for the program to be approved and implemented in the fall of 1972.

Rochester's Independent Studies Program (ISP) represented a pioneering initiative in problem-based learning. It antedated Harvard's New Pathway Program by over ten years and served as a model for the wave of problem-based learning initiatives being adopted by many medical schools across the nation and world-wide. The specific goals for the program (as adapted from those published in the 1972-73 Medical School Bulletin) were:

- To develop an individualized, student-learner-oriented program using a multidisciplinary approach for acquiring the knowledge and skills essential to the practice of medicine;
- To achieve a maximum degree of multidisciplinary learning through the participation of all faculty in the organization of basic science instruction;
- To recruit a multidisciplinary teaching team which would develop innovative approaches in philosophy and methodology for instruction in the basic sciences;
- To help students develop independent study techniques and attitudes, leading to a habit of life-long learning;
- To foster effective patterns of communication among students and faculty;
- To provide improved knowledge and assessment of student capabilities through close association among students and faculty members and to use information thus gained to develop the best educational program for each student;
- To make new concepts, methods, and skills of instruction and assessment developed in the Independent Studies Program available for use by all programs and faculty.

The opportunity to participate in the new program was made available to sixteen second-year students, chosen by lottery from among applicants. Two-thirds of the preceptors were basic science faculty; one-third came from clinical departments. The program was directed by Herbert R. Morgan, professor and former chair of Microbiology and associate professor of Medicine. Other early program leaders included Howard Harrison (Surgery), Martin Klemperer (Pediatrics and Medicine), David Goldblatt (Neurology), John Sandt (Psychiatry), Daniel Schuster (Psychiatry), R. Knight Steele (Medicine), Ian Stuard (Pathology), Peter Viles (Pediatrics), Donald Young (Medicine and Radiation Biology/Biophysics). (Stuard eventually succeeded Morgan as program director.) Others who became involved included George Abraham (Medicine and Microbiology), Marvin Amstey (OB-Gyn), Piero Balduzzi (Micro-

H. R.
Morgan,
*Director
of the
Independent
Studies
Program*

biology), J. Richard Ciccone (Psychiatry), Donald Greydanus (Pediatrics), Robert Klein (Medicine and Psychiatry), Susan Rosenthal (Oncology in Medicine), Donald Taves (Pharmacology and Toxicology, and Radiation Biology/Biophysics).

The Independent Studies Program featured seminars, clinical problem-based tutorials, and laboratory exercises. Students became actively engaged in their own learning, and for many the experience became the highlight of their basic science education. Alumni recall the program with enthusiasm; many report that learning became a pleasure, rather than a burden and resulted in skills that have stayed with them, no matter what directions their careers have taken. For example, an alumna recalls that the program was "freeing," enabling her to study independently where and when she chose to do so. The assignments, another said, "required one to do a lot more than rote memory—[they] forced you to do problem-solving on your own" and "it freed me from the daily grind of lectures." An alumnus said, "ISP was the most important thing to happen to me in medical school. I struggled during the first year, I wasn't engaged, but ISP changed all that." Another said: "It totally changed my way of thinking, and made me realize that just because things had always been done a certain way, it wasn't necessary that they had to be done that way forever after. It also influenced the way I now teach students myself."

The students who volunteered for the program were sufficiently self-aware to know that their personal characteristics made this kind of learning experience right for them. Faculty, too, were energized and challenged—even excited—by their involvement. They were gratified by the opportunity to work closely with a small band of bright students, and they learned a great deal outside their own areas of expertise. The opportunity to meet frequently for program planning and coordination brought faculty into close working relationships with colleagues in other disciplines, further enhancing the collegiality that had been a distinguishing mark of the school from its beginnings.

Although there had been anxieties about how labor-intensive the program would be and therefore how demanding on faculty time, these concerns never materialized, as shown by the program report published in the *Journal of Medical Education*.[5] When one factored in the time saved through student self-instruction and costs saved through eliminating faculty time spent in preparing and delivering lectures, program costs were quite reasonable, once the initial planning and implementation phases were over.

In many respects, Rochester's experience with an independent studies program anticipated the national experience that came later. Many of us felt, therefore, that it was very unfortunate that the program was abandoned in the

JULES COHEN

early 1980s, just as the national movement for problem-based learning was getting underway and before the program could be expanded and made available to all students. During the ten years of its existence, the Independent Studies Program was highly successful in preparing students for their clinical years, enhancing their satisfaction with basic science studies, and stimulating and broadening those faculty fortunate enough to be involved. Now the cycle of time is bringing problem-based learning back into Rochester's medical curriculum as a major undertaking of the new "Double Helix Curriculum."

Introduction to Human Health and Illness: A Program of Whole-Case Studies Based on the Biopsychosocial Model

As the revised Rochester medical school curriculum was being planned in the early 1980s, a central question was how to give expanded programmatic expression to the Biopsychosocial (BPS) model of medical education and practice. While the model already served as the orienting theme for the first- and second-year courses in Psychosocial Medicine, the curricular planners were determined that its presence be more widely felt throughout the curriculum.

To this end, a series of "whole case" conferences was developed. In a single comprehensive exercise, students would learn from *real* patients about the biology of their illnesses. They would also examine the personal issues and social forces influencing the presentation, diagnosis, course, and treatment of the patients' problems. The exercises were to go beyond the traditional basic science-clinical correlation format to a consideration of pathophysiology in systems-oriented terms. Students would consider patient-doctor, economic, ethical, and legal issues as they influence patients' health and/or illnesses. The course, called "Introduction to Human Health and Illness" (IHHI), ran as a course from 1985 until the introduction of the Double Helix curriculum in 1999.[6] Since then, many of the exercises continue to be presented as part of the expanded programs in Biopsychosocial Medicine.

Many institutions have introduced patient-centered interview instruction early in students' experiences and have exposed students to the community, ethical, and legal aspects of health care. To our knowledge, however, the IHHI program has been distinctive in bringing together students and patients in a single whole-class exercise, where the full range of biological and psychosocial influences on health and illness could be considered.

Beyond the broad objectives outlined above, the following objectives guided the program's implementation:

- Topics covered during IHHI sessions were chosen to parallel the content of basic science courses being taught concurrently, usually in the same week. For example: a session on scoliosis was taught when first-year students were dissecting the back in Gross Anatomy; a session on shock was taught when second-year students were studying the cardio-vascular system.

- IHHI sessions also reflected concepts covered in concurrently running first- and second-year courses in Biopsychosocial Medicine, the Medical Humanities Seminars, Ethics and Law in Medicine, Community Medicine, and Epidemiology. Thus, exposure to the patient-centered interview, issues in the doctor/patient relationship, ethical issues in patient care, and the economics and organization of health care as these affect individual patients were all reinforced in IHHI sessions.

  Topics of importance were included even when there was not a good fit with other courses in the curriculum. Examples include sessions on domestic violence, and smoking and health—multidimensional issues that have a significant impact on many patients and are clearly of major significance to public health.

- A third and particularly important objective of IHHI was to help students appreciate the powerful, personal impact of the physician in healing. As students heard patients' stories, they came to better understand how physicians' behavior and attitudes can influence patients' illnesses and their response to treatment. They came to appreciate the importance of physician credibility and compassion, as well as competence, as determinants in establishing patient confidence and compliance, as sources of both patient and physician satisfaction, and as influences on healing.

- A fourth objective of IHHI was to give students an additional opportunity to engage real patients directly, from the first weeks of medical school. They learned the importance of letting the patient "tell the story" in his or her own terms, how to ask questions sensitively, and how to interpret answers using data from the interview as part of the clinical reasoning process. All of these skills were reinforced in IHHI exercises, helping students appreciate the power of patient-centered learning. The exposure of *beginning* students to a broad range of concepts and an extensive base of information through the study of real patients was part of the course's power.

- A fifth specific objective of IHHI was to help students appreciate more fully the role played by other health professionals. For example, in a session on tuberculosis students heard from community health nurses and public health officials about their roles in caring for patients with TB and about viewing the disease as a community health issue.

Finally, the course enhanced faculty development. Rochester's increasingly specialized faculty were exposed to disciplines and orientations other than their own. Their knowledge was broadened by weaving interdisciplinary themes through their presentations and through working with their colleagues as they taught IHHI sessions together.

JULES COHEN

A partial 1997–98 schedule of IHHI topics is presented in Table 1; the relationship of the topics to the content of concurrent courses is specified. Topics remained relatively constant over the years but, as the specific content of basic science programs evolved, IHHI topics were adapted to parallel these changes.

TABLE 1

FIRST YEAR

Topic	Linkages to Basic Science/Other
Valvular Heart Disease	Gross Structure and Function(GSF)— Dissection of Thorax
Prostate Cancer	GSF – Dissection of Pelvis
Joint Replacement	GSF – Dissection of Extremities
Care of the Patient Living with HIV	Cell Structure and Function (CSF)— Histology of Lymphatic System, and Community Medicine
Diabetes Mellitus	CSF – Carbohydrate Metabolism
Russia: A Population's Decline in Life Expectancy	Community Medicine
Dialysis	Renal Physiology
Stroke	Neural Sciences
Congestive Heart Failure	Cardiovascular Physiology

SECOND YEAR

Topic	Linkages to Basic Science/Other
Down's Syndrome	Genetics
Pulmonary Embolism	Pathology – Thromboembolic Disease
A Completed Suicide	BPSM
Bone Marrow Transplantation	Immunology
Hyperlipidemia/Cardiac Risk Factors	Cardiovascular System
Smoking Cessation	Respiratory System
Liver Transplantation	Gastrointestinal System
Hemostasis	Hematology System
Male Infertility	Endocrine System
Head Trauma	Nervous System
Breast Cancer	Female Reproductive System

Whenever possible, teachers were selected for IHHI who had the experience and breadth to teach across disciplines and to engage biological, behavioral, and socioeconomic issues. For many sessions, however, more than one faculty member was needed to deal effectively with the full range of issues to be covered.

In a typical IHHI session, a faculty member might present a brief overview of the topic (15–20 minutes), then interview—with the class—one or two patients with the clinical disorder under review (45–60 minutes). The teacher then engaged the class in a general discussion illustrating various as pects of the case, including pathophysiological, psychological, economic, legal, and community health aspects, as appropriate (30–45 minutes). Patient interviews sometimes began the session. Whatever their timing, these interviews were key to the program's success. On occasion, patients would present their own case histories; when the patient was articulate, their stories were especially powerful. While most sessions were whole-class exercises, some small-group problem-solving sessions were led by student or faculty facilitators.

Three Examples of IHHI

The following typical IHHI sessions may serve as examples to illustrate how course objectives were met.

1. INTRODUCTORY SESSION—CORONARY HEART DISEASE. The very first IHHI session occurred at the end of orientation week for first-year students. The patient who participated each year, since the inception of the program, has coronary artery disease. Students brought to the session their general knowledge of the disorder, based on personal experience with family members and on what they had read in the lay press about this important clinical/public health/preventive medicine problem. They heard about the context in which the patient's symptoms began, learned about factors that influence his symptoms, observed the patient interacting with his physician in a patient-centered interview, and heard about the patient's experiences with other physicians. An edited conversation follows:

> Context for onset of illness:
> *Physician*: Tell us when this all began.
> *Patient:* Well, my wife had just finished a course of chemotherapy for breast cancer, and …

> Patient-doctor interaction:
> *Patient:* The doctor [a cardiologist] said, "I'll write it down for you. … I don't want to have to repeat what I'm telling you." He just didn't want to take the time to explain things to me or my wife … the chemistry just wasn't there.… My wife had to block the door to keep him from leaving until he explained what was going on.

> Risk-factor modification:
> *Patient:* It's chicken and fish, and fish and turkey, and fish and chicken.… Every so often I just have to cheat.

> Pathophysiology:
> *Patient:* If I walk in a cold wind or carry suitcases, especially after I eat, that's when I get uncomfortable … and especially when I get worked up, like at a school board meeting.

The students could ask questions about the patient's symptoms and personal experiences. During the course of the interview, question period, and discussion, the following issues were covered:

- Risk factors in the pathogenesis of the disease—both biological and behavioral;
- Factors important in the timing of the onset of symptoms, including psychological factors;
- Factors important in the pathophysiology of the disease, including ways in which psychological influences can produce or relieve symptoms;
- The power of the physician—for good or ill—as an element of treatment;
- The economics of the diagnosis and treatment of coronary artery disease, its economic impact on the community, and sources of payment for services;
- Shared decision-making by patients and physicians regarding choice and timing of treatment.

An emphasis of this session was the *patient*, his/her concerns and needs being the focus of medical care. This emphasis was integrated with a discussion of the basic biology of the disease process and how psychological and biological forces interact to produce symptoms and influence well-being.

2. THE PATIENT WITH HIV. A session for first-year students on *Care of Patients Living with HIV* was particularly powerful. This IHHI, coordinated by a member of the Infectious Diseases Unit, usually included two or three patients with HIV infection/AIDS and a nurse and social worker from the AIDS clinic. The session began with an overview of HIV infection, including information about prevention, pathophysiology, complications, and the natural history of the disease. Each patient then gave a brief synopsis of his/her experience with the illness. These presentations powerfully illustrated the personal impact of HIV infection. The nurse case-manager and social worker briefly reviewed their roles, illustrating the interdisciplinary team approach to patient care. The session concluded with questions from the students, to which patients and faculty responded.

Issues in diagnosis of HIV:
   Patient: When they told me that my test was positive, I said that it had to be a mistake. When the second test was positive, I was very scared and embarrassed.

Impact of support system on maintenance of health:
   Patient: I really wasn't sure what my dad would say or do after I told him I was HIV-positive. He drove the car to the side of the road, stopped the car, and hugged me. He said, "You'll always be my

son and I will always care for you no matter what happens." That reassurance has really helped me ever since in my dealing with the disease.

Issues at the end of life:

> *Patient:* Christmas is going to be here in three months, but every time I think about it I get very sad. Since I seem to be getting sicker every day, I am so really scared I won't be alive for Christmas.

Many of these patients were about the same age as the students themselves. Students often cried when they heard about the pain, fright, and embarrassment of receiving the diagnosis, the extraordinary difficulty of sharing this information with loved ones, the fear of death, and the importance of support from family, friends, and caregivers. While the biology of HIV is covered in detail, this session perhaps more than any other went far beyond biology in bringing home to students the power of the human dimension as an influence on the course of illness and on patients' sense of well-being.

3. SPINAL CORD INJURY. The final example is an IHHI exercise for first-year students which was presented at Family and Friends Weekend, an annual event which brings parents, other family members, and friends of first-year students to the campus each spring.

The patient was a young single mother of one, a cocaine addict who had been left quadriplegic as a result of a gunshot injury to her cervical spine. The wound had been inflicted during an attempted robbery as she was trying to buy drugs.

The patient died after electing to have her life-supporting respirator disconnected. The neurologist who presented the case reviewed the pathology and its clinical consequences. An attorney (Jane Greenlaw) and a philosopher-ethicist (Jeffrey Spike) from the Division of Medical Humanities reviewed and discussed the legal and ethical issues involved in the patient's right to discontinue her life support, as well as the impact of her decision on the man who fired the shot. Did she have the right to make this choice? Was this suicide? Can the man who fired the shot be charged with murder, since the injury he inflicted was fundamentally the cause of the patient's death?

Following the presentation, students and their families and friends met in small groups to discuss these issues for thirty to forty-five minutes. They then returned to the teaching auditorium for a whole-class concluding discussion. This session allowed for a comprehensive and challenging consideration of basic science, clinical science, ethics and law, and the interrelationships among them.

These examples illustrate the key IHHI principle: to help students appreciate the full range of issues that bear on the care of a single patient. Presenting these issues in the context of memorable and moving real patient experiences was powerfully effective in helping students appreciate the interplay of forces that influence a patient's health or illness. Perhaps most important, students came away from the IHHI sessions with a sense of the patient as *person*, rather than as "a case with disease X."

As we moved into an era of aggressive healthcare reform, IHHI sessions helped to bring into focus issues of healthcare organization and financing *as they affect individual patients*. Students learned first-hand about access to care, the impact of high costs on compliance, and the psychological distress that many patients feel as they cope with high costs and the complexities of insurance coverage or the lack thereof.

IHHI is described here in some detail because the program epitomizes the philosophical underpinning of the Rochester curriculum in the Biopsychosocial model, as developed here by George Engel and John Romano.

The Double Helix Curriculum *

A fifth major curricular change was introduced in September 1999 with the advent of the Double Helix curriculum. Seen by some as the most dramatic shift in medical education in more than half a century, the new model was forged over the preceding two years by Medical Center leaders, faculty in basic and clinical science, national education experts, students, and computer technology specialists.

The development of the new curriculum and its implementation were led by Edward M. Hundert, M.D., a psychiatrist and ethicist from Harvard University, who was recruited to Rochester to serve as Senior Associate Dean for Medical Education and to lead the evolution of the new Rochester curriculum for medical students, as well as to oversee residency programs.

The Double Helix curriculum represents a radical curricular change. It incorporates the latest research on how adults learn and takes seriously the logical conclusion of the information explosion in medical science—that the goal of medical education is not to learn medicine, but to learn *how to learn medicine*. The new approach recognizes that when students are hungry for information then they need to solve a problem; students who solve problems learn faster and retain facts longer than those "force-fed" through lectures alone. As a result, the curriculum confronts students with clinical problems *before* they are well advanced in their studies, forcing them to look for answers as they begin and progress through their four years of study.

"Today we know more about medicine than we can possibly teach in the years of medical school," Hundert says. "As a result, our ultimate goal is to teach students how to learn medicine now and throughout their careers."

---

*Adapted from the Medical Center's 1999 Report to the Community, prepared by Nancy Bolger based on an interview with Edward Hundert, M.D.

To this end, a novel six-week course entitled "Mastering Medical Information: Foundations for a Lifetime of Learning" begins and concludes first-year study.

While grounded in Rochester's hallmark Biopsychosocial model, the new paradigm breaks with tradition. The old "two–and–two" model—two years of largely classroom and laboratory study followed by two years spent in clinical settings—limited students' interactions with patients until they were thoroughly grounded in the concepts of basic science.

Case-based and classical problem-based learning was progressively introduced into the first two years of the program as part of the major Rochester curriculum change of the mid-1980s. In the Double Helix case-based approach, however, the basic and clinic sciences are completely integrated—woven together like strands of DNA—during all four years of study. From the first weeks of study, theory and practice are combined every day. For example, students learning the anatomy of the knee are instructed in how to examine an injured knee, how to help patients avoid knee injuries, and in the economic, ethical, and legal issues that may be related to the case under study.

The Double Helix curriculum is also supported by the university's multimillion-dollar investment in a new physical plant. The School of Medicine and Dentistry is strategically positioned as the link between the new Aab Institute of Biomedical Sciences and Strong Memorial Hospital. As a result, researchers and clinical faculty are in close contact with students; all share two new amphitheaters and a great hall/reception area.

Twelve state-of-the-art problem-based learning rooms have been created, each a combination classroom and physician's office. Information exchange is encouraged as small groups of students join the professor around a table in a room fully equipped with computers and video technology. A student learning to interview a patient, for example, can later watch—and learn—from a videotape of this essential engagement.

The new curriculum has required the school's leadership and faculty to devise new methods of testing student achievement during the four-year progression. At the end of the second and third years, all students will undergo an intensive two-week testing period. The comprehensive exam will cut across all basic and clinical sciences and measure and/or identify knowledge, skills, and attitudes. Each student will emerge from the testing period with an identified learning profile and an individualized study plan, both short and long term.

To ensure the robust advisory system needed to support the new curriculum, four advisory deans, diverse in gender, race, and specialty, have been appointed. Weekly and monthly meetings and "open-door" hours are built into the schedule to promote regular engagement between student and advisor.

While Rochester is well know for its interdisciplinary, collegial approach to education, patient care, and research, the Double Helix curriculum makes

JULES COHEN

special demands on those who teach. Gone is the old method, where a professor—acting as a "fount of knowledge"—stood at the head of the class and lectured. Now teachers themselves are involved in the learning process, guiding students through the complicated process of learning to find, filter, manage, and apply information. Workshops, seminars, and monthly meetings are presenting ways for faculty to work effectively within the Double Helix framework.

As the new century begins, the Double Helix curriculum promises to prepare physicians for careers that combine scientifically grounded, research-based medicine and sensitive patient care with valuable lessons from the past.

BUILDING A MEDICAL EDUCATION CONSORTIUM: THE ROLE OF THE AFFILIATED HOSPITALS

For over fifty years, the medical school and its affiliated hospitals have enjoyed a cooperative working relationship in education and clinical research which in many ways has been a model for the rest of the nation. Even before the term "consortium" became popularized to describe a cooperative approach to planning and managing graduate medical education (GME), Rochester developed just such a system.

The evolution of this cooperative model paralleled changes in medical practice and medical education that were taking place across the country. These changes included an increase in the number of medical students and residents; more dollars for GME; the development of medical specialties; increases in the number of highly specialized clinical faculty; and larger revenues from clinical services provided by these faculty. All these changes fueled the expansion of the educational system in Rochester's network of affiliated hospitals.

In the 1970s, as the hospital community began to feel increasing fiscal pressure, a decision was made to meet these growing challenges as a community, rather than as separate and competing entities (see chapter 9). It can be argued that this cooperative effort, which took place over many years, was an important cohesive factor in holding the community together, as institutions tried to solve their fiscal problems jointly. The cooperative nature of this relationship has become especially important to Rochester's health-care culture in recent years, as "health-care systems," which are inherently competitive, have developed and as pressures have increased to downsize graduate medical education.

How did this rich, highly integrated, and cooperative system come into being?

When Strong Memorial Hospital opened in 1926, and Rochester Municipal Hospital alongside it, the community already had other hospitals serving their own varied constituencies. Many first-rate physicians were associated with those hospitals and several of the institutions had excellent independent residency programs. At the time, many physicians in the community wondered why the medical school had elected to isolate itself from these clinical strengths. For years there were tensions.

Ultimately, leaders in the community hospitals and at the medical school recognized that mutual benefits could accrue from affiliating with each other for educational purposes. In 1945, the Genesee Hospital became the first to affiliate with the medical school. Ten years later Highland and Rochester General joined the affiliation; St. Mary's followed in 1967. That same year, through a contract with Monroe County, the University of Rochester assumed responsibility for professional services at Monroe Community Hospital, an institution dedicated to the care of the aged and chronically ill. In every case, the initiative for affiliation was generated by the community hospital, often spurred by physicians who were graduates of the medical school. Their purposes were straightforward: to improve quality of care through links with university-associated educational programs; to recruit high quality residents and attending physicians by linking with the school; to achieve a measure of pres-

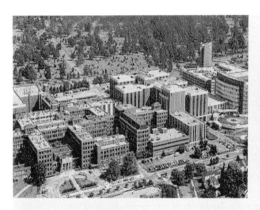 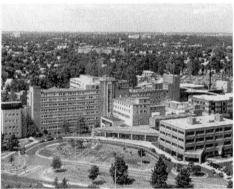
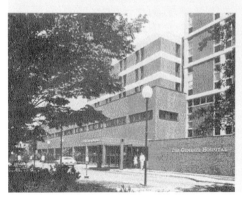 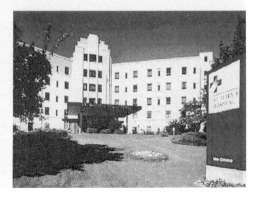

The four major affiliated teaching hospitals:
University of Rochester Medical Center (upper left), Rochester General Hospital (upper right), Genesee
Hospital (lower left), and St. Mary's Hospital (lower right)

JULES COHEN

tige through the academic connection; and, ultimately, to enrich the hospital culture by participating in medical education and in basic, clinical, and population-based research.

Both the medical school and the university knew that these benefits would also serve their own objectives. The affiliation would expand the population base and broaden the case mix for education, enriching the clinical experience of residents and medical students. The expanded population base would strengthen clinical research possibilities and enhance resources for both education and research. This would come about as relationships were developed with skilled practitioners and eventually with full-time academic faculty based in the affiliated hospitals.

Initially, connections among hospitals were limited to rotations of medical students. No full-time university faculty were based in the affiliated hospitals and all the residency programs in these institutions were free-standing. No university-appointed residents rotated to them.

This situation changed dramatically in the 1960s and 1970s. As public and private insurance and further state, federal, and foundation grant funding became available to support the growth of clinical programs, education, and research, the first full-time faculty were appointed to positions in affiliated hospitals. During the 1970s, the number of faculty increased substantially; as a result, more medical student experience in the affiliated hospitals became possible and attractive. The balance between the students' experience at Strong—highly oriented to specialty care—and their learning experience at the community hospitals has been extraordinarily valuable. (One student's comment on working in the community hospital where he was assigned is relevant: "You don't look up and see a lot of shoes of people who are more senior to you and who are going to get to see the patient first.") Integration began in graduate medical education programs, both residencies and fellowships, with highly successful integrations occuring in surgery and its subspecialties, as well as in pediatrics. Indeed, the growth of the surgical subspecialty programs—including some pioneering efforts nationally, such as in vascular surgery—was greatly facilitated by the expanded patient base, as well as funding that resulted from the affiliations.

The Associated Hospitals Program in Internal Medicine (now the Primary Care Program) was established by Lawrence Young after he stepped down as chair of Medicine. A high-quality university residency program in Family Medicine was established in 1967. These two programs gave expression to the medical school's commitment to education for primary care, as well as specialty care. They became models for educational links among affiliated institutions and for the wave of primary-care programs, especially in Internal Medicine, that appeared thereafter.

In 1980, based on a comprehensive review of the medical school's educational programs initiated by then Dean Frank Young, a policy decision was made—to work toward having all residency programs in the community be

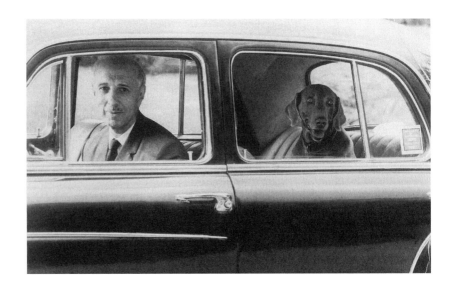

*Affiliated hospitals
teaching faculty leadership*

Top row, left to right: H. L. Segal *(Genesee)*,
S. B. Troup *(RGH)*, J. R. Hinshaw *(RGH)*

Middle row, left to right: T. Van Zandt *(RGH)*, A.
L. Ureles *(Genesee)*, M. LaForce *(Genesee)*

Bottom row, left to right: J. R. Jaenike *(Highland)*,
R. H. Sterns *(RGH)*,
N. Nadaraja *(St. Mary's)*,
R. J. Napodano *(St. Mary's)*

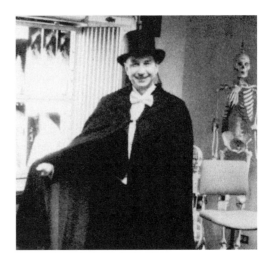

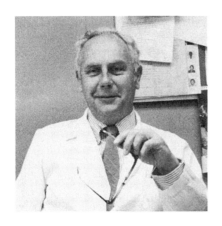

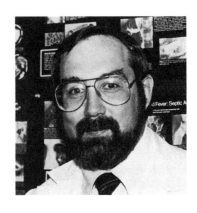

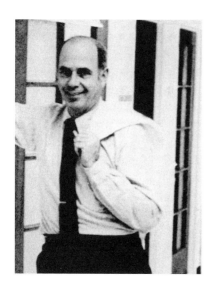

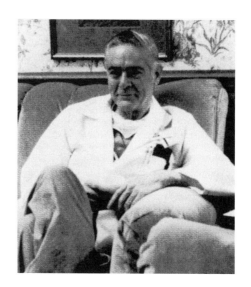

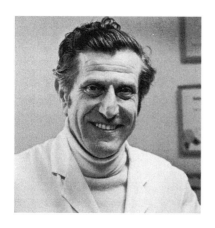

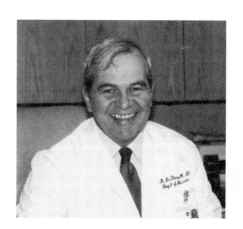

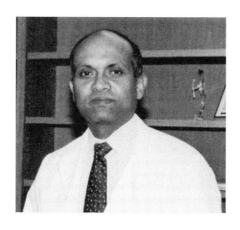

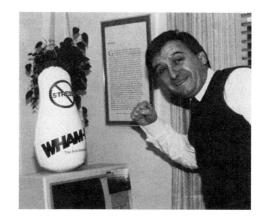

university-based and fully integrated. This objective has now largely been achieved.

Both community and medical school/university interests have been served by the development of this rich network of programs throughout the affiliated hospital system. Benefits include: improved quality of residents and practitioners; improved quality of care; growth of high-quality specialty services throughout the community, resulting in large part from the appointment of highly-specialized full-time and part-time medical school faculty in the associated hospitals; enhanced quality and range of educational experiences for medical students; and expanded influence of the medical school and university in the health affairs of the community. Thus, the original objectives of affiliation—for both the school and the participating hospitals—have for the most part been achieved and the benefits are mutually recognized.

Thus, from a combination of altruism, self-interest, and a commitment to community-wide planning for medical education, a true consortium of educational institutions has been developed. This community perspective survives—both in education and in organizing and financing health-care services—even though it is threatened by the present competitive environment. Orientation to cooperation and collaboration has a long history as a central element in the community's health-care value-system. There is reason, therefore, to hope and believe that it will continue to survive and thrive.

GRADUATE MEDICAL EDUCATION

When one reviews the history of graduate medical education (GME) programs at this institution, one is struck by several developments. Most of these of course reflect changes in the external environment, but several are "distinctively Rochester."

Growth and Development of GME at Rochester: A Balanced Agenda

In looking back through the medical school's history, one is struck by the enormous growth in the numbers of residents and the range of programs offered. In the very earliest years, only four clinical services (Medicine, Pediatrics, Obstetrics/Gynecology, and General Surgery) sponsored residencies and in each of these the numbers were small. In 1927–28 there were a total of about two dozen interns and residents in these services. In 1999–2000, 563 residents are working in thirty-two Medical Center programs. An additional 96 fellows are training in forty-one programs in the subspecialties.

What were the factors leading to this enormous growth? Most important was the development nationwide of specialty and subspecialty expertise, a change that reflects the evolution of medical knowledge and technical capacity over the years. The formation of national specialty accrediting bodies, and the leadership role played by Rochester faculty in these developments, fueled Rochester's interest to join the mainstream of GME in all fields. The creation of specialty divisions and departments and subspecialty units within the institution provided the organizational framework for the expansion.

After World War II, the availability of training grant funds and special research fellowships from the National Institutes of Health and various specialty societies further facilitated the growth of GME programs. When Medicare, Medicaid, and other insurance funds began to provide support for residents' salaries and benefits, for faculty efforts devoted to GME, and for dollars to support institutional indirect costs, the power of the purse as a stimulus to GME growth became substantial.

Further, it was a mark of departmental prestige to offer an approved residency or fellowship program. Skeptics say that the relatively inexpensive services provided by residents and fellows was an added inducement. Their services surely saved faculty time and energy, multiplied their productivity and their grant-getting and clinical income-generating potential, and enhanced their influence (some would say their political power). But one can also argue persuasively that the growth in GME programs has enriched the overall academic environment and enhanced learning all across the continuum—for medical students, faculty, nurses, and other health care professionals with whom residents and fellows interact.

Beyond simple growth in numbers and a richer mix of programs, other GME developments at Rochester have been equally striking. One of these has reflected the institutional agenda to insure programmatic balance between generalist and specialty fields. Beyond the generalist emphasis of several major clinical specialties (Medicine, Pediatrics, Obstetrics/Gynecology), several distinctive programs introduced over the years were designed to further the education of generalists.

One of the earliest was the two-year rotating internship, introduced in 1948 and inspired by John Romano. In this program interns rotated for six months on each of the following services: Medicine, Pediatrics, Psychiatry, and OB/GYN/Surgery. This nationally-recognized program helped ensure that residents had broad-based post-doctoral clinical training, whatever their ultimate career choice might be.

Under Lawrence Young's leadership, Rochester was one of the first medical schools in the country to offer a primary-care training program in Internal Medicine, as well as one of the early Medicine-Pediatrics residencies. Under the leadership of Eugene Farley, Rochester was one of the few, and earliest, research-intensive academic medical centers to offer a formal, high-quality Family Medicine residency. The Medical-Psychiatric Liaison Fellowship Program (see p. 31), developed under the leadership of George Engel, John Romano, William McCann, and Lawrence Young, achieved high prestige not only within the institution, but nationwide. The influence of Robert Haggerty, chair of Pediatrics, resulted in a strong generalist and community-oriented residency program in that department, as well as a first-rate program in Adolescent Medicine under the leadership of Stanford Friedman and his colleagues. Similarly, the formation of the General Medicine Unit of the Department of Medicine and its fellowship, again inspired by Lawrence Young and developed by Paul Griner and his colleagues, achieved national recognition and leadership in its field. These generalist-oriented and field-bridging traditions are continuing with the introduction of new collaborative residencies jointly offered by Medicine and Psychiatry and by Neurology and Psychiatry.

These initiatives have served to reinforce Rochester's commitment to generalism. We continue to prepare practicing and academic generalists, while ensuring that specialty graduates have had the broadest possible general professional education.

At the same time, we also prepare those seeking highly-specialized academic careers. This, too, has been an institutional emphasis, through our post-residency fellowship training programs and in the surgical subspecialties. Success in training for academic careers has been achieved, first, by designating this purpose as a central institutional objective, and then by building a substantive research experience into our specialty programs, often with external research support, while recruiting into these specialty programs trainees specifically committed to pursuing academic careers. It is no accident, therefore, that a high proportion of our graduates have had successful, research-oriented academic careers.

Rochester's Distinctive Contributions to GME Development

For the most part, Rochester's GME programs have been traditional in structure, content, and orientation. At the same time, several distinctive and trend-setting developments in GME have set the institution apart:

1. While the impact of the Biopsychosocial model (see p. 30) has been most powerfully felt in undergraduate medical education, its influence on graduate medical education has been substantial. Over the years, faculty skilled in biopsychosocial medicine have conducted formal teaching rounds for residents, as well as medical students, in Family Medicine, Internal Medicine, Obstetrics/Gynecology, Pediatrics, and Psychiatry. Through its overall influence on the educational culture of the institution, Biopsychosocialism—as I like to refer to it—has had an impact on residents in virtually all fields.

2. Rochester was one of the first medical schools to put into place dedicated, full-time directors of residency programs. William Morgan, in Medicine, was one of the first. Although he and his counterparts in several other

clinical departments had responsibilities beyond the residency program, most of these responsibilities related to the overall educational mission of the institution.

3. Rochester was one of the first medical centers to offer upper-level residents in generalist programs rotations in the subspecialties of their departments. As a result, graduates of these programs learned to handle complex clinical problems that might otherwise be referred to specialists. This initiative had a profound effect nationally on the education of broadly prepared generalists and, to some extent, changed the patterns and numbers of referrals made by generalists to specialists. While this may have limited the range of experiences available to post-resident fellows training in the specialties, patients have benefited from enhanced continuity of care and society has realized an economic benefit.

4. Rochester was one of the first institutions to put into place a "night-float" system to relieve residents of an over-burdensome schedule of working hours. The program began on the Internal Medicine service and in recent years has been embraced by Obstetrics/Gynecology and Pediatrics. In this system, residents are relieved at 10 p.m. by a "night-float" who follows patients through the night. As a result, residents can be fully alert and functional as they provide patient care and pursue educational activities throughout the day. The "night-float" attends to any problems that may come up during the nighttime hours, from addressing medical emergencies or answering patient-care needs (such as additional sedation) to providing simple diagnostic or treatment procedures. Thanks to the "night-float" system, it has been easier for the University of Rochester to meet recent regulatory requirements restricting residents' working hours, and the system has been a model for other institutions.

How Changes in the Health Care
System Have Affected GME

Advances in medical practice, changes in health-care organization and financing, and exponential growth in regulation, have had a profound effect on graduate medical education in all fields nationwide. Change, even change for the better, carries with it unintended and sometimes perverse consequences. This has certainly been the experience in medical education, especially graduate medical education. Rochester's GME programs have not been insulated from the impact of these changes but some of the adverse impact has been blunted by positive factors within the Rochester environment.

Advances in medicine and aging of the population have dramatically altered the mix, complexity, and severity of illness among hospitalized patients. Paradoxically, these changes simultaneously have both narrowed and broadened the range of residents' experience. While they have had fewer opportunities to see uncomplicated and as yet undiagnosed illnesses, they have been introduced to sicker hospitalized patients with more complicated conditions and to a range of drugs, medical treatments, and procedures never experienced—or even imagined—by their predecessors. Pressures to decrease hospital length-of-stay have put added work demands on residents and limited what George Engel liked to call the "digestion time"—the time a learner needs with patients in order to be able to fully understand the patient and his/her illness. Further, as one program director put it, residents have to spend more of their time "running around," organizing and chasing down the results of diagnostic procedures and laboratory tests, as well as working with consultants who are increasingly specialized.

Residents now have to deal with an array of new forces and regulations that affect the care of patients—managed care and other cost-containment efforts, medical-legal and ethical issues, new requirements for more extensive documentation and a higher level of supervision of their work, and a variety of care guidelines and protocols. Virtually all of these factors have been designed to improve the quality of patient care and contain costs, and in many respects they have succeeded. But they have also put added pressures on residents, negatively affected patient-centered decision-making flexibility, reduced residents' autonomy, and slowed the growth of their capacity to function independently and with self confidence.

While major competitive pressures involving the organization and financing of health care are at work in Rochester, a fundamental cooperative spirit remains. Graduate medical education is still strongly supported by all teaching hospitals. Many practitioners give willingly and generously of their time, serving as teaching attendings on in-patient services and welcoming residents (and medical students) into their offices. These experiences in ambulatory settings ensure that learners are exposed to a broad range of clinical problems. Despite time and economic pressures, full- and part-time faculty in all Rochester hospitals and health-care systems remain deeply committed to education. Their involvement and generosity have been critically important in ensuring that the clinical education of residents, fellows, and medical students remains broad-based and of good quality. This has not been the case everywhere. The medical school and the medical center are deeply appreciative of these efforts by clinical faculty.

A GROWING COMMITMENT TO PUBLIC HEALTH

One of medicine's traditional goals has been to provide the best possible care for each patient. Medical education programs are designed to teach students the most effective ways to meet that goal. Here at Rochester, and at medical schools across the nation, we have been largely successful in this undertaking. We have been less successful in providing a similarly high level of quality care to our communities, especially for those who are less fortunate socially and economically. In the early 1980s, medical school leaders around the country began to appreciate more fully the importance of this orientation to "population health" and they began building this new emphasis into medical education programs.

The transition came easily at Rochester for several reasons. The University of Rochester's first commitment to serve the poor was made as early as 1925, when the Rochester Municipal Hospital was moved from its former location and rebuilt as an adjunct to the new Strong Memorial Hospital.

A second commitment came later, when the university supported the development of teaching affiliations with other Rochester hospitals, alliances designed to enhance the quality of care throughout the community. As discussed earlier, these affiliations are based on the belief that the presence of academic/teaching programs in a patient-care environment enhances the quality of that care, a concept widely endorsed both by the academic center and the partnering hospitals. Arguably, the most important value of affiliation has been that it adds a *community* orientation to the quality, organization, and financing of care provided to the sick—all to the benefit of the public's health.

A third level of commitment came in the 1960s with the recruitment of Robert Berg and his colleagues and the establishment of a Department of Community and Preventive Medicine. This innovative move was critically important in imprinting on the school's teaching programs a commitment to community health. An early result of the new emphasis was the development and introduction of the course "Patient, Physician, and Society." Through small group discussions, students were introduced to issues relating to the organization and financing of medical care. They learned how the interactions of physicians with their patients around these issues

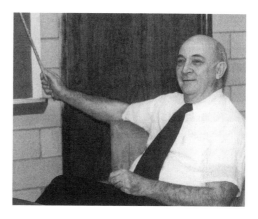

R. L. Berg, *Community and Preventive Medicine*

influenced patients' health care—and their health. The course "Epidemiology," with its orientation to population health, also was introduced in the early 1960s, another creation of the Department of Community and Preventive Medicine.

Finally, the roles that Berg and his colleague Ernest Saward played in developing the Regional Medical Program (a cooperative community-wide effort to enhance the education of all health-care providers) and the network of community health centers were influential in creating an educational environment in which orientation to the health of the community was a central feature. With this new environment in place, it became relatively straightforward to expand attention to the health of the community within our medical education programs.

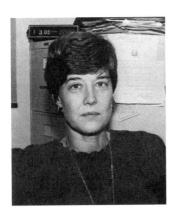

Kathryn
Montgomery
(Hunter),
*founding
Director of
the Division
of Medical
Humanities*

Changes in the Formal Curriculum

Over the years, the "Patient, Physician and Society" course was transformed into an enriched program in the Medical Humanities. In addition, a separate course, "Ethics and Law in Medicine," was introduced and the program in Community Medicine dealing with issues of health-care organization and financing was strengthened. With the strong support of Dean Robert Joynt, a new Division of the Medical Humanities was created, under the leadership of Kathryn Montgomery (Hunter), and later, Jane Greenlaw; the new division was given responsibility for teaching the history and philosophy of medicine and medical practice, medical ethics, and legal medicine. Seminars in medical law/ethics were introduced into the third-year Clinical Clerkship programs and the fourth-year Senior Seminar program. An ethics consultation service was created, and students were able to elect rotations with this service. All these innovations helped focus informed interest on community health-care issues.

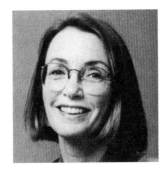

Jane
Greenlaw,
*current
Director of
the Division
of Medical
Humanities*

Engaging Medical Students in Community Outreach

In an effort to expose students more directly to the needs of Rochester's disadvantaged, a program of voluntary outreach activities was created under the leadership of Joan Hensler and later, Nancy Chin. This program—Students of Rochester Outreach (SRO)—has introduced students to the needs of the homeless, single-parent families, substance abusers, the disadvantaged elderly, new immigrants, and other underserved members of the community. Students volunteer as tutors in the school system, as health screeners, counselors/mentors, and just plain friends to those in need. The SRO program was begun with generous gifts from private donors, two local foundations, and the Josiah Macy, Jr.,

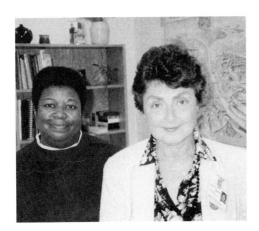

Cathy Collins *and* Joan Hensler: *Students of Rochester Outreach*

Foundation in New York City; in more recent years it has been supported largely by institutional resources.

The satisfaction reported by students who volunteer in these varied settings has been key to the program's success. Thousands of medical students, nursing students, and undergraduates have enrolled in these service activities, giving generously of their time, energy, and experience to benefit our community—while reaping educational benefits and personal satisfaction. Equally important, the program has brought the Medical Center into direct contact with agencies that serve the disadvantaged, making clear that the institution is committed to the community it serves and from which it draws support.

Building Partnerships in International Health

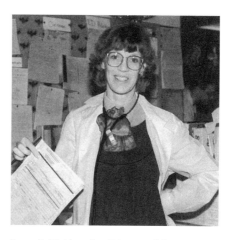

Lynn S. Bickley, *first Director of the program in International Health*

As a companion to the SRO program, the medical school during the early 1980s established a formal program in International Health, which quickly became one of the leading programs of its kind in the nation. Conceived and initially directed by Lynn S. Bickley, the program sent Rochester medical students to Third World countries where they could experience first-hand the health-care problems and needs of seriously disadvantaged populations. International fellowships funded by private donors made these educational opportunities possible. Later, successful grant applications to the US Agency for International Development (USAID) enabled us to develop a major program in Bamako, Mali, one of Rochester's Sister Cities and the capital of one of the poorest countries in the world. The program focused on improving the health of children and enhancing the training of health-care professionals; Rochester students played a key role in these efforts. Mali benefited from their service, and the students' educational experience was enriched.

More recently, inspired by Daphne Hare and supported by USAID, a program was developed by Bickley and our International Health Office to work with five medical schools in the former Soviet Union to improve their medical education programs. Under the leadership of Ralph Jozefowicz from the Department of Neurology and the USAID Project team at the University of Rochester, these initiatives have benefited our own programs, as well as those in Russia and the Ukraine.

While Mali, Russia, and the Ukraine have represented the major sites of our involvement, students have been awarded fellowships to serve throughout the world—in Asia, South America, the Middle East, and Africa—to their enormous benefit. Each student who receives a fellowship is required to conduct a research project as part of the experience and to submit a written (and sometimes published) report, an exercise that adds to the value of the experience. One hoped-for outcome of these international experiences is that students will gain knowledge and skills that can be applied to disadvantaged populations in this country.

These educational undertakings—Community Medicine, Epidemiology, Medical Humanities/Ethics and Law, Students of Rochester Outreach, and the International Health Program—have greatly enriched the community/population orientation of our medical education programs. Students not only learn a different perspective about health care through these programs, but their lives are touched by their contacts with those who are hurting, here at home and around the world.

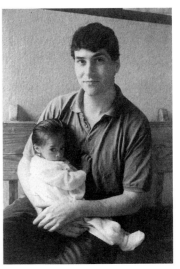

Learning to understand people is an important part of becoming a doctor. At Rochester, two organizations play an important role in this effort. SRO (Students of Rochester Outreach) and a wide variety of International Medicine Programs enable students to work with disadvantaged and underserved communities at home and around the world. Through these experiences, illustrated here and on the following pages, students come to understand the ways in which social forces influence health and illness.

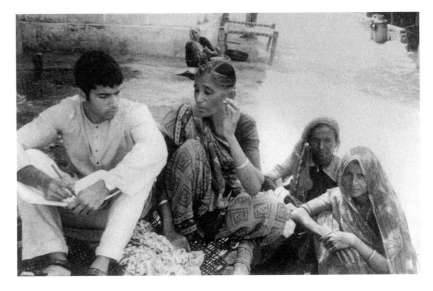

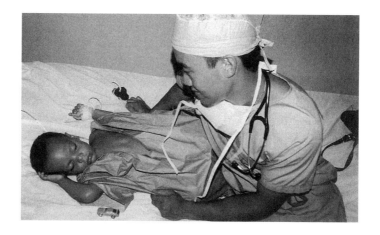

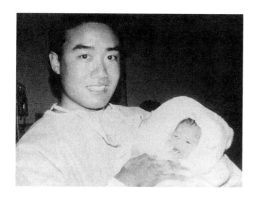

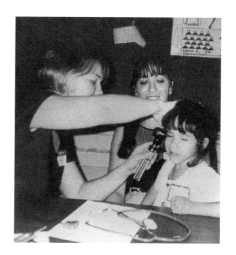

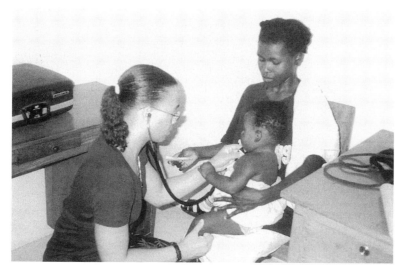

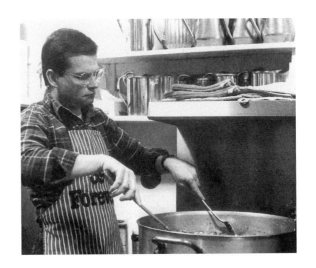

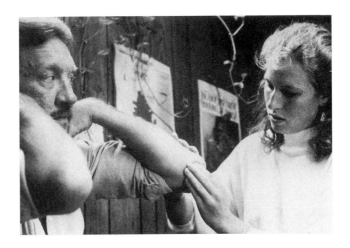

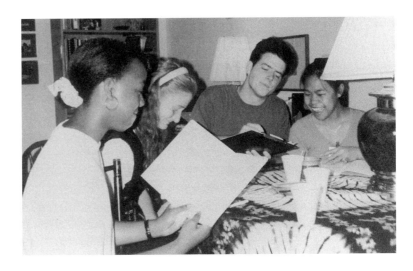

Jules Cohen

"TO EACH . . .": HELPING STUDENTS PREPARE FOR CAREERS AS GENERALISTS, SPECIALISTS, AND IN ACADEMIC MEDICINE

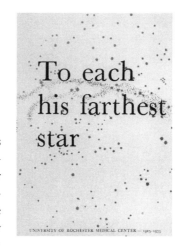

The cover of To Each His Farthest Star, *published on the occasion of the Medical Center's 50th anniversary, 1975*

One of the great strengths of Rochester's medical education program has been an operating philosophy that allows each learner to reach for his or her highest career aspiration. In earlier times, this was known as the "To Each His Farthest Star" credo, but now the farthest stars are within the reach of both men and women equally.[7] This philosophy of opportunity has been expressed repeatedly in the writings of those who helped shape Rochester's educational culture and its programs, starting with Whipple himself. Consider these phrases drawn from our institutional past: "individualized attention to every student," "no tracking," "the object is to produce among graduates the undifferentiated physician, able to pursue any career path of his or her choosing." Achieving that educational objective is not as easy as it sounds. To state this objective meant the school had to consciously design and put into place curricular structures and program content which would express this commitment to balance. The school also had to provide a range of opportunities outside the formal curriculum that would enable each student to pursue his or her individual interests.

Several key elements of strategy were adopted to achieve these goals. First, those in leadership positions have repeatedly emphasized that this educational philosophy is an institutional priority. Whipple, Corner, Fenn, Bloor and Stotz, Frank Young, Herbert and William Morgan, Orbison, McCann, Larry Young, Morton, Mahoney and Schwartz, Clauson, Haggerty, Forbes and Bradford, Berg, Joynt, and of course Romano and Engel—all these and many other institutional leaders have by precept and example expressed the critical importance of attending to the individual needs of students in order to help them achieve their highest aspirations. The direct engagement of chairs and other senior leadership as educators and mentors has set an important example for other faculty.

A second factor was the determination to keep the student body small, so that students could be individually nurtured professionally and encouraged by committed faculty mentors. The ability and willingness of school leaders to resist political and economic pressures to increase the size of the student body has been very important in ensuring the continued collegiality of students and faculty. Alumni and faculty repeatedly emphasize the value and power of smallness as they have reflected on the Rochester tradition of student-faculty engagement. The faculty's "open door" policy is a tradition at Rochester. In recent years, this tradition has been challenged by the increasing pressure on clinical faculty to generate more practice revenue, and on both clinical and basic science faculty to generate research grant income. These pressures have, of course, been felt by faculty at many other schools. But the tradition of engagement with students—a hallmark at Rochester from the beginning—although threatened, remains alive and well.

An equally important strategy to encourage individualized achievement can be found in the nature of the curriculum itself, which features exposure to scientific academic values and role models, as well as a full range of practicing generalists and specialists. This educational system exposes students to the full range of career opportunities, presenting them as equally valued.

Exposure to the Sciences and to Research

From the school's early days, and at the time of every major curricular change, a conscious determination has been made to expose *all* students to the full range of the sciences basic to medicine, biomedical and behavioral. Even where lecture and laboratory hours have been reduced and other modes of instruction and learning introduced, the school has insisted that all students have this broad exposure. This educational principal in and of itself has been important in emphasizing to students the value the school places on the sciences and the valued role that full-time academic faculty, scientifically oriented, play in medical education. As a result, scientists have been important role models for our students from the first days of the institution.

Students have had many opportunities over the years to engage in research with faculty mentors. The M.D./Ph.D. Program, established in the mid-1960s (see chapter 2), provides a rich opportunity for students to enter academic career paths. In addition, the funded "Year-Out" fellowship program, which goes back to the first days of the school and which has attracted six to ten students (or more) every year since its inception, provides students with similar opportunities. Both programs enable students to sample academic life while they work closely with faculty mentors, developing warm, productive, and lasting personal relationships with them. Often students have begun a substantive research project of their own, and some have earned master's degrees in their chosen fields. As a result of these opportunities, many of our students have pursued successful academic careers. The Student Summer Research Fellowship (which high proportions of the students pursue, often for more than a single summer) has had a similar impact.

At the GME level, initiatives such as the Clinical Investigator Train-

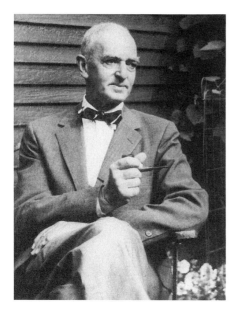
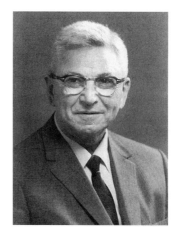

Distinguished Rochester practicing internists L. A. Kohn *(left) and* J. D. Goldstein *(above)*

ing Program, which flourished here during the 1960s, and special academic career preparation opportunities within various departments have made important contributions to an educational environment that encourages students, residents, and fellows to pursue academic careers. It is no surprise that for years Rochester has ranked among the top ten schools in the nation in the proportion of graduates who have gone on to serve as full-time medical school faculty.

Exposure to Clinical Practice

At the same time, it is no accident that Rochester has ranked among the top research-intensive medical schools in the proportion of its graduates who become primary-care practitioners. Beginning with their first two years of study, Rochester students work with generalist and specialist clinicians whose principle responsibility is the care of patients. No less "scientific" in their orientation, these practitioners become important role models for our students. Opportunities to work with practitioners in their offices, or to be supervised by them in the care of inpatients, reflect the importance the school places on the work of practicing clinicians, a value established during the school's earliest days.

The importance of the generalist orientation has also been reflected in the institution's residencies and fellowships, as mentioned earlier. Over the years the pediatric residency program has embraced a strong orientation both to generalism and to community service. The internal medicine residency emphasizes a balanced commitment to those who will practice as generalists and to those aspiring to academic specialty careers. Generalist fellowship programs are part of the structure of both departments. In the late 1950s and early 1960s the school sponsored a unique two-year rotating internship which attracted outstanding physicians. After he retired as chair of Medicine in the early 1970s, Lawrence Young established and developed one of the nation's first and most prestigious internal medicine primary care programs. For over 25 years the school has sponsored a high-quality family medicine residency, while a mixed medicine-pediatrics residency leads to board certification in both disciplines. The presence of these first-rate residencies has been an important influence in orienting medical students to generalism. The high place that clinical *generalism* and *generalists* have enjoyed in the life of the institution is "Distinctively Rochester."

In summary, each of the following has been critically important in creating opportunities for students to achieve their highest individual aspirations:

- A school philosophy and an educational environment which features individualized attention to each student;
- A determination to keep class size relatively small, to make possible this individualized attention;
- A conscious effort to construct a formal curriculum characterized by balanced, in-depth exposure to the full range of medical sciences, as well as to a full range of clinical specialties and generalist fields;
- A determination to expose students and postgraduate physicians to role-modeling academic research scientists and clinicians *and* to community-based generalist practitioners;
- An openness to the development of faculty-inspired special programs and professional experiences which give students and postgraduate physicians a chance to sample the full range of career options.

The learner-centeredness of the school's programs and the traditional willingness of faculty to welcome students as professional colleagues into their laboratories and offices and to mentor them individually—these have been key to helping fulfill the mission celebrated in the phrase "To each (his/her) farthest star."

Advisors to our students, helping them to reach their farthest stars

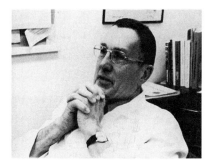

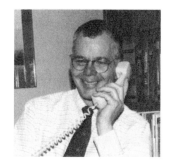

William T. VanHuysen

C. Douglas Angevine

Above and right: 1960s–1997, Associate Deans for Student Affairs

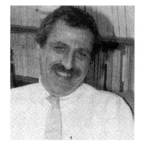

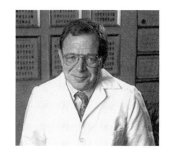

Laurence Jacobs

J. Franklin Richeson

1997– Present, Associate Deans for Advising

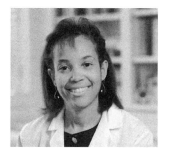

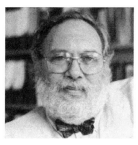

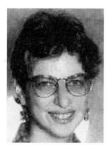

Tana Grady-Weliky, *Assoc. Dean for Undergraduate Medical Education*

Laurence B. Guttmacher

Elizabeth H. Naumburg

J. Franklin Richeson *(pictured above)*

Assistant Deans

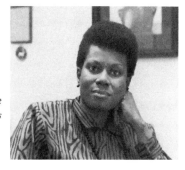

Brenda D. Lee *(left), 1987–Present*

Karen C. Pryor *(right), 1993–1997*

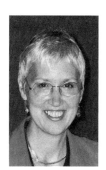

RECOGNIZING FACULTY
CONTRIBUTIONS TO TEACHING

We have referred to the value that Rochester faculty place on their role as teachers and as mentors, rather than reluctant instructors. The seeds of this value system were sown by the first faculty; recall Whipple's words: "I would be remembered as a teacher."

Belief in the importance of this faculty responsibility has been reinforced in many ways over the years. Junior faculty have seen that even the most senior faculty—those who carry especially heavy clinical, research, and administrative responsibilities—are actively involved in teaching at both undergraduate and graduate levels. There is enormous power in this role-modeling. Close attention and time repeatedly given to educational planning, especially in the last forty years, has sent an additional, powerful message to faculty about the value the institution places on teaching. The willingness of school leaders to recognize with tenure appointments and promotions those faculty whose contributions have been distinctive in education, as opposed to clinical service and research achievements, sends an important message to faculty aspiring to academic advancement. A host of school-wide and departmental teaching awards, based on feedback from medical students and postgraduate learners, has provided added reinforcement.

And yet Rochester medical faculty (like those at all other medical schools and those involved in higher education generally) have often felt they have not received rightful recognition of their teaching efforts. In particular, it has seemed that research achievement—as measured by numbers of papers published and the number and size of research grants received—is a more important determinant of recognition. These feelings among faculty are particularly acute at times of planned curricular change, when the pedagogic changes proposed seem to be more labor-intensive than established teaching methods.

In an effort to address these faculty concerns directly, the school has introduced over the past twenty-five years a number of new programs and approaches that recognize teaching efforts. First, several named teaching awards, now endowed by grateful donors, recognize teaching excellence in each year of the curriculum. Endowments for the Manuel D. Goldman Prize for excellence in first-year teaching, the Herbert W. Mapstone Prize for second-year teaching, the Harry L. Segal Award for third-year teaching, and the Keith Miner-Ford Award for fourth-year teaching are fully funded. Each carries a substantial and meaningful monetary award. Other faculty, also chosen by the students, receive commendations for teaching excellence. Further, the Graduate Student Society Faculty Award and the Alumni Award for excellence in graduate medical education also recognize faculty efforts.

In addition to these awards, a major endowment, amounting now to over one million dollars, was developed with the encouragement and support of Dean Robert Joynt to fund the designation each year of several Dean's

Teaching Scholars. These awards go to as-yet-untenured faculty who are making high-quality contributions to teaching, while continuing their research or patient care. Awardees are selected by a small committee of highly respected senior faculty, based on nominations from departments, letters from colleagues, student comments, and, most valuable, the nominees' self-assessment of their contributions to teaching, research, and/or patient care. Each award carries with it a substantial three-year salary supplement. The endowment—inspired by a major gift from the Class of 1957 in memory of one of its most distinguished members, Lowell A. Glasgow—has grown through contributions from grateful patients, alumni, current and former faculty, and foundations. Individual awards are named for distinguished former faculty members, in memory of patients, or in the name of the foundations supporting the awards. In recent years, several Senior Dean's Teaching Scholars also have been recognized, with funding provided by a grant from the Robert Wood Johnson Foundation. These are fully tenured senior faculty who have made outstanding contributions to teaching during their many years of service to the school. The Dean's Teaching Scholar Awards are prestigious, sending a clear message to the faculty of the school's commitment to teaching.

Still another initiative has been the creation of the annual medical school Convocation, which opens the academic year. This gathering, conceived and introduced by Dean Frank Young to celebrate student and faculty achievement, is always attended by hundreds of students and faculty. This is the occasion where medical and graduate student awards for outstanding performance are given, where faculty teaching awards are presented by the students, where the new Dean's Teaching Scholars are announced, and where newly designated Chairs are presented. This celebration is another statement of the importance that the school places on education and on faculty teaching contributions.

Perhaps most important of all has been a change in the way faculty are evaluated for promotion. There is now a very explicit requirement that faculty members' contributions to teaching be specified and evaluated by the nominating department and supported by letters of referral, as well as the faculty member's own self-assessment. The ad hoc committees and school-wide Executive Committee that evaluate proposed promotions are explicitly charged with considering teaching efforts. Recommended promotions do not go forward unless data about the quantity and quality of teaching and prior teaching awards are included in the recommendations. As faculty have come to understand that these changes in the promotion process represent a meaningful application of new standards, it becomes clear that the school and its students truly value their teaching contributions.

These tables list the faculty honored through the years as Dean's Teaching Scholars, Senior Dean's Teaching Scholars, and Recipients of the Gold Medal awarded by the Medical Alumni Association. The tributes reflect the contributions these faculty have made to the life of the institution, especially to medical education.

"And gladly wolde he lerne and gladly teche . . ."
Geoffrey Chaucer, Prologue to the Canterbury Tales

Dean's Teaching Scholars Award

1987
Philip M. Dvoretsky, M.D., *Andrew W. Mellon Dean's Teaching Scholar*

1988
Martha L. Blair, Ph.D., *Andrew W. Mellon Dean's Teaching Scholar*
Ralph F. Jozefowicz, M.D., *Andrew W. Mellon Dean's Teaching Scholar*

1991
Edgar R. Black, M.D., *Lawrence E. Young Dean's Teaching Scholar*
John G. Frelinger, Ph.D., *Andrew W. Mellon Dean's Teaching Scholar*
J. Franklin Richeson, M.D., *DeWitt Brower Dean's Teaching Scholar*

1992
David A. Baram, M.D., *George L. Engel & John Romano Dean's Teaching Scholar*
Francis Gigliotti, M.D., *Lowell A. Glasgow Dean's Teaching Scholar*
John Olschowka, Ph.D., *George W. Merck Dean's Teaching Scholar*
Charles H. Packman, M.D., *William S. McCann Dean's Teaching Scholar*
Otto Thaler, M.D., *Robert Wood Johnson Senior Dean's Teaching Scholar*

1993
Lynn S. Bickley, M.D., *George W. Corner Dean's Teaching Scholar*
David L. Felten, M.D., Ph.D., *Robert Wood Johnson Senior Dean's Teaching Scholar*

1994
Suzanne Y. Felten, Ph.D., *Robert Wood Johnson Senior Dean's Teaching Scholar*
Karl Kieburtz, M.D., M.P.H., *George W. Merck Dean's Teaching Scholar*
Richard E. Kreipe, M.D., *Andrew W. Mellon Dean's Teaching Scholar*
Lawrence A. Tabak, D.D.S., Ph.D., *Robert Wood Johnson Senior Dean's Teaching Scholar*

1995
Donald R. Bordley, M.D., *Lawrence E. Young Dean's Teaching Scholar*
Ronald M. Epstein, M.D., *George Engel & John Romano Dean's Teaching Scholar*
James E. Melvin, D.D.S., Ph.D., *Andrew W. Mellon Dean's Teaching Scholar*
John T. Hansen, Ph.D., *Robert Wood Johnson Senior Dean's Teaching Scholar*

1996
J. Peter Harris, M.D., *Gilbert B. Forbes Dean's Teaching Scholar*
David G. Hicks, M.D., *Andrew W. Mellon Dean's Teaching Scholar*
Michael Kerry O'Banion, M.D., Ph.D., *George W. Corner Dean's Teaching Scholar*
Seymour J. Schwartz, M.D., *Robert Wood Johnson Senior Dean's Teaching Scholar*

1997

Laurence Guttmacher, M.D., *George Engel & John Romano Dean's Teaching Scholar*
William C. Hulbert, Jr., M.D., *George W. Merck Dean's Teaching Scholar*
Michael P. McDermott, Ph.D., *Andrew W. Mellon Dean's Teaching Scholar*
Dennis J. McCance, Ph.D., *Robert Wood Johnson Senior Dean's Teaching Scholar*

1998

Denise A. Figlewicz, Ph.D., *DeWitt Brower Dean's Teaching Scholar*
Diane M. Hartmann, M.D., *Lowell A. Glascow Dean's Teaching Scholar*
Jeffrey M. Lyness, M.D., *Jules Cohen Dean's Teaching Scholar*

1999

Mary T. Caserta, M.D., *Gilbert B. Forbes Dean's Teaching Scholar*
Barbara J. Davis, Ph.D., *George W. Corner Dean's Teaching Scholar*
David R. Lambert, M.D., *Lawrence E. Young Dean's Teaching Scholar*
Andrew J. Swinburne, M.D., *Robert Wood Johnson Senior Dean's Teaching Scholar*

Medical Alumni Association Gold Medal Recipients

In recognition of integrity, inspiring teaching, and devotion to medical students

1952	Samuel W. Clausen	1976	Arthur J. Moss
1953	George H. Whipple	1977	William T. VanHuysen
1954	William B. Hawkins	1978	Victor E. Emmel
1955	Karl M. Wilson	1979	Ruth A. Lawrence
1956	Lawrence A. Kohn	1980	Otto F. Thaler
1957	Paul H. Garvey	1981	Robert M. McCormack
1958	Wallace O. Fenn	1982	Gilbert B. Forbes
1959	William S. McCann	1983	Paul N. Yu
1960	William L. Bradford	1984	David Goldblatt
1961	John J. Morton Jr.	1985	Jules Cohen
1962	Ralph E. Jacox	1986	Victor DiStefano
1963	Charles E. Tobin	1987	William L. Morgan Jr.
1964	Edward F. Adolph	1988	Milton N. Luria
1965	Henry A. Blair	1989	Robert J. Joynt
1966	Wilbur K. Smith	1990	Richard Satran
1967	E. Henry Keutmann	1991	Magaret T. Colgan
1968	J. Lowell Orbison	1992	Eric A. Schenk
1969	Earle B. Mahoney	1993	Chloe G. Alexson
1970	Harold Hodge	1994	John R. Devanny
1971	John Romano	1995	John T. Hansen
1972	George L. Engel	1996	William Hall
1973	Lawrence E. Young	1997	Robert F. Betts
1974	Jacob W. Holler	1998	Ralph F. Jozefowicz
1975	Theodore E. VanZandt	1999	J. Franklin Richeson

REFERENCES

1. Engel G.L. The Need for a New Medical Model: A Challenge for Biomedicine. Science 196:129–136, 1977.
2. Peabody F.W. The Care of the Patient. JAMA 88:877–882, 1927.
3. Morgan W.L., Engel G.L. The Clinical Approach to the Patient. WB Saunders Co. Philadelphia. 1969.
4. Morgan W.L., Engel G.L., Luria M.N. The General Clerkship: A Course Designed to Teach the Clinical Approach to the Patient. J. Med. Educ. 47:556–63, 1972.
5. Geertsma R.H., Meyerowitz S., Salzman L.F., Donovan J.C. An Independent Study Program within a Medical Curriculum. J. Med. Educ. 52:123–32, 1977.
6. Cohen J., Krackov S.K., Black E.R., Holyst M. Introduction to Human Health and Illness: A Series of Patient-Centered Conferences Based on the Biopsychosocial Model. Academic Medicine 75:390–396, 2000.
7. To Each His Farthest Star. The University of Rochester Medical Center 1925–1975. Romano J., Senior Editor. WF Humphrey Press. Geneva. 1975.

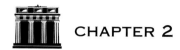

CHAPTER 2

Graduate Education in Biomedical Sciences: Partners in Inquiry

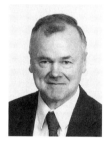
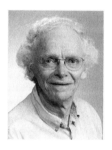
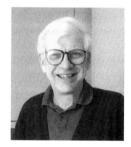

GEORGE A.
KIMMICH, PH.D.

VICTOR G.
LATIES, PH.D.

ROBERT E.
MARQUIS, PH.D.

A strong spirit of interdisciplinary endeavor is a hallmark of graduate education at the University of Rochester Medical Center. Our faculty is justifiably proud of this tradition. In conversations with prospective students or faculty members and other visitors to the campus we are quick to mention the low barriers among departments and ease of building collaborative research and teaching relationships. This tradition has served us well and surely will be a strength in the future.

No two individuals have precisely the same views concerning the origins of our unusual spirit of interdepartmental collegiality. Two aspects deserve mention as important catalysts in enabling the tradition of cooperation to take root and flourish. One relates to the fact that all basic science departments in the Medical Center are under one roof. As a result, there is—and always has been—easy access among and between the faculty and facilities of different departments. Another aspect of this collegiality is possible due to the proximity of the Medical Center to the University's River Campus with its strong programs in natural science. Interactions at a distance are difficult and erode any sense of common interest; at Rochester, each department, on either campus, has expertise that can be valuable to all other departments, which either share the same building or are only a pleasant, five-minute, cross-campus walk away. The ease with which joint research efforts involving close neighbors are made has undoubtedly been a primary catalyst for encouraging the low-barrier tradition.

As a medium-size university, we are fully competitive with much larger institutions in garnering research funds from public and private funding agencies. Historically we have placed among the top twenty-five medical schools nationally, and current research funding to the School of Medicine and Dentistry, sponsored by outside agencies, exceeds $100 million annually. In part, our research funding success is a direct result of strong interdisciplinary collaborative activity in the laboratory and the classroom.

From 1919 to 1975

The development of graduate education at the Medical Center during this period has been thoroughly reviewed by J. Newell Stannard in his chapter "Zealous Companions in Research—The Graduate Studies Program" in *To Each His Farthest Star*, published on the occasion of the institution's fiftieth anniversary. Stannard points out that the school of Medicine and Dentistry awarded a Ph.D. degree in 1925, four years before the first class of medical students received their M.D. degrees.

Emphasis on graduate education at the medical school has always been strong. In Stannard's 1975 article there is a table summarizing the ratio of Ph.D. to M.D. students in residence from 1931 through 1974. The ratios remained below 20 percent until 1949, then rose gradually until 1974. That year there were 381 medical students in residence and 222 students enrolled in doctoral programs, for a ratio of 58 percent. By late 1999, when there were 410 medical students and 317 Ph.D. students, the ratio had risen to 77 percent.

An overview of the doctoral programs throughout our history is given in Table 1. The first column summarizes the distribution of Ph.D. degrees awarded before the war and shows that Biochemistry and Physiology were dominant in the early years. Of the fifty-eight doctorates awarded between 1925 and the end of 1941, only nine were earned in other fields. (Note that the figure for Physiology includes degrees awarded through the Department of Vital Economics which merged with the Department of Physiology.)

The school was well on the way to becoming a major player in graduate education in the period before World War II, Stannard concluded. During the war, Rochester was highly active in research associated with the Manhattan Project. This connection with the U.S. Atomic Energy Commission (AEC), which evolved into the U.S. Department of Energy (DOE), greatly influenced graduate education at Rochester. When the war ended, the AEC continued to fund research at Rochester and the Department of Radiation Biology was created. Soon it was offering the first Ph.D. in that subject in the world. The department also was empowered to expand the school's

GEORGE A. KIMMICH, VICTOR G. LATIES, ROBERT E. MARQUIS

research activity in biophysics. By 1965, with flourishing doctoral programs in both fields, the name was changed to the Department of Radiation Biology & Biophysics (RB&B). William Neuman and Aser Rothstein served as co-chairs of the department. The scope of the new department's research was further broadened to include aspects of toxicology beyond that directly related to radioisotope exposure.

At that time, in close cooperation with the Department of Pharmacology, chaired by Harold Hodge, and with leadership provided by Thomas Clarkson, an interdisciplinary research cluster gained a major training grant from the National Institutes of Health to provide support for doctoral candidates in Toxicology. This group of faculty comprised a division within RB&B, but evolved into the Department of Environmental Medicine.

With continued outside support, RB&B prospered and at its peak had more than forty-five faculty members with primary appointments and as many as 125 doctoral candidates enrolled in three doctoral programs, almost half the number of Ph.D. candidates in the medical school. Because the department had no formal commitment to teach medical students, activities focused on basic research and graduate education. Its faculty played a key role in organizing a set of interdepartmental (IND) courses that served to expand opportunities offered by the various graduate programs in the Medical Center. The original four courses were in Cell Biology, Molecular Genetics, Biomacromolecules, and Ultrastructure. Because the purpose of these courses was to introduce graduate students to the most current thinking and techniques in basic research, teaching necessarily included faculty from a number of departments. Thus, the IND courses were a major force in bringing about cooperative faculty interactions in the classroom.

In time, other IND courses were added to the basic set. Perhaps the most notable of these courses was IND 401 Biochemistry, begun in 1970. With its introduction, separate biochemistry courses were in place for graduate and medical students. This development was much needed; the growing interest and research capability in molecular biology required an intensive, molecular approach for graduate students, with less emphasis on clinical biochemistry.

IND 401 was organized as a graduate course, but was open to upper-level undergraduate and non-matriculated students who had achieved satisfactory performance in appropriate pre-requisite courses. This dual role resulted in total enrollments of more than one-hundred students. Later development of the Rochester Plan, and subsequently the Program in Biology & Medicine, further enhanced the course's value, bringing together students from the two campuses. For many years, IND 401 was a required component in all Ph.D. programs at the Medical Center and also for the Ph.D. in Biology, forming another link between the Medical Center and the River Campus.

The second column of Table 1 summarizes the number of Ph.D. graduates from 1925 through the academic year of 1972–73. The doctoral programs in Biochemistry, Biophysics, Pharmacology, Physiology, and Radiation

Biology had then been in place for a generation. During the 1950s and '60s, graduate education had grown in other departments as well: Bacteriology (which became Microbiology in 1961 and then Microbiology & Immunology in 1987), Anatomy (Neurobiology & Anatomy after 1985), and Pathology (Pathology & Laboratory Medicine after 1985). By the early 1970s, after the Center for Brain Research moved from the River Campus to the Medical Center, and the Department of Anatomy had begun to focus its research on the nervous system, most of the currently active programs were in place. By the end of 1973, the School of Medicine and Dentistry had awarded more than 500 Ph.D. degrees and was a major player in American graduate education in biomedical sciences.

From 1976 to 1999

Although in the pre-war years education in the biomedical sciences at the university was largely a school-by-school endeavor, post-war growth involved increased interaction between the Medical Center and the River Campus. The principal interactions in graduate education between the two campuses involved Biology, Psychology, and Chemistry, but also included departments in the College of Engineering and Applied Science. Initially these interactions were informal and depended mainly on shared interests among faculty members. Formal programs also developed, however, such as the program in Biomedical Engineering, which continues as a strong, well-funded intercollege program for both undergraduate and graduate education.

In the early 1970s, with the introduction of the Rochester Plan, supported by the Commonwealth Fund, formal interactions between the two campuses increased. The major objective of the Rochester Plan was to better prepare students for careers in the health professions, with emphasis on pre-medical and medical education. An example of one of the bridging programs is the Early Admission Program, which allowed outstanding undergraduates to enter medical school at the end of their sophomore year and to integrate their preclinical studies in the Medical Center with advanced courses in the Colleges of Arts and Science or Engineering and Applied Science. This brought faculty from both sides of Elmwood Avenue into more frequent contact and diminished the separation between college and medical school education. For Rochester Plan students, the four years spent on the two campuses became a single educational experience. For example, undergraduates could develop research opportunities that continued through the last two years of undergraduate education and the first two years of medical education.

Further expansion only required an infusion of funds. Providently, at just that time, the National Institutes of Health (NIH) instituted a set of new training programs, mainly for graduate education, in specific but broad areas of biomedical science. The Rochester teams, brought together in response to the NIH initiative, were highly successful in gaining training grants. Success depended very much on developing interdepartmental programs, in, for ex-

GEORGE A. KIMMICH, VICTOR G. LATIES, ROBERT E. MARQUIS

ample, Genetics, Neuroscience, Cell and Developmental Biology, Microbiology and Immunology, and Physiological and Pharmacological Sciences. The result was enhanced, cooperative curricular and research activity among departments in the Medical Center, and also between the Medical Center and the River Campus.

The 1970s was also a time of major growth in combined graduate-professional training programs, especially the MD/PhD program, funded in large part by Medical Scientist Trainee awards from the NIH. The program's development resulted directly in the growth of graduate education but also added another, new dimension. Previously, the M.D. and Ph.D. degrees had to be obtained separately. The new program required integration of the two, with research being carried out during the time in medical school, on either a part-time (while taking the regular curriculum) or a nearly full-time (during the interim years of graduate study, usually between the basic-science and clinical-science years of the medical curriculum) schedule.

In 1980, mainly through the initiative of then Provost Richard D. O'Brien, the Program in Biology and Medicine (PBM) was established. The PBM was designed to formalize interactions between the Medical Center and the River Campus developed during the Rochester Plan, and to implement a university-wide approach to biomedical education. Educational cooperation, it was hoped, would lead to increased interactions in research and other scholarship.

The opening, defining statement of the official description of the PBM states: "There shall be a Program in Biology and Medicine whose objectives shall be to coordinate the various activities in basic biology in the University in order to provide the best possible programs for undergraduate and graduate teaching and for research." Although Provost O'Brien came to Rochester from Cornell University, where he had helped to integrate programs in Biology and the Division of Biological Sciences, his work at Rochester was different, in part because of our strong departmental structure. Consequently, the founding document for the PBM states clearly that "there will be no change in the departmental status of the departments and individuals involved in the program." Robert Marquis from the Department of Microbiology and Immunology was appointed the first director of the PBM.

In the first years of the PBM, a major effort was made to build strong and integrated undergraduate curricula in biomedical sciences. Two kinds of degrees were instituted at Rochester and officially approved by the State of New York: The B.A., which provided a broad education in modern biological sciences, and the B.S., offering specialized training in several tracks, initially in Biochemistry, Cell and Developmental Biology, Microbiology, Molecular Genetics, Neuroscience, and Population Biology. The basic curricular plan remains intact in the Undergraduate Program in Biology and Medicine (UPBM).

The PBM enhanced undergraduate education in major ways. It brought Medical Center faculty into formal, well-defined education programs for un-

TABLE 1

A Visual History of the Graduate Degree Program of the School of Medicine and Dentistry
Ph.D. Degrees Awarded

"25" refers to 1924–25, etc.

	25–41	25–73	74	75	76	77	78	79	80	81	82	83
Anatomy	2	30	1	4	2	2	2	3	4	2	1	2
Biochemistry	29	110	4	2	2	5	4	6	3	3	4	2
Biophysics		57	8	4	2	9	9	15	13	5	11	5
Genetics												
Health Services Research												
Microbiology & Immunology*	3	38	3	5	4	7	1	7	9	8	5	6
Neuroscience**		11	1	1	3	2	3	5		5	1	5
Pathology	3	26	2		1				2	1		
Pharmacology		47	3	2	4	4	2	6	4	1	3	5
Physiology***	20	104	3	2	3		5	2	1	1	5	2
Radiation Biology****	1	73	4	6	2	4	1	3	1	1	2	3
Toxicology		7	1	3	3	4	4	2	7	4	4	4
TOTAL	58	503	30	29	26	37	31	49	44	31	36	34

*Includes 16 Bacteriology degrees awarded before 1961.
**Includes 1 Neurobiology & Anatomy degree awarded in 1970.
***Includes 51 Vital Economics degrees awarded before 1956.
****Includes one radiology degree awarded in 1936.

dergraduates. Many new courses were introduced, including laboratory courses in biochemistry and in microbiology, many of which also served graduate students. Indeed, the course offerings for graduate students were greatly augmented as a result of the growth in the undergraduate enterprise. This was perhaps most notable in the College of Engineering and Applied Sciences, especially in the fields of biomedical engineering and biotechnology. All biomedical science undergraduates had—and still have—the opportunity to be involved in independent study courses that enable them to share in basic research activity which provides them with first-hand experience and insight into the nature of a research career. Every semester as many as seventy-five biology undergraduates take independent research courses at the medical school. River Campus students are also offered the opportunity to earn a degree with distinction in research, which requires a written research summary. Medical Center faculty and graduate students continue to play major roles in this worthwhile effort.

Currently, the largest undergraduate tracks in the Medical Center are those leading to the B.S. degree in biology, with specialization in either biochemistry or in microbiology & immunology. About 40 students per class,

GEORGE A. KIMMICH, VICTOR G. LATIES, ROBERT E. MARQUIS

	84	85	86	87	88	89	90	91	92	93	94	95	96	97	98	99	25–99
Anatomy	2	1	2	2	1	2	5	3	2	3	2	3	1	1	2	3	88
Biochemistry	1	3	6	2	2	6	5	5	3	9	10	4	13	3	4	10	231
Biophysics	2	6	5	2	4	3	3	5	2	1	4	3	2	2	7	4	193
Genetics														3	2		5
HSR																1	1
Microbiology	3	7	4	5	3	11	5	7	4	6	7	10	12	12	9	8	206
Neuroscience	1	2	5	3	2	4	2	3	3		3	6	6	2	2	3	84
Pathology			1			1					1	2	1	2	2	2	44
Pharmacology	2	2	2	4	2	4	4		4	5	1	5	2	2	2	2	124
Physiology		1	2	1		1			2			3	1	2	1	1	143
Radiation Bio.	2		1	1	3	1			2								110
Toxicology	4	6	5	4	3	2	5	3	6	3	3	4	4	2	5	5	107
Total	17	28	33	24	20	34	30	26	28	27	31	40	42	31	36	39	1336

out of a total number of 150 graduates with majors in biological sciences, choose these tracks. They take courses with graduate students and most work in research laboratories along with graduate students.

From the beginning, the PBM had a graduate committee, and the PBM Graduate Fellowship Program was established in 1982. The first competition led to the award of seven fellowships, four for Medical Center students, two for River Campus students, and one in the Center for Brain Research, which at the time was an inter-divisional center.

In the fall of 1988, university funds were committed to expanding the PBM to offer new opportunities to graduate students, while continuing the undergraduate programs. This commitment followed the appointment of George Kimmich as the new PBM director in 1987. Three years later, Kimmich took on the additional responsibility of serving as the school's senior associate dean for graduate studies. He succeeded Irving Spar, who had served the school for fourteen years in that role.

Beginning in 1987, students applying to doctoral programs in the biological sciences were given a new option: admission free of constraints imposed by traditional departmental boundaries. Applicants could apply either to the graduate program in Biology & Medicine or to a specific department. Successful PBM applicants were admitted uncommitted to a particular degree program or a specific department. During their first year, they took courses suitable for any one of the several participating Ph.D. programs or courses to satisfy specific degree requirements. Students also completed at least three research rotations, choosing each research mentor from a list of more than 220 faculty members in twelve participating programs in the Medical Center and River Campus. The experience of interacting with faculty and students in multiple departments during laboratory rotations enhanced awareness of research opportunities available in various scientific disciplines and departments and, as a result, students were better able to select specific programs and mentors to meet their individual career goals.

During the 1990s, Microbiology & Immunology was the department producing the largest number of Ph.D.s (80), followed by Biochemistry (66), Toxicology (40), Biophysics (33), Neuroscience (30), Pharmacology (27), and Neurobiology & Anatomy (25). The decade also saw departmental mergers that produced the Departments of Biochemistry & Biophysics, and Pharmacology & Physiology, with each new department continuing to administer both of the original doctoral programs.

By the end of 1999, the School of Medicine and Dentistry (SMD) had awarded more than 1,300 Ph.D degrees. The final column in Table 1 shows how degrees were distributed among fields. Almost half (44%) were in Biochemistry (233), Microbiology & Immunology (216), and Biophysics (192). The rest were in Physiology (143), Pharmacology (124), Radiation Biology (111), Toxicology (107), Anatomy (88), Neuroscience (75), and Pathology (44). A small number of students have earned doctorates in the recently established programs in Genetics and Health Sciences Research.

Graduate Education of Dental Fellows

Early in its history, SMD training in dentistry focused on the graduate education of dentists who already possessed their professional degree. In 1930, a grant from the Rockefeller Foundation enabled the school to found the Dental Fellowship Program, which supported students who worked for a Ph.D. in any of the basic science departments. The program was an instant success and attracted subsequent support from both the Markle and Carnegie Foundations. For the last 30 years, most of the training funds for this program have come from the National Institute of Dental Research. Dr. William Bowen, who chaired the Department of Dental Research from 1982 to 1995, was instrumental in building a department in which basic research would be the cornerstone for pursuing problems in oral biology. Under his leadership several NIH training grants were funded that allowed dentists to pursue opportunities for Ph.D. training in a wide variety of research specialties. Students funded by these programs completed Ph.D. work in their chosen discipline while also fulfilling graduate dentistry clinical/curricular requirements.

They provided additional strength to already vigorous SMD graduate training programs.

About sixty-five Ph.D. degrees have been awarded to dental scientists so far, approximately 5 percent of those listed in Table 1, with dental students working in almost every graduate program. The addition of a research doctoral to the dental degree proved to make these students much valued in the marketplace. About 20 percent went on to become deans of dental schools, and at least two rose to be university presidents. Others became directors of dental institutes or professors in our own and other academic institutions.

The Role of Women in Graduate Education

Women have constituted almost half the SMD graduate student enrollment during the academic years between 1995 and 1999, comprising between 44 percent and 48 percent of the total. This percentage had been between 40 and 41 percent during each of the five previous years. These numbers illustrate considerable progress in the participation of women in our programs.

The first women Ph.D.s from each doctoral program are listed in Table 2, which also presents the first of either gender to earn each degree. Note that a woman was either first or tied for first in five of the twelve programs. Vincent

TABLE 2

First Recipients of Ph.D. Degrees

Program	First Recipient (year)	First Woman (year)
Anatomy	Adrian Buyse (1933)	Dorothy L. Oder (1950)
Biochemistry	Warren M. Sperry (1925)	Ruth H. Snider & Frances L. Haven (1935)
Biophysics	William F. Bale (1936)	Florence K. Millar (1953)
Genetics	Linda J. Metheny (1996)	Linda J. Metheny (1996)
Health Services Research	Sharon K. Palmiter (1998)	Sharon K. Palmiter (1998)
Microbiology & Immunology*	Clarence F. Schmidt (1932)	Jane P. Welton (1944)
Neuroscience	David L. Robinson (1972)	Susan M. Stine (1978)
Pathology	Frieda S. Robscheit-Robbins (1934)	Frieda S. Robscheit-Robbins (1934)
Pharmacology	Margaret W. Neuman (1943)	Margaret W. Neuman (1943)
Physiology**	Vincent du Vigneaud & M. Elizabeth Marsh (1927)	M. Elizabeth Marsh (1927)
Radiation Biology	William J. Bair (1954)	Alison P. Casarett (1957)
Toxicology	John E. Ballou & Tor Norseth (1969)	Barbara M. Davis (1972)

*Includes Bacteriology
**Includes Vital Economics

Du Vigneaud, who went on to win a Nobel Prize, was apparently the first to finish the requirements in 1927 and he is usually described as having earned our second Ph.D. Elizabeth Marsh and he were, however, voted their degrees at the same meeting of the trustees in 1927. In several of the other fields, a woman earned the degree within a few years of the first male recipient.

The Future: Graduate Education in the Biomedical Sciences

During the last two decades, a striking transformation has occurred in the biomedical sciences. Sweeping advances in technology have made it possible to view the functioning of biosystems at the molecular and atomic levels, with detail only dreamed about a few years ago.

As a result, graduate education in biomedical sciences is moving in two opposing directions. On the one hand, it is becoming more and more specialized with the growth of detailed knowledge of biological systems and the development of new specialties, such as bioinformatics. The internet has become a major tool in graduate education for day-to-day classroom teaching, for transfer of information developed in research projects, and for carrying out a variety of tasks, including genome searches, literature searches, and molecular modeling. On the other hand, there has been a call for increased flexibility in education so that graduates can adjust readily to changes in research focus and methods in academe, in governmental and funding agencies, and in industry. The current trend for more of our graduates to go into industrial jobs is likely to continue, maintaining the high demand for Ph.D. graduates in biomedical science. In addition, many Ph.D. graduates in biomedical sciences are going into new types of careers—in advertising, patent and intellectual property law, regulatory activities and finance—using the skills learned in scientific research in a variety of new applications.

A plan was developed to meet these new challenges by interdepartmental committees organized by Shey-Shing Sheu, who became senior associate dean for graduate studies in 1997. The plan resulted in the development of a new interdisciplinary Graduate Program in the Biomedical Sciences Program (GEBS). The program's hallmark is a set of research clusters, each of which is comprised of faculty drawn from several different departments. Faculty apply and are admitted to the one or two clusters most closely aligned with their research activity. Ten research clusters were established at the inception of GEBS: Biochemistry, Molecular Biology and Genetics; Cell Regulation and Molecular Pharmacology; Microbiology, Immunology, and Vaccine Biology; Integrative Biomedical Science; Molecular Biophysics and Structural Biology; Molecular Toxicology and Environmental Medicine; Neuroscience; Oral Biology; and Pathobiology and Molecular Medicine.

Each cluster is responsible for recruiting first-year students and for supervising their activity during the first year of study. Laboratory rotations may be taken in any of the cooperating laboratories, regardless of the depart-

GEORGE A. KIMMICH, VICTOR G. LATIES, ROBERT E. MARQUIS

mental affiliation of the mentor for that rotation. After each student identifies a permanent graduate mentor, primary supervision is transferred to the department responsible for overseeing the program in which the student is pursuing a degree.

The GEBS program is related loosely to the Medical Center's Aab Institute of Biomedical Sciences, which in turn is designed to expand significantly the research enterprise of the Medical Center. The expansion is enhanced by the recent completion of a new building, the Arthur Kornberg Research Center, and by the recruitment of a large number of new faculty and other researchers to staff the institute. Interactions with faculty at the River Campus continue under GEBS. The GEBS program also includes three new first-year courses: biochemistry, cell biology, and molecular biology. These courses, along with a course in bioethics, are core requirements for all first-year students, who then take upper-level courses in their specific biomedical disciplines.

In September 1999, the first group of sixty doctoral candidates was accepted into the GEBS program. During the prior year, proposals for training grants to supplement the current set of awards were submitted. In essence, the move is designed to expand the partnership between the university and federal and other sponsors of research training to allow for the full growth of the GEBS program and to ensure that Rochester remains at the forefront in graduate education.

TABLE 3
Comparison of Degrees Granted, 1975–99

Notice that the number of Ph.D.s awarded varies between a third and almost a half of the number of M.D. degrees. The total number of graduate students in residence is greater than the number of medical students because the average time required to complete the doctorate is often more than four years.

Year	M.D. Degrees	Ph.D. Degrees	Ph.D. , M.D.
1975	93	29	.31
1980	96	44	.46
1985	101	28	.28
1990	99	30	.30
1995	95	40	.42
1999	98	39	.40

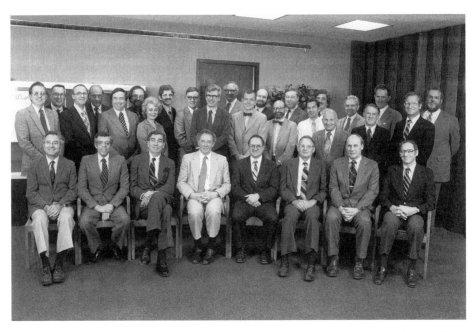

Medical Center Advisory Board, 1980. Among those seated in the first row are members who played key roles in the development of graduate education in basic science. Second from the left (between Louis Lasagna *and* James Bartlett*) is* Irving Spar, *who served as Senior Associate Dean for Graduate Education; fourth from the left is* Richard O'Brien, *Provost and initiator of the University Program in Biology & Medicine; next to him is* Frank Young, *Dean of the School of Medicine & Dentistry and later Commissioner of the U. S. Food & Drug Administration; next to him is* Robert Sproull, *President of the University, for whom the Sproull Graduate Fellowships are named; at the right end of the row is* Marshall Lichtman, *who became Dean of the School of Medicine & Dentistry.*

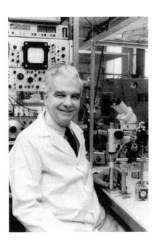

Paul Horowicz, Ph.D.—*Department of Physiology, Professor and Chair, 1969–1996; Director of Graduate Training Program in Systems and Integrative Biology, 1974–1984*

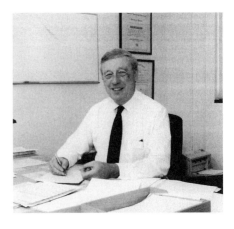

Paul LaCelle, M.D.—*Departments of Medicine and of Radiation Biology and Biophysics, 1967– 1977; Chair, Department of Biophysics, 1977– 1996; Senior Associate Dean for Academic Affairs and Research, 1993–1998*

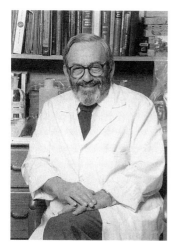

Leon Miller, M.D., Ph.D.—
Departments of Biochemistry and of Radiation Biology and Biophysics (1948–1978); Professor Emeritus, Biochemistry and Biophysics, 1978–present. Leon received an M.D. with honors from SMD in 1945 and continues daily participation as a faculty member.

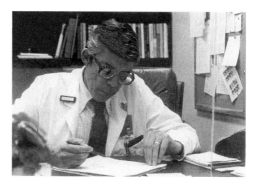

Irving Spar, Ph.D.—*Department of Radiation Biology and Biophysics, 1952–1985; Senior Associate Dean for Graduate Studies, 1975–1989; Professor Emeritus, 1992–1996*

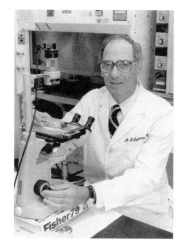

Marshall Lichtman, M.D.—
Department of Medicine (Hematology), 1965–present; Senior Associate Dean for Academic Affairs and Research, and then Academic Dean, 1979–1989; Dean, School of Medicine and Dentistry, 1990–1995

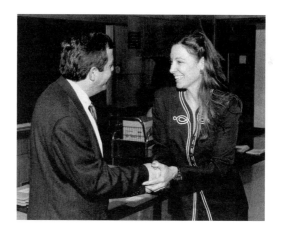

Dayle Daines, Ph.D.—*shown during her graduate work in Microbiology and Immunology, receiving the Melville Hare Teaching Award from Senior Associate Dean* Edward Hundert.

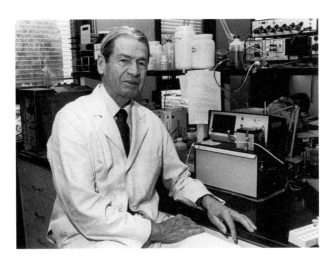

Harold Hodge, Ph.D.—*Chair,
Department of Pharmacology,
1958–1970*

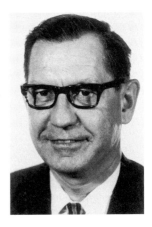

William (Bill) Neuman,
Ph.D.—*Department of
Radiation Biology and
Biophysics; Department
Chair, 1965–1975; Aser
Rothstein served as co-chair
with Bill from 1965–1972.*

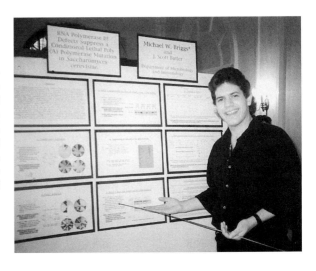

Michael Briggs,
Ph.D.—*shown
during his graduate
work in
Microbiology and
Immunology, giving
a poster presentation
during the annual
Genetics Day
activities. Mike is
now a post-doctoral
fellow with Dr.
Dennis McCance.*

GEORGE A. KIMMICH, VICTOR G. LATIES, ROBERT E. MARQUIS

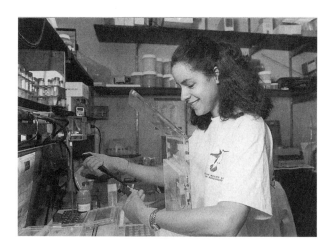

Aida Casiano-Colón, Ph.D.—*shown during her graduate work in Microbiology & Immunology, setting up a chemostat for continuous culture of oral bacteria. Aida is now an Assistant Professor in the Microbiology laboratory at Genesee Hospital*

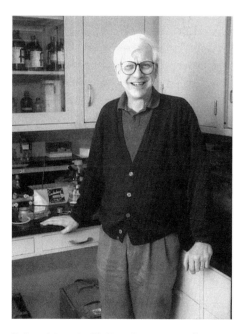

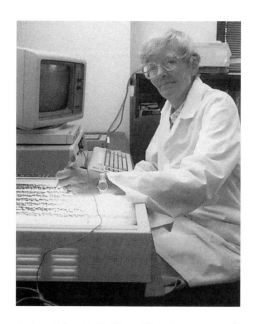

Robert Marquis, Ph.D.—*Department of Microbiology and Immunology, 1963–present; First Director of University Program in Biology and Medicine, 1980–1987*

Barbara Iglewski, Ph.D.—*Chair, Department of Microbiology & Immunology, 1986–present; Vice-Provost for Research and Graduate Education, 1996–1998*

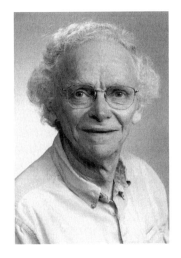

Victor Laties, Ph.D.—*Professor Emeritus, Department of Environmental Medicine; Director of Toxicology Training Program, 1978–1991; 1995–1996*

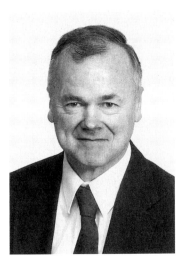

George Kimmich, Ph.D.— *Department of Radiation Biology and Biophysics, 1968–1982; Biochemistry and Biophysics, 1983–present; Director, University Program in Biology and Medicine, 1987–1989; Director, Graduate PBM, 1990–1996; Senior Associate Dean for Graduate Studies 1990–1996*

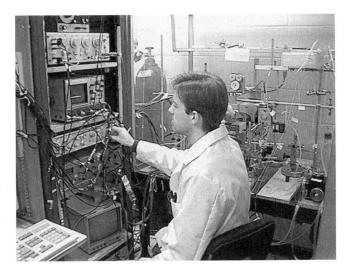

Michael Aschner, Ph.D.— *Graduate student, Neurobiology and Anatomy, 1980–1985; Postdoctoral Fellow, Toxicology, 1986–1987; Associate Professor, Department of Physiology and Pharmacology, Wake Forest University School of Medicine*

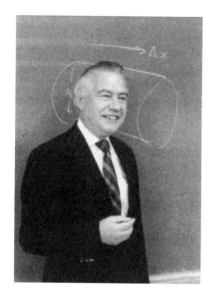

Thomas Clarkson, Ph.D.—*Director,
Toxicology Training Program, 1967–
1975; Chair, Division of Toxicology,
1980–1986; Environmental Health
Sciences Center, 1987–1991;
Department of Environmental Medicine,
1992–1998; elected to Institute of
Medicine, National Academy of Sciences,
1981*

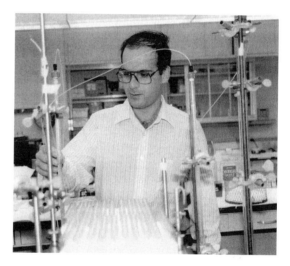

Andrew Custer, M.S.—*Graduate Student
with Dr. Peter Shrager. Andrew is studying
proteins associated with ion channel
clustering during axonal development.*

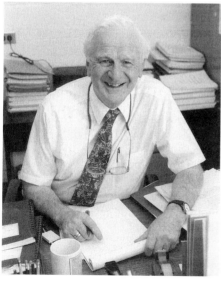

William H. Bowen, B.D.S.,
Ph.D.—*Welcher Professor of
Dentistry in the Center for Oral
Biology; Chair, Department of
Dental Research, 1982–1995;
Director, Rochester Caries Research
Center, 1984–1995; Director,
Cariology Training Program, 1985–
present; elected to Institute of
Medicine of the National Academy
of Medicine, 1997*

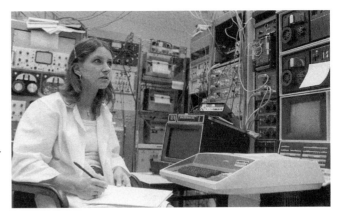

Debra Cory-Slechta, Ph.D.—*as a Post-Doctoral Fellow in the Division of Toxicology, 1979–1982; Chair, Department of Environmental Medicine, 1998–present*

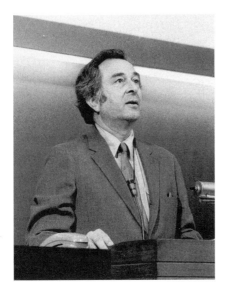

Louis Lasagna, M.D.—*Chair, Department of Pharmacology, 1970–1980; elected to Institute of Medicine of the National Academy of Sciences, 1971*

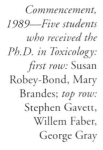

Commencement, 1989—Five students who received the Ph.D. in Toxicology: first row: Susan Robey-Bond, Mary Brandes; *top row:* Stephen Gavett, Willem Faber, George Gray

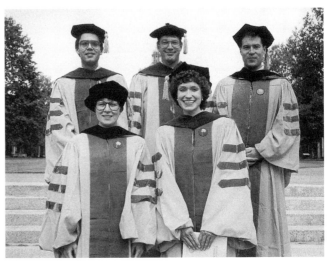

GEORGE A. KIMMICH, VICTOR G. LATIES, ROBERT E. MARQUIS

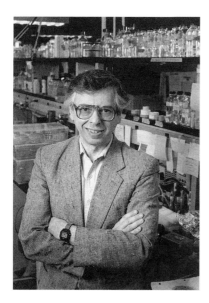

Fred Sherman, Ph.D.—*Department of Radiation Biology and Biophysics, 1961–1997; Chair, Department of Biochemistry, 1982–1998; elected to the National Academy of Sciences, 1985*

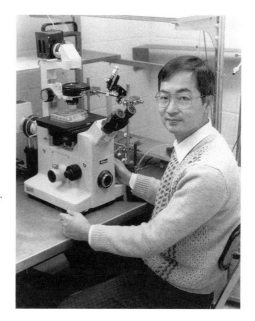

Shey-Shing Sheu, Ph.D.—*Departments of Pharmacology and Physiology, 1983–present; Senior Associate Dean for Graduate Studies, 1997–2000*

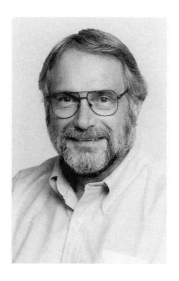

M. W. Anders, D.V.M., Ph.D. —*Lewis Pratt Ross Professor and Chair, Department of Pharmacology and Physiology (formerly Dept. of Pharmacology), 1982–2000; Director, Pharmacological Sciences Training Grant, 1992–1998*

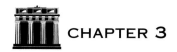

CHAPTER 3

Distinction in Research

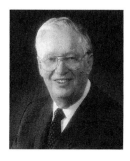

GILBERT B. FORBES, M.D.

Scholars' pens carry farther, and give a louder report than thunder.
—Sir Thomas Brown, 1642

From the beginning of the medical school, scientific research was of paramount importance. The very first building to be constructed on the new medical school/hospital campus was a research laboratory in 1922, just a year after George Whipple's arrival in Rochester as dean. The first three professorial appointees (George Whipple, Pathology and dean; George Corner, Anatomy; and Walter Bloor, Biochemistry) had already begun research careers.

Other decisions served to foster a climate for research. A first-class medical library was developed, offering complete sets of a number of foreign journals. Pre-clinical teaching schedules were arranged to provide ample research time for the faculty. "Year-out" fellowships for students allowed them to spend significant time doing research with a member of the faculty (a review some years ago, of the careers of "year-out" fellows, showed that a high proportion of them had indeed achieved academic positions).[1] Graduate students in the basic sciences were recruited, a trend well established by 1931, when the ratio of graduate to medical students was about 0.15 (later to rise to 0.5 or more).

More evidence of the supportive climate for research at Rochester can be cited. The very first Ph.D. degrees to be awarded by the University of Rochester were in biochemistry (Warren Sperry, 1925) and in vital economics

(Elizabeth Marsh, 1927 and Vincent du Vigneaud, 1927). An important decision was made early on to allocate medical school funds, albeit in rather meager amounts, for faculty research and graduate students' stipends. Finally and most importantly, the decision was made to build the medical school and hospital under one roof, so that medical science and clinical care were firmly established as true partners in the education of future physicians and scientists. To quote from the first bulletin of the medical school, written by George Corner and dated 1925–26: "Therefore the schedule [of instruction] will provide for elective studies or independent work, and in all work, prescribed, elective and independent, the relation of teachers and students will be those which would be naturally expected in a graduate school of arts and sciences."

In consideration of his role as first dean of the medical school, his prodigious research production over many years, and as Nobel laureate, it is entirely fitting to begin the following series of personal sketches with George Whipple.

REFERENCES, GILBERT B. FORBES, M.D.

1. Fenninger, Leonard. The Rochester Student Fellowship Program. Jour Med Education, 33, 207–210, (1958).

George Hoyt Whipple, M.D. (1878–1976)
At Rochester 1921–1976

Architect of Science and Learning

George Whipple was no stranger to research and scholarship. As a young instructor in pathology at Johns Hopkins, he published a fascinating report of a case of intestinal lipodystrophy, now known as Whipple's disease.[1] Well worth reading for its clarity and thoroughness, this report presents the clinical, biochemical, and pathological findings of what was then a new disease.

Whipple's interest in the metabolism of bile acids, begun at Johns Hopkins, was continued when he became professor of Experimental Medicine and director of the Hooper Foundation for Medical Research at the University of California in San Francisco in 1914. It was there that he began his work on blood protein formation and erythrocyte regeneration, in the midst of studies on the intoxicating effects of intestinal obstruction.

By 1920, he had become Dean of the University of California Medical

School. But that year also brought an offer from President Rush Rhees to form a new medical school at the University of Rochester. Aided by the existence of a generous endowment (funded by George Eastman and the Rockefeller Foundation) and encouraged by a personal visit from President and Mrs. Rhees (four days travel by railroad each way), Whipple was persuaded to come to Rochester as professor of pathology and dean. He made it clear to President Rhees, however, that his acceptance of the deanship at Rochester was contingent on his ability to continue to do research. Upon his arrival in Rochester in 1921, he not only saw to it that his Berkeley dog colony was maintained (with the help of funds from Rochester), but that plans for constructing a laboratory and animal house would have priority. Indeed, this was the very first building to be constructed on the new medical school campus!

Under the watchful eye of his assistant, Frieda Robscheit-Robbins (who was to collaborate with him for many years), the experimental dog colony was transported to Rochester late in 1922 so that Whipple's research on bilirubin production and red blood cell regeneration could continue. Whipple's unswerving dedication to scientific research is clearly evident from the fact that his research activities continued in the midst of the many chores involved in organizing this new medical school, designing its buildings, and recruiting its faculty.

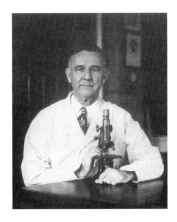

Dean Whipple

The experimental dog colony was to provide the mainstay of his subsequent research on hemoglobin regeneration and on plasma protein metabolism. For this purpose, the animals' plasma protein was depleted by periodic bleeding and then reinfused with erythrocytes. Within two and a half years, Whipple and Robscheit-Robbins had established the favorable influence of feeding liver, heart, and skeletal muscle, on the blood regeneration of dogs made anemic by bleeding.[2] George Corner in his biography of Whipple states that "this report with its unequivocal emphasis on liver feeding . . . is the most important single paper as regards George H. Whipple's world reputation as a scientist, in the whole of his immense lifetime list of more than 300 publications."[3] This paper caught the attention of George Minot in Boston, who went on to show that either raw or cooked liver was effective in the treatment of pernicious anemia.

Work on the plasma proteins continued, culminating in Whipple's hypothesis of a dynamic equilibrium between blood and tissue proteins, a significant contribution to our understanding of the fundamental nature of protein metabolism.[4]

Whipple and his colleagues were among the first to seize on the new technique of isotopic tracers. It happened that Ernest O. Lawrence (the inventor of the cyclotron) attended a meeting of the National Academy of Sciences held in Rochester in the autumn of 1937 where he met George Whipple and promised him a supply of the newly discovered ^{59}Fe (the work of Martin Kamen, who later discovered ^{14}C). The result was an epoch-making study of the use of radioactive iron as a tracer.[5]

Whipple continued to do research and to publish scientific papers throughout World War II, the last appearing in 1959 when its author was eighty-one. He served as dean of the medical school until he was seventy-five, dealing with the accelerated wartime curriculum for medical students and the loss of faculty to the Armed Forces. Summations of his work can be found in several publications.[6,7,8]

But what about Whipple the man? We students were rather in awe of him in the classroom, but his penchant for austerity could be breached (save for the financial kind!) at times. Personal conversations were pleasant, and, contrary to legend, he did not always object to early marriage—indeed, he attended the wedding of one of my classmates. His "year-out" student fellows, four to six being selected at the end of the second medical school year, discovered that his austerity had a "soft side"; he was a jovial host at parties in his home and he was capable of many acts of kindness. Every Wednesday evening, after dinner in the hospital dining room, student fellows and the entire Department of Pathology faculty gathered together in the laboratory, where they sat on hard stools and discussed the microscopic sections from the preceding week's autopsy and surgical material. Whipple's student fellows found their "year-out" to be most instructive, and most participated in his ongoing research projects.

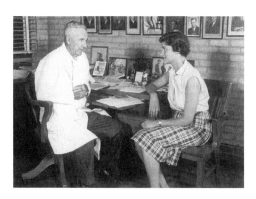

Dean Whipple *in his office, with student*

Austerity was, however, evident everywhere within the school. Mechanical microscopic stages were purchased by most students to help orient the slide, but they were not provided for the pathology faculty, who were obliged to hold down and move the slide with their fingers. Whipple refused to have the walls and ceilings of the medical school painted, as shown in the accompanying photograph of the dean's office (although, the wall of his office displayed a photograph of Julie Andrews!). Faculty salaries were maintained at embarrassingly low levels, and the personnel of the dean's office consisted of one executive secretary (the indomitable, highly efficient Hilda DeBrine, who recognized and at times counseled all the students) plus a typist or two. The end result of this frugality was the accumulation by 1953 of a sizable fund for scholarships and faculty support, a sum augmented by Eli Lilly and Company in payment for testing liver extracts.

GILBERT B. FORBES

Many honors were to come Whipple's way. In addition to the Nobel Prize (1934), he was elected to the National Academy of Sciences, to the American Philosophical Society, and to the Board of Trustees of the Rockefeller Foundation. In 1935, he turned down an offer to be the director of the Rockefeller Institute, but for many years he served on the Board of Scientific Directors of the Institute.

In reviewing his long and productive career, Whipple stated, "I would say that teaching and research represent the ultimate in pleasure and satisfaction in my career. Perhaps research may give a greater sense of accomplishment, but teaching carries greater personal happiness. . . . Administrative duties are important and, at times, stimulating, but these tasks must not absorb too much time and energy, else the research program will wither away. . . . I believe a good medical teacher must be an investigator, philosopher and/or clinician. I would be remembered as a teacher."[9]

REFERENCES, GEORGE HOYT WHIPPLE, M.D.

1. Whipple GH. A hitherto undescribed disease characterized anatomically by deposits of fat and fatty acids in the intestinal and mesenteric lymphatic tissues. Johns Hopkins Hospital Bull 18, 382–91 (1907). This disease is now known to be due to infection with a bacterium, appropriately named tropheryma whippelii (M. N. Swartz, New Eng Jour Med 342, 648–50 (2000)).

2. Whipple GH and Robscheit-Robbins FS. Blood regeneration in severe anemia. II. Favorable influence of liver, heart and skeletal muscle in diet. Am Jour Physiol 72, 408–18 (1925).

3. Corner GW. George Hoyt Whipple and his friends. pp. vi, 335, Lippincott Co., Philadelphia (1963).

4. Holman RL, Mahoney EB, and Whipple GH. Blood plasma protein given by vein utilized in body metabolism. II. A dynamic equilibrium between plasma and tissue proteins. Jour Exp Med 59, 269–82 (1934).

5. Hahn PF, Bale WF, Lawrence EO, and Whipple GH. Radioactive iron and its metabolism in anemia. Its absorption, transportation, and utilization. Jour Exp Med 69, 739–53 (1939).

6. Madden SC and Whipple GH. Plasma proteins: their source, production and utilization. Physiol Rev, 20, 194–217 (1940).

7. Whipple GH. Hemoglobin regeneration as influenced by diet and other factors. Nobel Prize lecture. Jour. Am. Med. Assoc., 104, 791–93 (1935).

8. Miller LL. George Hoyt Whipple 1878–1976, Biographical Memoirs, Vol. 66, pp. 3–25, 1995, National Academy Press.

9. Whipple GH. Autobiographical sketch. Perspectives Biol Med 2, 253–89 (1959).

George Washington Corner, M.D. (1889–1982)
At Rochester 1924–1940

Isolating Progesterone

George Washington Corner, whose studies of mammalian reproduction processes have had an important impact on medical science, was one of the most gifted men to grace the University of Rochester faculty. An historian, a classicist, and an educator, he was also a scientist *extraordinaire.*

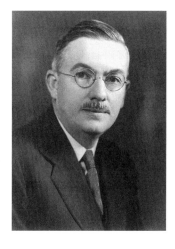

George W. Corner, M.D., Professor and Chair, Anatomy

Corner did not decide to study medicine until September of 1909, whereupon he applied to Johns Hopkins and was immediately accepted into the class of 1913(!). His interest in biology was sparked in college, and resulted in his early publication of a brief account of the life cycle of the protozoan *Cothurnia.*

At Hopkins (perhaps the best medical school of its time) Corner came under the influence of notable medical scientists and teachers. Upon graduation, he worked as an assistant with Dr. Franklin Mall, who suggested he study the corpus luteum of the sow. A subsequent internship in obstetrics and gynecology under the tutelage of Dr. Howard Kelly further stimulated his interest in reproductive physiology.

A four-year stint at the University of California at Berkeley, where Corner worked with Herbert Evans and Philip Smith, resulted in his long and definitive paper on the corpus luteum, a paper that includes his early speculations about the function of this part of the ovary.[1]

Corner was then called back to Hopkins to join the Department of Anatomy, where he continued his study on ways in which the sow's ovary and uterus change during the reproductive cycle. He timed ovulation by observing sows in the stockyard's holding pens and marking those who appeared to be in heat. He then solicited the help of the slaughterhouse personnel in seeing to it that the marked animals were killed at the right time. A paper written during this time uses the term "progestational proliferation" and notes that this is the prime function of the corpus luteum.[2] Corner had correctly deduced the corpus luteum's function and established the relation of ovulation to its disappearance. He described the process: "The schedule of estrus, ovulation, the fate of the unfertilized ovum, the rise and fall of the corpus luteum, and the progestational change in the uterus." His detailed description was the first of its kind to focus on a large domestic animal.

In 1923, when Corner was thirty-four, he was recruited by President Rush Rhees and Dean George H. Whipple to join the new medical school at Rochester as head of the Department of Anatomy. During their visit to Baltimore, Rhees and Whipple assured Corner that Rochester's slaughterhouses could provide him with all the sows' ovaries and uteri he would need for his research. They also assured him he would have a role to play in selecting faculty and organizing the medical curriculum.

Since neither the school nor the adjacent hospital had yet been built, Corner, his wife, and their two children spent the academic year 1923–24 in Europe, at the University of Rochester's expense. While in London, at Whipple's request Corner interviewed Wallace Fenn, then on a Rockefeller Foundation-funded travelling fellowship; Fenn later came to Rochester as head of the Department of Physiology.

By this time, Corner had extended his observations of the reproductive cycle to primates, hoping to discover a relationship between ovulation and menstruation. Using young female monkeys, provided by the Philadelphia Zoo, he painstakingly detailed their reproductive cycles. He was able to show that ovulation occurs at the midpoint of the interval between two menstrual periods, and that the corpus luteum remains intact for about two weeks if the ovum is not fertilized.

The very first building erected at Rochester's new medical school site was the animal house, completed in November 1922, only fourteen months after Whipple's arrival in Rochester. Facilities for a monkey colony were provided, so that Corner could continue his research.

During these early years at Rochester Corner decided to make a serious attempt to find the means (probably a hormone, he hypothesized) by which the corpus luteum exerts its effect. To this end he offered a "year-out" fellowship to medical student Willard Myron Allen, and, in 1927, they began work on isolating—and eventually purifying—the hormone which we know as progesterone. (It should be noted that the discipline of endocrinology was developing during the early 1920s with the discovery of two hormones, insulin and estrone.)

To test the potency of extracts they had made from sows' ovaries, they devised the "Corner and Allen test" for use with rabbits: "Mate your doe to a fertile male; eighteen hours later remove both ovaries (easier than digging out the corpora lutea separately), inject your extract daily for five days, kill the doe, prepare a cross section of the uterus, put it under your microscope. If the progestation change has occurred, you have a potent extract. This is the routine test. . . . If you want to make it deluxe, you may wash the tiny embryos out of the uterus and rejoice at the sight of them."[3]

The results were exciting. Corner and Allen were able to show that the administration of extracts of the corpus luteum could carry pregnancy to term in rabbits whose ovaries had been removed after fertilization.[4] They correctly deduced that the corpus luteum elaborated a hormone whose action was distinct from that of estrogen. Then came the troublesome process of purifying the extract and isolating the hormone.[5] Their success in 1933 was the culmination of a concept first formulated in 1918–19.

At Rochester, gross anatomy was taught in the dissecting room and lectures were infrequent. There were only two examinations, both oral, but each student had to prepare a paper on a topic of his choosing; papers were carefully read and graded by Corner himself. Late in the fall of 1936, Corner made a trip to England where he was to give the Vicary Lecture, honoring Thomas Vicary, a sixteenth-century surgeon. Those of us engaged in gross anatomy missed him and wanted to tell him so. One of our classmates, who had majored in Latin at Yale, drafted a letter in Latin, a copy of which was posted on the department's bulletin board; in due course, Corner replied, also in Latin, and a translated copy was added to the bulletin board.

George Corner left Rochester in 1940 to become director of the Department of Embryology at the Carnegie Institute in Baltimore. With the departure of his chief, Willard Allen also left Rochester in 1940 to become chair of Obstetrics and Gynecology at Washington University School of Medicine, a position he held for many years.

In 1955, Corner was recruited to write the history of the Rockefeller Institute for Medical Research. In 1960 he became executive officer of the American Philosophical Society, a post which he held for seventeen years. One of the benefits of this position that Corner most enjoyed was the opportunity to use a desk that had belonged to Benjamin Franklin.

At the request of Rochester's Medical Alumni Association and with financial help from Eli Lilly and Co., Corner wrote a biography of George Whipple that includes much valuable information about the early days of the Medical School.[6] Corner's autobiography provides a full description of his stellar career, and a vivid description of the problems and joys of his scientific accomplishments.[7]

REFERENCES, GEORGE WASHINGTON CORNER, M.D.

1. Corner GW. On the origin of the corpus luteum of the sow from both granulosa and theca interna. Am. Jour. Anatomy 26, 117–83 (1919).

2. Corner GW. Cyclic changes in the ovaries and uterus of the sow, and their relation to the mechanism of implantation. Carnegie Inst. Wash., pub. 276 Contributions to Embryology No. 64, 117–46 (1921).

3. Corner GW. The Seven Ages of a Scientist: An Autobiography, p. 233 Phil., U. Penn. Press (1981).

4. Corner GW and Allen WM. Physiology of the corpus luteum; 2 Production of a special uterine reaction (progestational proliferation) by extracts of the corpus

luteum. Amer. Jour. of Physiol. 88, 326–39 (1929); 3 Normal growth and implantation of embryos after very early oblation of the ovaries, under the influence of extracts of the corpus luteum, ibid. 88, 340–46 (1929).

5. Wintersteiner OP and Allen WM. Crystalline progestin. Jour. Biol. Chem. 107, 321–36 (1934).

6. Corner GW. George Hoyt Whipple and his Friends. Phil., Lippincott Pub. (1963).

7. See note 3.

Wallace Osgood Fenn, Ph.D. (1893–1971)
At Rochester 1924–1971

Physiologist Par Excellence

What is the measure of a man? The answer was provided by the late W. Allen Wallis, former Chancellor of the University of Rochester, in his remarks at the Fenn Memorial Service in 1971: "To have known Wallace Fenn is an experience from which all of us will always derive inspiration and pleasure. . . . [Dr. Fenn] told Dean Orbison there had never been a day when he had come to the University without looking forward with pleasure and keen anticipation to that day's work."

Fenn's father was dean of the Harvard Divinity School and for a time he thought of entering the ministry. He took a Ph.D. degree in plant physiology at Harvard, then spent several years as instructor in Dr. Walter B. Cannon's physiology department at Harvard. The fact that several of his early publications dealt with the effects of electrolytes and pH on the properties of gelatin prophesied his later important work on the reaction of biological tissues to such influences.

A special Rockefeller Traveling Fellowship enabled the young scientist to go to England to work with Professor A.V. Hill at Manchester University. Hill had set up a laboratory in the cellar of his house, where the ambient temperature was 6–8° C, in order, he said, "to avoid the electrical and mechanical disturbances which infested the laboratory in Manchester."

Dean George Whipple had been alerted by Cannon about this promising young man, and Whipple asked George Corner, newly appointed chair of the Department of Anatomy at Rochester, to interview Fenn in London in 1923. That same year, he had John R. Murlin, chair of the Department of Vital Economics, query Hill about Fenn at the International Congress of Physiologists in Edinburgh. So, in a way, Whipple did have a "committee" to advise him in selecting the chair of Physiology: Cannon, Corner, and Murlin.

But it was not until Fenn stepped off the train in Rochester in 1924 that Whipple actually met the much-heralded young man. Only thirty-one years old at the time, the medical school's youngest department head proved to be one of the most scientifically productive members of the faculty. He went on to achieve an international reputation as a scientist, as well as gaining fame as a superb teacher of medical and graduate students.

Fenn's scientific career encompassed and defined several branches of physiology. Beginning in A.V. Hill's laboratory he studied the oxygen consumption of nerve and muscle, relating this to the work performed. He showed that when a muscle shortens it produces more heat than with an isometric contraction; hence, shortening is an active process, not passive, as one would expect from a pre-stretched spring.[1] Hill referred to this as "the Fenn Effect," a term still used today.

During Fenn's early years at Rochester he extended his basic studies to include human muscle physiology. In addition to finding that the force-velocity relationships of human muscle are similar to that of frog muscle, he described the biomechanics of running. For this study he borrowed cinephotographic equipment from Eastman Kodak Company. As the film speed in the camera was unreliable, he included in the pictures of the runners a falling shotput to mark the exact time of the frame. His conclusion that the major work and limitations of sprint running are in the repetitive acceleration and deceleration of the upper and lower extremities has been confirmed many times.[2]

The next phase of Fenn's research involved studies of the electrolyte composition of muscle. He demonstrated that ions such as potassium were not locked up in muscle, as had been previously thought, but could move in or out under appropriate circumstances. He found that certain stimuli produced a loss of potassium from muscle and a gain in sodium, together with a change in pH; these changes were reversed slowly during recovery. While he had shown that sodium could under appropriate circumstances enter tissue cells and that radiosodium regularly did so under normal circumstances, some explanation had to be sought for the fact that tissue levels of this ion were low in the face of a high extracellular fluid concentration. This led one of his students, R.B. Dean, to postulate the existence of a sodium "pump," which has subsequently been shown to be an energy-requiring enzymatic process.[3] Indeed, a sizable share of the energy expenditure of organisms is used to run the sodium pump.

(It seems appropriate, if parenthetical, to point out that the analysis of tissue and body fluids at that time was done by cumbersome chemical techniques requiring many hours for completion. Only later, with the invention of the flame photometer, could Na and K analyses be done with relative ease.)

In the 1930s the university constructed a cyclotron capable of pro-

GILBERT B. FORBES

ducing a number of artificial radioisotopes, among them radioactive potassium. Fenn was quick to use this isotope to trace the course of potassium through the body, its absorption, excretion, and distribution in various tissues.[4] He is credited by some with virtually creating the field of potassium metabolism. The isotope used (^{42}K) has a half-life of only twelve hours, which meant that it had to be delivered promptly to Fenn's laboratory from the cyclotron located about half a mile away. Nobel laureate Dr. Carlton Gadjusek once told me that, during his student days at Rochester, he was the courier

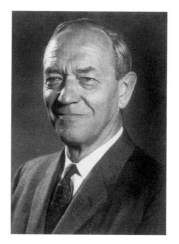

Wallace O. Fenn, Ph.D., *Professor and Chair, Physiology*

who ran with the newly radioactive samples to the physiology laboratory.

It is worthy of note that the Geiger counter used by Fenn and his associates to assay radiopotassium was constructed by a fellow faculty member, Dr. William Bale. A high degree of technical expertise was required to build the detection tube and its associated electronics, but the effort was in keeping with the rather parsimonious attitude which emanated from the dean's office: home-made apparatus is always preferable!

The result of all this was a clear understanding of the physiological significance of potassium and its metabolism in the body. Fenn showed that nearly all muscle potassium is exchangeable with radiopotassium, thus proving that intracellular potassium is not maintained by binding or sequestration, but by active energetic process.[5,6] Others would show that estimates of total body potassium in humans could be made with administrated radiopotassium.

With the coming of war in 1941, Fenn offered to help the Army Air Force address problems encountered in high-altitude flight. For this purpose, and for the very first time, he was granted outside funding. All his previous work had been accomplished with medical school funds. The specific question addressed by Fenn and his associates was this: Would breathing oxygen under pressure enable our pilots to fly higher than enemy aircraft?

In the process of answering this question Fenn's team described the three components—elastic, viscous, and turbulent—involved in the work of breathing, and they formulated the pressure-volume diagram of the lungs and thorax, a concept which enjoys wide usage.[7,8] For this purpose they used a chamber made by a Rochester firm for large chemical processes and equipped it with an old air suction pump. Using this simple equipment Fenn and his associates made many simulated high-altitude flights, sometimes to the point of hypoxic-induced loss of consciousness. (Hearing about this, Dean Whipple forbade Fenn's further participation: he didn't want to lose the services of this esteemed member of his faculty.)

These activities led to his involvement in the space program. Shortly after stepping down from the chairmanship of the Department of Physiology in 1959 Fenn was named a Distinguished University Professor and director of the University Space Program, a position he held for four years.

Fenn's later investigations targeted the mechanisms of oxygen toxicity and the effects of hydrostatic pressure upon biological processes. The former reflected the concern (at that time) about the damaging effect of oxygen on the retina of premature infants.

In addition to this long and highly productive research career, Dr. Fenn was renowned as a teacher. He enjoyed teaching medical students, and he mounted a vigorous graduate program; at one point, twenty-five graduate students worked in his department. He published several scientific articles in German, and one in Italian. He liked to be active, both mentally and physically. Though his office was located on the fourth floor of the medical school, he rarely took the elevator; when asked about this, he replied "I'm exercising my coronaries!" He also taught Sunday School at the First Unitarian Church in Rochester for many years.

Dr. Fenn was awarded several honorary degrees from institutions both here and abroad. He served as president of the American Physiological Society, the American Institute of Biological Sciences, and the XXIV International Congress of Physiological Sciences. He received a number of awards, including one from the Accademia Nazionale dec Lincei in Rome, and one from the German Physiological Society. He was active in the affairs of the National Institutes of Health, and he was very proud of his membership in the National Academy of Sciences.

Wallace Fenn had very definite ideas about the proper function of a medical school. I quote here from an article he wrote on medical education:

> A medical school must do much more than train medical students. It must serve as a center of learning and research in the medical sciences. As such, the heads of its several departments must be so trained as to cover the whole broad field of the medical sciences; since the progress in medical science is based on progress in chemistry, physics, and biology, there must be some departments that maintain strong contacts with these fields. Every preclinical department in its teaching must correlate both forwards into the clinic and backwards into the basic sciences. Similarly the clinician must correlate his teaching backwards into the preclinical sciences and forwards into the life of the practitioner. Both the forward and the backward correlations are important, but of the two the backward correlation is ultimately more essential for the enduring vitality of the medical school. Without this the medical school is no longer part of the continuum which is science but becomes an isolated applied branch of science. Like the leaves of a tree, the clinic cannot flourish in the long run if the flow of sap from the roots is cut off and the roots of medical science should remain firmly embedded in the departments of physics, chemistry, and biology. The

pre-clinical professors and departments must serve as conduits for the transfer of new concepts and new knowledge from the basic sciences into the clinic.[9]

Wallace Fenn was truly a man for all seasons: alumni who were his students consider themselves privileged to have been touched by him, while those who matriculated after his death can still benefit from his wisdom by reading his works. His scientific integrity, his wisdom, and his scientific initiative should serve as a beacon to us all.

REFERENCES, WALLACE OSGOOD FENN, PH.D.

1. Fenn WO. A quantitative comparison between the energy liberated and the work performed by the isolated sartorius muscle of the frog. Jour. Physiol (London) 58, 175–203. (1924).

2. Fenn WO. Frictional-kinetic factors in the work of sprint running. Am. Jour. Physiol. 92, 583–611; 93, 433–462 (1930).

3. Dean RB. Theories of electrolyte equilibrium in muscle. Biol. Symposia III, p. 331 (1941).

4. Fenn WO and Cobb DM. Electrolyte changes in muscle during activity. Am. Jour. Physiol. 115, 345–56 (1936).

5. Fenn WO. The role of potassium in physiological processes. Physiol. Rev. 20, 377–415 (1940).

6. Fenn WO, Noonan TR, Mullins LJ, and Haege LF. The exchange of radioactive potassium with body potassium. Am. Jour. Physiol. 135, 149–63 (1941).

7. Rahn H, Otis AB, Chadwick LE, and Fenn WO. The pressure volume diagram of the thorax and lung. Am. Jour. Physiol. 146, 161–78 (1946).

8. Otis AH, Fenn WO, and Rahn H. Mechanics of breathing. Jour. Appl. Physiol. 2, 592–607 (1950).

9. Fenn WO. An adaptation of comments made in a presentation to the Medical School Alumni Association, October 1957.

Harold C. Hodge, Ph.D. (1904–1990)
At Rochester 1931–1971

Groundbreaking Pharmacologist:
From a Dental Research Classic to the Manhattan Project

Educated at Illinois Wesleyan University and State University of Iowa (Ph.D. Chemistry 1930), Harold Hodge was recruited to Rochester in 1931 as a Rockefeller Fellow in Dentistry with an appointment in Biochemistry. At the time, Dean George Whipple was interested in expanding the school's activities in dental research; earlier, he had considered, then rejected, the idea of running a dental school. Hodge was an early recruit to what was to become a full-fledged postgraduate program in dental research, an outstanding program which has produced professors of dentistry and deans who serve, or have served, at dental schools across the country.

In 1929, the Rockefeller Foundation awarded the school money to provide fellowships for dentists. The grant's purpose was two-fold: to support dental research and teacher training and to investigate the biological background of dental health and disease. Yale and Rochester were to share equally. No doubt George Eastman's well-known philanthropy in the field of dentistry was an important factor in Rochester's being chosen to receive the grant. Rockefeller advisor Abraham Flexner, on his first trip to Rochester in 1920 to discuss the possibility of building a new medical school here, met with both University of Rochester President Rush Rhees and George Eastman. He also visited the Dental Dispensary on East Main Street, which had opened in October 1917, financed by Eastman. While Dr. Whipple scrupulously recused himself when Flexner's proposal was being considered by the Rockefeller board of directors, the fact that he himself was a member of the Foundation could hardly have hurt Rochester's chances.

Whereas most of the early Fellows had been trained as dentists, Hodge was an exception; he was a chemist. He was to profit from his fellowship since the program offered opportunities to consult and collaborate in a number of research venues, and also offered specialized training in areas of interest. He early became interested in the structure of teeth and rather quickly produced an important study on the structure and metabolism of tooth and bone. Together with colleagues from radiology, he participated in the development of a technique for the quantitative analysis of tooth structure.[1] The University of Arizona Press has reprinted the paper as a "Classic in Radiology."

Perhaps I may be permitted a personal reminiscence. As an undergraduate at the University of Rochester, I was privileged to attend a special session,

GILBERT B. FORBES

held on Washington's birthday in 1933, devoted to recent scientific advances by members of the faculty. I clearly remember Harold Hodge's presentation of his work on tooth hardness, using a special diamond-tipped scribe. It was a brilliant presentation, made clear for undergraduates and appropriately illustrated, that presaged his later teaching prowess with medical students.[2] Hodge also made chemical analyses of dental enamel and dentine and soon was to observe the effects of fluorine in preventing dental caries.[3] His work on this element, its metabolism, distribution in the body, and anticariogenic properties, attracted wide attention, and he was asked to contribute the definitive chapter on fluorine in a multi-volume work on mineral metabolism.[4]

In the mid-thirties, the faculty decided to institute formal course work in pharmacology for medical students. Hodge was chosen for this task and quickly set up a full-fledged course for second-year students, complete with lectures, an experimental laboratory, and a series of special projects to be carried out by small groups of medical students. Project results were presented by the students to the entire class. In 1938, I was asked to be the spokesperson for my group, and I remember well Hodge's insightful comments, his personality and wit, and the kindness that shone forth during those two days of presentations.*

While medical student teaching in pharmacology continued, another twenty years were to pass before this discipline achieved departmental status, with Hodge named Professor and Chair. In the meantime he saw to it that graduate students were attracted to work in areas having to do with mineral metabolism, especially as it pertained to tooth and bone. One of his students, William Neuman, became world-famous for his work on bone metabolism; another, Frank Smith, studied fluoride metabolism in great detail.

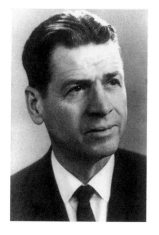

Harold C. Hodge, Ph.D., *Professor of Pharmacology and Radiation Biology and Biophysics*

During World War II, the medical school became involved in the so-called Manhattan Project, as part of the Manhattan District, designed to create the atomic bomb. One of the responsibilities of the Rochester contingent was to study the toxicology of uranium and beryllium, both of which had to be handled by the workers in the course of constructing the bomb. A top-secret laboratory was set up for this purpose, and Hodge was appointed to direct the project. During the war years he and his team did a masterful job in evaluating the toxicity of uranium compounds, especially after inhalation. This culminated in a massive work, generally conceded to be the most extensive and thorough study ever done on the pharmacology and toxicology of any substance.[5] The Rochester Project was also involved in mea-

---

*Students liked Hodge very much, in part because he kept *au courant.* At one time he even grew a marijuana plant in his office.

suring radiation intensity of toxic dusts and in developing standards for radio-active safety.

The end of the war saw the formation of the U.S. Atomic Energy Commission, which took over the facilities and programs of the Manhattan District. Rochester was selected as one of two sites (along with Vanderbilt University) to develop a school to train medical scientists in the new field of radiation biology. At Rochester, a new department was created for this purpose, and Hodge added the title of Professor of Radiation Biology and Biophysics to his name.

Hodge played a pivotal role in encouraging others to help create the "bible" used (in successive editions) by poison control centers throughout the country.[6] This compendium provides ready access to information about the ingredients of the myriad of potentially toxic substances to which humans, especially children, can be exposed. Hodge's co-author, Marion Gleason, was able to persuade manufacturers to provide a list of their products' ingredients, information usually closely guarded. With this book at hand, staff at poison-control centers could quickly assess a situation involving exposure to a commercial product and determine proper treatment.

Hodge was pleased to be chosen as the first president of the newly formed Society of Toxicology in 1961. He served as president of the International Association of Dental Research in 1947; in 1966 he was named president of the American Society for Pharmacology and Experimental Therapeutics. He was elected Fellow of the Royal Society of Medicine (London), and received the first prize in Prevention Odontology by the Swedish Medical Research Council in 1988. His publication record encompasses 286 papers and five books.

Hodge retired from Rochester in 1970, moving to the University of California at San Francisco where he served as Professor in Residence for another thirteen years. He will always be remembered as an exceptional scholar, a man of great wisdom who endeared himself to his students. He made his mark at Rochester and in the scientific world at large.

REFERENCES, HAROLD C. HODGE, PH.D.

1. Warren SL, Bishop FW, Hodge HC and VanHuysen G. A quantitative method for studying roentgen-ray absorption of tooth slabs. Am. Jour. Roentgen Radium Therap. 31, 663–72 (1934).

2. Hodge HC and McKay H. The microhardness of teeth. Jour. Am. Dent. Assoc. 20, 227–233 (1933).

3. Hodge HC and Finn SB. Reduction in experimental rat caries by fluorine. Proc. Soc. Exp. Biol. Med. 42, 318 (1939).

4. Hodge HC. Fluoride, in Mineral Metabolism, Volume II A, Chapter 24, ed. by CL Comar and F Bronner. NY, Academic Press, pp. 573–602 (1964).

5. Voegtlin C and Hodge HC (eds). The Pharmacology and Toxicology of Uranium Compounds, 4 Volumes. NY, McGraw-Hill Book Co. (1949, 1953).

GILBERT B. FORBES

6. Gleason MN, Gosselin RE, and Hodge HC. Clinical toxicology of commercial products: acute poisoning (home and farm). Baltimore, Williams and Wilkins, pp. xv, 1160 (1957).

Leon Miller, M.D., Ph.D. (b. 1912)

At Rochester 1938–Present

Charting Liver's Role in Metabolic Functions

A native Rochesterian educated at Cornell University (B.A., M.A. 1934, Ph.D. Chemistry 1937), Leon Miller was recruited by Dean George H. Whipple in 1938 to join his research group, then studying protein metabolism. This was a propitious time for Miller's arrival. He was able to further the work of Whipple and his colleagues by employing the newly-discovered radioisotopes, principally iron and carbon-14. Later he developed and perfected a technique for perfusing the isolated rat liver, a device which he used to significantly advance our knowledge of protein and amino acid metabolism.

During his early years at Rochester (and while continuing a busy laboratory schedule), Miller worked toward the medical degree that was awarded him in 1945. After teaching biochemistry at Jefferson Medical College, he returned to Rochester in 1948. Rochester had just been chosen by the Atomic Energy Commission (AEC) as a training site for scientists working in the new discipline of radiation biology and the medical school's Department of Radiation Biology was being formed, funded by and under the auspices of the AEC.

Dr. William Bale, a section leader in the new department, recruited Miller and saw to it that he was supplied with funds to support his research. He was given a joint appointment in Biochemistry and Radiation Biology and allowed to continue his research with George Whipple. The one proviso: he should use radioactive isotopes frequently enough to justify the AEC's continued support.

Miller's early work at Rochester focused on the uses of radioactive isotopes. A chance encounter between Whipple and the inventor of the cyclotron, Ernest O. Lawrence, in 1937 led to a gift by the latter of a supply of radioactive iron. Miller demonstrated that administered radioactive iron was incorporated into the hemoglobin of red blood cells.[1] He also studied factors which promoted the hepatic toxicity of chloroform; he showed that susceptibility to chloroform damage was greatly increased by protein malnutrition and that methionine was the limiting amino acid.[2]

Miller also was involved in canine studies that demonstrated that

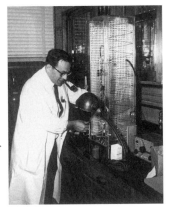

Leon Miller,
M.D., Ph.D.,
*Professor of
Biochemistry*

parenterally administered amino acids and peptides were well utilized and could keep the animals healthy for some time. In effect, this was the culmination of past work in Whipple's laboratory. Miller's findings encouraged those physicians who wanted to try a similar technique in treating malnourished patients.

Soon after his return to Rochester in 1948, the thirty-six year-old Miller began what would become the most important work of his career: developing and perfecting a new technique to perfuse the isolated rat liver.[3,4,5] Although it was known that the liver performed a number of metabolic functions, the procedure of isolating this organ from the rest of the body would provide a better understanding of its unique and manifold functions.

Miller devised and made an ingenious apparatus that could control, among other things, temperature, perfusion pressure, pH, oxygen and CO_2 partial pressures. He had determined that anticoagulants were required to prevent clotting, (the perfusate contained blood) antibiotics to prevent infection, and cortisone and insulin to provide a proper hormonal milieu. Using his new device, he succeeded in maintaining the vitality of liver preparations for 12 hours, and sometimes as long as 24 hours.

In the book edited by Bartosek, Guaitani, and Miller,[6] Miller describes the apparatus and techniques in some detail. The method enabled him and his associates to study lipogenesis, protein and glycogen synthesis, and the effects on them of various hormones. The technique has been widely used by investigators both here and abroad.

Miller's publications have documented liver's role in a host of metabolic phenomena. In addition to showing that both thyroidectomy and hypophysectomy significantly reduce protein turnover by the liver, he presented evidence that x-radiation interferes with a number of synthetic processes, that cirrhosis induced by diet interferes with hepatic hormone metabolism, and that the liver is the site of amino acid interconversions and the synthesis of clotting factors. (See note 7 for a description of one of his early studies.)

In 1977, Dr. Miller was named Emeritus Professor. He maintains an office at the medical school and continues to be involved in research. Author and co-author of 151 papers and book chapters, teacher of medical students and graduate students, Leon Miller has made his mark on biological science.

References, Leon Miller, M.D., Ph.D.

1. Miller LL, Hahn PF. The appearance of radioactive iron as hemoglobin in the red cell. Jour. Biol. Chem. 134, 585–90 (1940).

2. Miller LL, Whipple GH. Chloroform injury increases as protein stores decrease. Studies in nitrogen metabolism in these dogs. Am. Jour. Med. Sci. 199, 204–16 (1940).

3. 3 papers in Isolated Liver Perfusion and its Applications, ed by L Bartosek, A Guaitani, and LL Miller. New York, Raven Press (1973).

History of isolated liver perfusion and some still unsolved problems. pp. 1–10; Techniques of isolated rat liver perfusion pp. 11–52; Some effects of perfusate pH on amino acid and protein metabolism in the isolated perfused rat liver (with EE Griffin) pp. 139–146.

4. Miller LL, John DW. Nutritional, hormonal and temporal factors regulating net plasma protein biosynthesis in the isolated perfused rat liver, in Plasma Protein Metabolism, N.Y., Academic Press, pp. 207–22 (1970).

5. Miller LL. Protein and amino acid metabolism studies with the isolated perfused rat liver. Nutrition Reviews 17, 225–28 (1959).

6. See note 3.

7. Miller LL, Bly CG, Watson ML, Bale WF. The dominant role of the liver in plasma protein synthesis. A direct study of the isolated perfused rat liver with the aid of lysine - ε - C^{14}. Jour. Exp. Med. 94, 431–53 (1951).

David Hamilton Smith, M.D. (1932–1999)
At Rochester 1953–1958; 1976–1983

PORTER W. ANDERSON, PH.D. (b. 1937)
At Rochester 1977–1994

Creating the Hib Vaccine for Bacterial Meningitis

David H. Smith, M.D., seemed destined to succeed. A research partnership with his Harvard colleague, Porter Anderson, Ph.D. (later his teammate at Rochester), led to a stunning breakthrough: the development of a vaccine to prevent *Haemophilus influenza* type b infection, a deadly pediatric disease that in the 1960s was reaching alarming proportions.

A brilliant undergraduate at Ohio Wesleyan University where he was president of the student body in his senior year, Smith was elected to Alpha Omega Alpha while a medical student at the University of Rochester, went on to a coveted internship at the Boston Children's Hospital, and from there to a faculty position at Harvard Medical School. During his medical student days in Rochester, he took a "year-out" fellowship to work on the cytopathogenic effects of viruses under the direction of Dr. Herbert Morgan, chair of the Department of Microbiology, a hiatus he later described as "life-changing."

Except for service in the U.S. Air Force and as invited professor at the University of Geneva in Switzerland, Smith would spend the next eighteen years in Boston, first as an intern and chief resident at Boston Children's Hospital, and then as assistant/associate professor of Pediatrics at Harvard Medical School. During this time he came under the mentorship of Dr. Charles Janeway, chair of Pediatrics, who suggested that the young doctor look into the possibility of developing a vaccine against bacterial meningitis (*Haemophilus influenza* type b, or Hib). The Hib organism was responsible for a large percentage of the meningitis cases seen at Boston Children's Hospital and had reached near-epidemic proportion nationwide, affecting 10,000 children a year resulting in death, deafness, and/or mental retardation. During the 1940s, sulfonamides and penicillin were proving effective in treating children with Hib, but recovery rates were disappointing. A variable proportion, particularly young infants, were left with neurological deficits.

In his capacity as chief of the Division of Infectious Diseases at Boston Children's Hospital, Smith trained a number of Fellows and mounted a vigorous research program which included antibiotic action on bacterial DNA metabolism[*] and the phenomenon of transferable drug resistance.

In the early 1970s, Smith and Anderson were immunizing house staff and faculty at Boston Children's Hospital with a polysaccharide vaccine they had developed.[1,2] It became quickly apparent that developing a vaccine for infants, the ones at highest risk, would not be easy. Indeed, it would take more than a decade of hard work to develop an appropriate vaccine for infants.

For his research efforts at Harvard, Smith received the E. Mead Johnson Award for Research in Pediatrics in 1976 and the Distinguished Scientist Award by the Medical Society of Czechoslovakia in 1972.

In 1976 Smith was recruited to chair the Department of Pediatrics at the University of Rochester School of Medicine and Dentistry. He quickly set about to build on the Department's strengths in epidemiology and community-oriented research by emphasizing wet-bench laboratory research: laboratory space was quadrupled and new faculty were hired. Among his recruits were Anderson,[**] and Richard Insel, M.D.,[***] another Harvard colleague.

In the midst of a busy schedule (department chairmanships at academic medical centers everywhere were becoming "administrative nightmares"), Smith never lost sight of his goal of devising an effective Hib vaccine. While overseeing manifold departmental functions—including teaching medical students and house officers, managing the budget, recruiting and mentoring new faculty, serving on committees, and so on—Smith, Anderson, and Insel quietly continued their efforts on the vaccine front.

---

[*]In the laboratory of Dr. Bernard Davis, Department of Microbiology at Harvard.
[**] Now retired and living in Florida.
[***] Professor of Pediatrics and Director of the Strong Children's Research Center.

GILBERT B. FORBES

It was Porter Anderson who decided to explore the possibility of altering the capsular polysaccharide of the bacteria, first by reducing its size (hence the name oligosaccharide), and then co-valently bonding it to a protein to produce a conjugate vaccine. Based on work by others at the Rockefeller Institute and Harvard, Anderson chose a mutant form of diphtheria toxin, which was known to be non-toxic while retaining its immunogenic properties. This original combination containing the polysaccharide was duly shown to produce an antibody response in adults.[3] But the question remained about its effectiveness for infants, those most at risk from this organism.

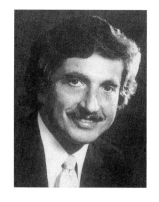

David H. Smith, M.D., *Professor and Chair, Pediatrics*

Early in the 1980s, Anderson and Smith took the bold step of giving the conjugate vaccine (this time with the oligosaccharide) to two infants, daughters of faculty members Keith Powell and Marvin Miller; the injections were given by Insel. The antibody response to this homemade vaccine was so good, and continued to be so effective in other infants, that Smith was emboldened to try his hand at commercial production, which required the creation of off-campus facilities.

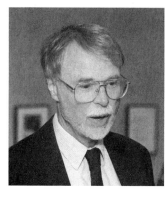

Porter W. Anderson, Ph.D., *Professor of Pediatrics*

There was great urgency surrounding the project. Smith knew that John Robbins and Rachel Schneerson had developed a conjugate vaccine at the National Institutes of Health and that a group of Canadian investigators was also working on a vaccine. Connaught Laboratories and Merck Sharp and Dohme had conducted trials of their vaccines in Alaskan Inuits only to be disappointed at the results. On the other hand, Smith and his collaborators, including practicing pediatricians in Rochester, had inoculated several hundred infants with their vaccine, had determined that antibodies persisted for up to two years, and could report that the vaccine was very well tolerated.[4]

The great question was: How to proceed? Should the Rochester team license the vaccine to a pharmaceutical house who would then produce it commercially, or should they form their own manufacturing facility? When Smith failed to interest pharmaceutical houses in the earlier vaccine, he decided to create his own pharmaceutical company and shepherd the vaccine through FDA approval. He resigned his professorship, formed Praxis Biologics, Inc., raised venture capital, mortgaged his house, hired personnel, and set up shop in the former St. Agnes School on the University of Rochester's south campus. He also acquired a manufacturing facility in

Sanford, N.C. Common stock was issued and listed on the "over-the-counter" market.

Success came swiftly. The non-conjugate vaccine was licensed by the FDA in 1985 for use in children over two years of age; the conjugate vaccine for infants was licensed five years later. Proceeds from the sale of the vaccine for children and adults enabled the fledgling company to continue to work on the conjugate vaccine for young infants. In 1990, Praxis Biologics was bought by the American Cyanamid Corporation for $232 million; the Monroe County component continues under the name of Lederle-Praxis Biologics.

This conjugate vaccine was the first FDA-licensed vaccine for young infants since the advent of the polio vaccine three decades earlier. Its widespread use has literally changed the face of pediatrics, virtually eliminating the incidence of *Haemophilus influenza* type b meningitis and other diseases caused by this organism.

The story is a fascinating one: the combined efforts of a perceptive, innovative basic scientist and a bold entrepreneur-visionary clinician/scientist have wrought a remarkable achievement in medical science.

In 1996, Smith and Anderson received the prestigious Albert Lasker Medical Research Award (along with Robbins and Schneerson) for their work on the Hib vaccine. In 1999, the University of Rochester Medical Center inaugurated the David H. Smith Center for Vaccine Biology and Immunology in the new Arthur W. Kornberg Medical Research Building, as well as the David H. Smith Research Laboratories at Strong Children's Research Center.

Dr. Anderson, now professor emeritus, is enjoying a busy retirement; "I still have some research findings to write up and publish," he says.

Dr. Smith died in 1999 from invasive malignant melanoma.

REFERENCES, DAVID HAMILTON SMITH, M.D.

1. Anderson P, Peter G, Johnston RB Jr., Wetterlow LH, and Smith DH. Immunization of humans with polyribophosphate, the capsular antigen of Haemophilus influenza type b. Jour Clin. Invest. 51, 39–44 (1972).

2. Anderson P, Insel RA, Smith DH, et al. A polysaccharide-protein complex form Haemophilus influenza type b. vaccine trial in human adults. Jour. Infect. Dis. 144, 530–38 (1981).

3. See note 2.

4. Madore DV, Johnson CL … and Smith DH. Safety and immunologic response to Haemophilus influenza type b oligosaccharide–CRM 197 conjugate vaccine in 1–6 month old infants. Pediatrics 85, 331–37 (1990). (CRM stands for cross reactive material.)

Robert Ader, Ph.D., M.D. (b. 1932)
At Rochester 1957–Present

Father of Psychoneuroimmunology

Few scientists can be credited with laying the foundation for a new branch of subspecialty study. Robert Ader, Ph.D., M.D., has done just that, in a body of innovative work that has proved incontrovertibly that our immune system is inextricably connected with the workings of our minds and bodies.

Robert Ader was granted a Ph.D. in psychology by Cornell University in 1957. When he came to Rochester looking for a job, he was immediately hired by John Romano as a research instructor in the Department of Psychiatry; from there, he proceeded up the academic ladder. On the retirement of George Engel in 1983, he inherited Engel's position as director of the Division of Behavioral and Psychosocial Medicine and was named George L. Engel Professor of Psychosocial Medicine. Though not a physician (his M.D. degree was granted *honoris causa* from the University of Trondheim in Norway), he has continued to oversee the activities of this Division since that time.

Housed as they were in the same department, Ader was to be greatly influenced by the ideas and opinions of George Engel, a strong advocate of the role of psychological factors in physiological functions; for it was at this time that Engel was formulating the concept of the Biopsychosocial model of human disease.

Dr. Ader's early work was concerned with factors that influence the development of gastric erosions in the rat. Physicians have always been curious about the etiology of peptic ulcers in human patients and, prior to the advent of specific inhibition of histamine-stimulated gastric acid secretion, in factors contributing to a cure. In the laboratory, Ader studied the effect of various social factors that might influence the rats' susceptibility to gastric erosions. He found, for example, that most animals develop ulcers when they are immobilized for twenty-four hours; in addition, his research showed that the incidence of ulcers is inversely proportional to cage volume. In a related finding, Ader and his team showed that handling young animals offers some degree of protection against the effect of immobilization, as does individual as compared to group housing.[1]

In collaboration with Stanford Friedman and Lowell Glasgow, Ader studied the effect of social factors on the susceptibility of mice to experimental infections. For example, the mortality rate from malaria was higher in mice housed in groups than among those in single-animal cages, whereas (unexpectedly) the reverse was true for mice infected with encephalomyocarditis virus.[2]

During the 1970s, Ader became interested in the possibility that the immune system could be classically conditioned—that there was "an intimate and virtually unexplored relationship between the central nervous system and immunologic processes."[3] In this endeavor, he had as collaborator Nicholas

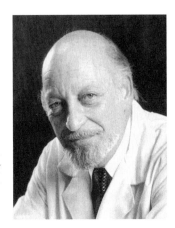

Robert Ader,
Ph.D., M.D.,
*George L.
Engel Professor
of Psychosocial
Medicine*

Cohen, a member of the Department of Microbiology and Immunology. This research came about as a result of studies of taste-aversion learning in rats. When the animals are presented with a stimulus in the form of saccharin solution paired with an injection of the noxious and immunosuppressive drug cyclophosphamide (CY), the animals soon learn to avoid the former. However, conditioned animals subjected to repeated exposure to saccharin began to die, which suggested to Ader and Cohen that this presumably benign material might have begun to mimic the immunosuppressive effect of CY.

Ader and Cohen went on to show that animals conditioned by exposure to saccharin and CY demonstrated a reduced antibody response to the antigen (sheep red blood cells) when they were re-exposed to the conditioned stimulus (saccharin). They then looked at a fatal autoimmune disease (systemic lupus erythematosus) in mice, in which the progress of the disease can be retarded by CY. They found beneficial effects when they substituted the conditioned stimulus (saccharin) for actual drug on some scheduled treatment days; such effects were noted only in mice that had been conditioned.[4]

About this time, team member David Felten proved the existence of networks of sympathetic nerve fibers that were in direct contact with lymphocytes and macrophages. This cumulative body of evidence led Ader to coin the term "psychoneuroimmunology," which he used in his presidential address before the American Psychosomatic Society in 1980.[5]

In 1993, Ader founded the Center for Psychoneuroimmunology Research; he continues to serve as its director. An adjunct of the Department of Psychiatry, the Center has a vigorous research and teaching program and a large number of publications.

Robert Ader is a very busy man who has received numerous honors. He is past president of the American Psychosomatic Society (1979–80), the Academy of Behavioral Medicine Research (1984–85), the International Society for Developmental Psychobiology (1981–82), and the Psychoneuroimmunology Research Society (1993–94). He was a visiting professor at the University of Utrecht (1970–71) and a fellow of the Center for Advanced Study in Behavioral Sciences, Stanford University (1992–93). In 1996, he received the Scientist of the Year Award from the International Center of Epistemology, Harvard University; a Research Scientist Award from the National Institute of Mental Health (1969–99); and the Arthur Kornberg Research Award from the University of Rochester Medical Center.

Dr. Ader has advanced the discipline of Psychoneuroimmunology with vigor and determination, with the result that the immune system can no longer be considered autonomous: "homeostatic mechanisms are the product of an integrated system of defenses of which the immune system is one component."[6] He is the avowed leader of a discipline which has extended the role of the central nervous system beyond behavior and hormonal function into the realm of the immune system and its bearing on host defenses.

REFERENCES, ROBERT ADER, PH.D., M.D.

1. Ader R. Experimentally induced gastric lesions: Results and implications of studies in animals. Advances in Psychosomatic Medicine 6, 1–39 (1971).

2. Friedman SB, Glasgow LA, Ader R. Psychosocial factors modifying host resistance to experimental infections. Ann. NY Academy of Sciences 164, 381–92 (1969).

3. Ader R, Cohen N. Behaviorally conditioned immunosuppression. Psychosomatic Med. 37, 333–40 (1975).

4. Ader R, Cohen N. Behaviorally conditioned immunosuppression and murine systemic lupus erythematosus. Science 215, 1534–36 (1982).

5. Ader R (ed). Psychoneuroimmunology. NY, Acad. Press (1981).

6. Ader R. Historical Perspective on Psychoneuroimmunology in Psychoneuroimmunology, Stress and Infection, ed. by H. Friedman, TW Klein, AL Friedman. Boca Raton, CRC Press, pp. 1–24 (1995).

Fred Sherman, Ph.D. (b. 1932)
At Rochester 1960–Present

A Father of Yeast Molecular Genetics

"Skeptics concerned about the future of genetic engineering should stroll through the barnyard," Fred Sherman once advised an interviewer. "That prize cow that gives so much rich milk was genetically engineered over hundreds of years of scientific breeding. The difference is now we can speed change by several orders of magnitude." Sherman's work in the laboratory has been instrumental in facilitating that rate of change.

Educated at the University of Minnesota and University of California at Berkeley, Sherman came to Rochester in 1960 after postdoctoral training at the University of Washington and the Lab Genétique, Gif-sur-Yvette in France. While his original appointment was in the Department of Radiation Biology and Biophysics, he gradually moved up the faculty ladder to become chair and professor of Biochemistry in 1982, a position he held until 1996. Having relinquished his administrative post, he continues his professorship in the department now known as Biochemistry and Biophysics.

It is worth noting that Sherman's Ph.D. work at Berkeley was in the field of biophysics. It was not until late in the course of this work that he developed an interest in genetics (despite never having had a course in this field!). Watson and Crick had published their discovery of the structure of DNA in 1953, the year of young Sherman's undergraduate degree, and the new science of molecular genetics was just getting underway.

His specific interest was sparked by a study of mutations in yeast induced by elevated temperatures. Further work with yeast in his postdoctoral years helped to convince him that this organism provided an ideal species for genetic analysis and manipulation. Yeast, a eukaryote with a nucleus and chromosomes, will grow anaerobically as well as aerobically; its haploid cells can grow as well as diploid cells. As a result, yeast has an advantage over the organism long favored by geneticists, *Escherichia coli*. Several species can serve as experimental organisms, one of which is responsible for the bread we eat, and another for the beer and wine we drink.

During his postdoctoral years, Sherman happened on a yeast mutant deficient in the compound common to all eukaryotes, namely cytochrome c, which facilitates the electron transport system. This protein is easily purified, has a low molecular weight, and thus lends itself to amino acid sequence analysis. He devised an ingenious spectroscopic method that allows for easy identification of yeast colonies containing cytochrome c mutants.

Sherman and his associates discovered two isoenzymes of cytochrome c, mapped deletion sites, transformed defective mutants using synthetic oligonucleotides, determined the structural properties of iso-1-cytochrome c, and studied the regulatory mechanism for maintaining elevated proportions of the iso-1 enzyme. Much of this work involved cloning the gene and identifying chromosomal positions of regulating signals, using recombinant DNA techniques.[1] He has also studied a yeast pathogenic for man, *Candida albicans*.

For seventeen years, Sherman taught a summer course in yeast genetics at the Cold Spring Harbor Laboratory in Long Island, while continuing to supervise graduate students at Rochester. His teaching partner has written an account of those interesting years.[2] In 1982, Sherman was persuaded to become chair of the Department of Biochemistry at Rochester, a post he held for 14 years. Although not particularly fond of administration, he managed to carry out these duties while maintaining an active research program. Indeed, during a recent (1999) interview he exclaimed, "Now I'm sixty-seven and raring to go! Ready for new challenges, now that I'm free of administration!"

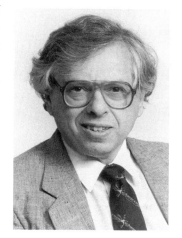

Fred Sherman, Ph.D., *Professor and Chair, Biochemistry*

Many honors have come Sherman's way. He was elected a fellow of the American Academy of Microbiology; he has served on the Committee on Chemical Environmental Mutagens of the National Research Council, and on study sections of the American Cancer Society and of the National Institutes of Health. In 1985 he was elected to the National Academy of Sciences, and later was elected chair of its section on genetics.

Fred Sherman is generally recognized as one of the fathers of yeast molecular genetics. A conference held in his honor at Rochester in the fall of 1999 attracted some 150 scientists, many from abroad. He is fond of reminding us that this lowly organism offers a wonderful opportunity to study how genes work, for it undergoes biological processes in much the same way as human cells do.

Recently, Sherman and his Rochester colleague David Pearce have found similarities between certain yeast genes and the gene abnormalities in a human condition known as Batten Disease, a progressive neurodegenerative condition in which the cytoplasm of neurons accumulate deposits of ceroid lipofuscin.[3,4] This exciting discovery will most certainly stimulate wide use of yeast as a means of studying other human diseases. One can safely predict that Fred Sherman and his associates will be in the forefront of such endeavors.

REFERENCES, FRED SHERMAN, PH.D.

1. Sherman F. My life with cytochrome c., in The Early Days of Yeast Genetics, ed. by MN Hall and P Linder. Cold Spring Harbor Laboratory Press, pp. 347–357 (1993).
2. Fink GR. The double entendre, in ibid. pp. 435–444.
3. Pearce DA and Sherman F. A yeast model for the study of Batten Disease. Proc. Nat'l Acad. Sci. 95, 6915–18 (1998).
4. Pearce DA, Ferea T, Nosel SA, Das B, and Sherman F. Actions of BTNl, the yeast orthologue of the gene mutated in Batten Disease. Nature Genetics 22, 55–58 (1999).

William H. Bowen, B.D.S., Ph.D. (b. 1933)
At Rochester 1956–1959; 1982–present

Unlocking the Secrets of Dental Caries

Educated in Ireland and England, William Bowen spent three years as a research fellow at Rochester's Eastman Dental Center, earning a masters degree, before returning to England to pursue a doctoral degree. In 1973 he was appointed chief of the Caries Prevention and Research Branch of the National Institutes of Health. In 1982 he returned to Rochester, this time as professor of dentistry and chair of dental research.

William Bowen is an important part of the continuum of dental research activity and post-graduate dental education begun by Harold Hodge in 1930, which has earned the medical school the right to include the words "and Dentistry" in its title.

Bowen's distinguished career has combined expertise in basic and clinical science. Much of his research has targeted those factors that promote the formation of dental plaque and the role plaque plays in dental decay. He and his associates have described the function of the glucosyltransferases that are responsible for the formation of the bulk of the carbohydrate polymer of which dental plaque is composed. They have demonstrated that glucosyltransferases represent a primary virulence factor of cariogenic streptococci.[1] These enzymes, shed from bacteria, become firmly attached to the tooth surface in active form. The researchers have shown that the polymer which these enzymes produce when sorbed to a solid surface is markedly different in structure and more "sticky," for cariogenic bacteria, than the polymer which forms when the enzyme is in solution.[2,3]

GILBERT B. FORBES

Bowen has developed animal models (monkey, rat) for the study of experimental caries in its various aspects, with emphasis on bacterial factors. He has proposed that exposure to heavy metals, such as lead, accounts for the unusually high incidence of dental decay among children who live in inner cities.[4] Recent epidemiologic evidence supports this hypothesis.

Most recently, Bowen has suggested that the decline in dental decay can be attributed not only to fluoride but also to the increased usage of food preservatives, such as benzoate. Such preservatives function as weak acids that enter oral bacteria, rendering them less tolerant of low pH. This research suggests the possibility of discovering novel antimicrobial agents.

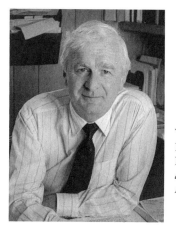

William H. Bowen, B.D.S., Ph.D., *Professor and Chair, Dental Research*

The author or co-author of some 200 publications in the scientific literature, Bowen has been awarded four honorary degrees (all from abroad) and has served as president of the International Association for Dental Research and the American Association for Dental Research. He is a fellow of the Royal College of Surgeons, England, and a member of the Institute of Medicine of the National Academy of Sciences. In 1997 he was awarded the coveted Yngve Ericsson Prize in Preventive Odontology by the Swedish Medical Research Council; this award has been termed the "Dental Nobel Prize."

He has served as advisor to nine masters and five Ph.D. students at Rochester, as well as to several post-graduate students abroad. He has been a visiting professor at a number of institutions both here and abroad, and has given numerous lectures at other institutions.

Although he retired as chair of dental research in 1995, Bowen continues to pursue an active research program and to train dental researchers. Dental caries is an almost universal disease of mankind. More scientific work in this area is needed, especially the kind of research expertise and insight that is the hallmark of William Bowen's career.

REFERENCES, WILLIAM H. BOWEN, B.D.S., PH.D.

1. Yamashita Y, Bowen WH, Burne RA, and Kuramitsu HK. Role of the Streptococcus mutans gtf genes in caries induction in the specific-pathogen-free rat model. Infect. Immun. 61, 3811–17 (1993).

2. Schilling KM and Bowen WH. Glucans synthesized in situ in experimental salivary pellicle function as specific binding sites for Streptococcus mutans. Infect. Immun. 60, 284–95 (1992).

3. Kopec LK, Vacca-Smith AM, and Bowen WH. Structural aspects of glucans

formed in solution and on the surface of hydroxyapatite. Glycobiology 7, 929–34 (1997).

4. Watson GE, Davis BA, Raubertas RF, Pearson SK, and Bowen WH. Influence of maternal lead ingestion on caries in rat pups. Nature Medicine 3, 1024–25 (1997).

Thomas W. Clarkson, Ph.D. (b. 1932)
At Rochester 1957–Present

Toxicology Research and Environmental Health

Thomas Clarkson, an internationally known toxicologist with a particular interest in mercury, has developed Rochester's Environmental Health Sciences Center (EHSC) as a first-class facility for toxicology research. Under his leadership, the Center has achieved its own international status and has become a splendid resource for specialists and clinicians.

Born in England, Clarkson earned a Ph.D. in biochemistry at the University of Manchester. He came to Rochester in 1957 as a postdoctoral fellow in Biophysics and Toxicology, and except for a year at the Weizmann Institute in Israel and two years as scientific officer for the Medical Research Council in England, he has spent his entire career at Rochester. He was named to a full professorship in 1971, became head of the Division of Toxicology in 1980 and director of the EHSC in 1986. In 1992, he was appointed chair of the newly created Department of Environmental Medicine, a post from which he retired in 1998. He continues to teach graduate students and pursue research.

Clarkson's interest in mercury as a toxic agent came about at the request of his mentor, Aser Rothstein, professor of Radiation Biology. Rothstein had been asked by the Atomic Energy Commission (AEC) for information about the possible toxicity of this liquid metal. As work progressed in building the hydrogen bomb, large mercury columns were being used to separate isotopes of lithium. The process was essential to the project but the AEC was rightfully concerned about worker safety. Convinced that mercury was worth investigating as a potential environmental hazard, Clarkson set about studying in great detail the metal's metabolism and toxicity, in particular two of its compounds, phenyl mercury and methyl mercury.

In the 1960s, Clarkson's research was stimulated by a tragic occurrence—a widespread "epidemic" of methyl mercury poisoning in Iraq. Imported grain, treated with methyl mercury (a fungicide) and intended for planting, was instead widely consumed (despite warnings on the shipping containers).

Soon thousands of Iraqi, including pregnant women and infants, came down with symptoms of mercury poisoning.

Clarkson organized a team of Iraqi and American scientists to help those afflicted and to study the toxic effects. He developed techniques for analyzing absorbed mercury in snippets of single strands of hair and used this to date the time of ingestion of the compound. Since levels of mercury in hair reflect the absorbed dose, Clarkson and his colleagues were able to establish a dose-response relationship between the prevalence of neurological symptoms in adults and the absorbed dose. The Iraqi studies also demonstrated a quantitative relationship between mercury levels in the mothers' hair and the frequency of adverse developmental effects in their offspring.

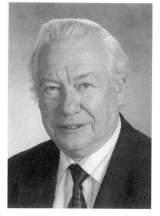

Thomas W. Clarkson, Ph.D., *Chair, Department of Environmental Medicine*

This technique was also used by the Clarkson team to study populations exposed to methyl mercury in Canada and Peru, and children exposed to phenyl mercury in Argentina.

A Clarkson-led study which has attracted wide international interest targets a group of women of child-bearing age and their offspring who live in the Seychelles, an archipelago off the coast of East Africa, and whose consumption of ocean fish is particularly high. Ocean fish are invariably contaminated with methyl mercury, as they ingest naturally occurring mercury which has been methylated by the action of bacteria and other organisms. The study's goal is to determine the lowest possible level of mercury that can occur in women of childbearing age without adversely affecting the developmental health of their children.

Clarkson and his associates have just completed a five-year longitudinal study of several hundred Seychellois children, including measures of child development and periodic analyses of maternal and child hair for the presence and amounts of absorbed methyl mercury. Using standard measures of child development, these studies failed to reveal an adverse effect of methyl mercury exposure, either *in utero* or during childhood. Over a range of less than 3 ppm to 25 ppm Hg exposure, no downward trend in developmental scores was detected (indeed there was a very slight upward trend). The result: clear evidence that—at least in the Seychelles—a diet comprised of plentiful amounts of ocean fish does not affect child development.

Other research efforts target a recent flurry of concern about possible toxic effects from amalgam dental fillings. The trauma of chewing dislodges tiny bits of mercury used in the amalgam, debris that is then ingested along with the masticated food. Dr. Clarkson currently is collaborating with dentists in assaying urine samples from children who have such fillings.

The Clarkson bibliography is a large one, as is the level of outside research support (in excess of a million dollars a year in the past three decades). Among Clarkson's many honors: an honorary degree from University of Umea, Sweden; a Merit Award from the Society of Toxicology; appointment to the Institute of Medicine of the National Academy of Sciences; and a number of visiting professorships, both here and abroad.

Clarkson's work has provided fundamental insight into the mechanism of mercury toxicity and into the epidemiology of exposure factors of this environmentally ubiquitous metal. He and his associates also have studied the mechanism responsible for converting metabolic mercury to mercuric ion in the body, factors influencing the uptake of mercury by the central nervous system, the binding of methyl mercury to cysteine which facilitated its entry into cells, and the turnover of mercury in adult subjects.

His work has helped put the discipline of Toxicology on firm ground, and has become a model for the study of other intoxicants. His achievements through the years have been truly outstanding.

To quote fellow faculty member Richard Miller, "Environmental exposures and the resultant toxic effects on all species, including man, have confounded us for generations. Industrial pollution with heavy metals, especially mercury, has produced such toxic endpoints as neurological disease, birth defects and mental retardation. The assessment of these endpoints utilizing a dose-response relationship has been extremely difficult to establish in man.

"Professor Clarkson, through a combination of basic and clinical investigations, established the toxicities, mechanisms of action and dose-response relationship for methyl mercury. Through Professor Clarkson's efforts, we now can assess risk for methyl mercury exposures to adults, children, but most importantly [to] the pregnant woman and babe *in utero*. Without his laboratory and field studies throughout the world, environmental medicine and toxicology would still be trying to understand animal dose extrapolation to the human for methyl mercury. Methyl mercury is the first environmental teratogen in humans where we have such dose-response relationships," and the first time a dose-response relationship had been established for human prenatal effects.

REFERENCES, THOMAS W. CLARKSON, PH.D.

1. Bakir F, Damluji SF ... Clarkson TW. Methylmercury poisoning in Iraq. Science 181, 230–41 (1973).
2. Marsh DO, Clarkson TW, et al. Fetal methylmercury poisoning: Relationship between concentration in simple strands of maternal hair and child effects. Arch. Neurol. 44, 1017–22 (1987).

GILBERT B. FORBES

3. Cox C, Clarkson TW, et al. Dose-response analysis of infants prenatally exposed to methylmercury: An application of a single compartment model to single-strand hair analysis. Environ. Res. 49, 318–32 (1989).

4. Davidson PW, Myers GJ … Clarkson TW. Effects of prenatal and postnatal methylmercury exposure from fish consumption on neurodevelopment. JAMA 280, 701–07 (1998).

We now continue with photographs and brief captions for other faculty members who have made significant contributions to research while at Rochester. Unfortunately, space does not permit the inclusion of many others whose research efforts were noteworthy.

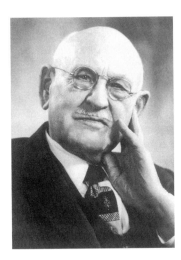

John R. Murlin, Ph.D.,†
Professor and Chair, Vital Economics.
Early work on insulin, discovered glucagon

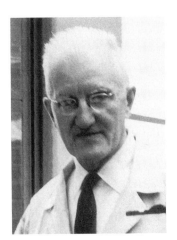

Edward F. Adolph, Ph.D.,†
Professor of Physiology.
Water balance, physiological regulations

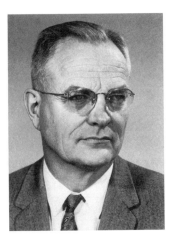

Alexander L. Dounce, Ph.D.,†
Professor of Biochemistry.
Early work on the nucleotide genetic code

† deceased

GILBERT B. FORBES

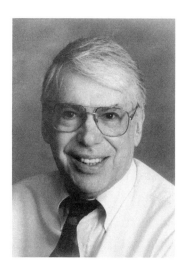

Paul D. Coleman, Ph.D., *Professor of Neurobiology and Anatomy. Neurons, dendritic extent, normal aging, Alzheimer's disease*

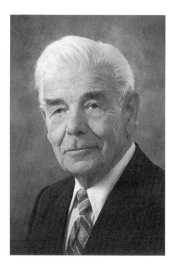

Burtis Breese, M.D.,† *Clinical Professor of Pediatrics. Research in the setting of private practice*

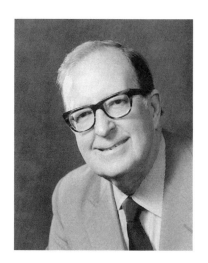

Frank Disney, M.D., *Clinical Professor of Pediatrics. Research in the setting of private practice*

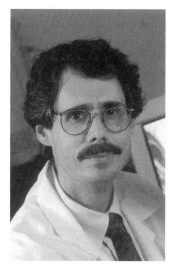

Howard J. Federoff, M.D., Ph.D., *Professor of Neurology and Medicine, Director of Center for Aging and Developmental Biology, Molecular Neurobiology*

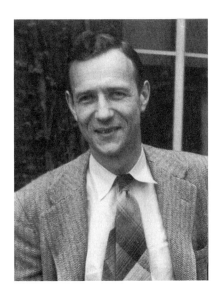

Hermann Rahn, Ph.D.,†
Associate Professor of Physiology.
Respiratory physiology, high
altitude flight

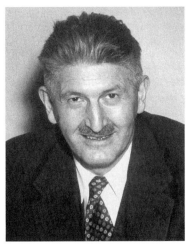

Stafford Warren, M.D.,†
Professor and Chair, Radiology.
Toxicity electromagnetic radiation,
Head Section on Health, the
Manhattan Project, Dean of UCLA
School of Medicine

William F. Neuman, Ph.D.,†
Professor of Biochemistry, Professor
and Co-Chair, Radiation Biology.
The inorganic phase of bone

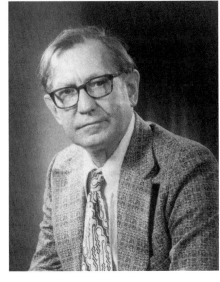

GILBERT B. FORBES

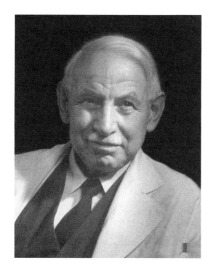

Walter R. Bloor, Ph.D.,†
Professor and Chair, Biochemistry.
Metabolism fat and related
compounds

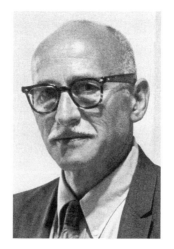

Sidney A. Weinberg,†
Research Associate in Radiology.
Gastroscopic photography, cine fluorography
development

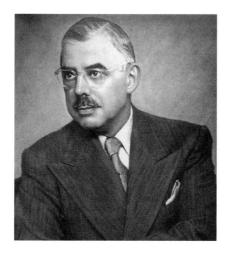

William Van Wagenen,
M.D.,†
Associate Professor,
Neurological Surgery.
Section of corpus callosum
for epilepsy

The next group of photographs depicts some of our illustrious alumni/ae. Some have distinguished themselves by research, others by highly significant clinical and administrative efforts. The available space allows for only a few among the many who deserve recognition.

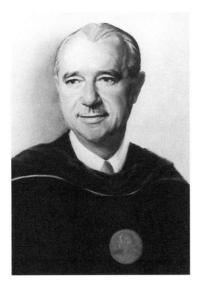

Vincent du Vigneaud,† *Ph.D. 1927, Nobel Prize 1955. Chair of Biochemistry, Cornell University Medical School. Synthesis of pitressin, oxytocin*

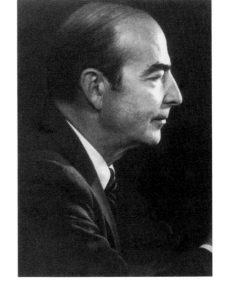

Arthur Kornberg, *M.D. 1941, Nobel Prize 1959. Currently Professor of Biochemistry, Emeritus, Stanford University. DNA Synthesis*

GILBERT B. FORBES

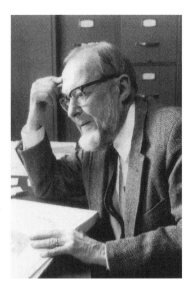

James V. Neel,† *M.D. 1944.*
Professor of Genetics, University of
Michigan. Genetics sickle cell disease,
radiation damage atomic bomb

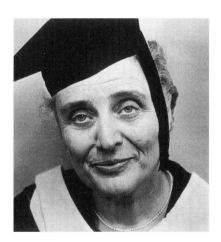

Mary Steichen Calderone,†
M.D. 1939. Medical Director,
Planned Parenthood, Co-founder
Sex Information and Education
Council

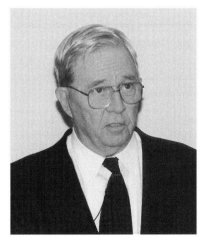

Donald Henderson, *M.D. 1954.*
Dean Johns Hopkins School Public Health.
Smallpox eradication

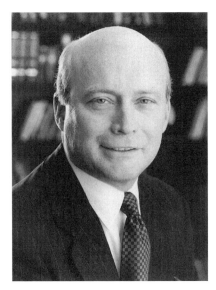

John W. Rowe, *M.D. 1970.*
President of Mount Sinai
Medical Center

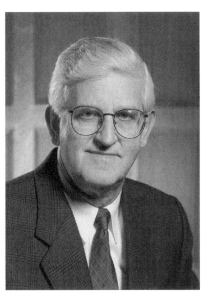

Joseph B. Martin, *Ph.D. 1971*
(M.D., University of Alberta).
Dean, Harvard Medical School.
Studies in neuroendocrinology;
studies of the brain peptides

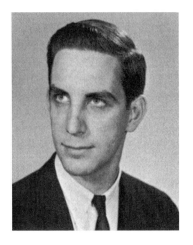

Edward D. Miller, *M.D. 1968.*
CEO, Johns Hopkins Medicine,
Dean of the School of Medicine

GILBERT B. FORBES

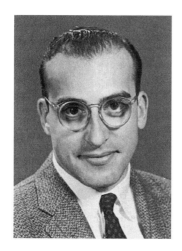

William Peck, *M.D. 1960.*
Dean and Vice-Chancellor,
Washington University
School of Medicine.
Studies of bone cell function

Robert L. Brent, *M.D. 1953, Ph.D.*
1955, D.Sc. 1988.
Long term Chair of Pediatrics,
Thomas Jefferson University.
Causation congenital malformations

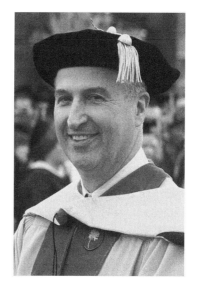

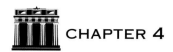

CHAPTER 4

Achievements in the Basic Biomedical Sciences

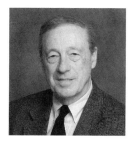

PAUL L. LaCELLE, M.D.

When the development of a medical school at the University of Rochester was contemplated, University of Rochester President Rush Rhees and George Eastman of Eastman Kodak Company stipulated that the school should be of highest quality. The appointment of George H. Whipple, M.D., as dean and architect of the school, assured that quality. Dean Whipple emphasized research as well as education, and viewed the relation between the two as essential. Further, in research endeavors, he transcended departmental boundaries, bringing together individuals from a variety of disciplines for successful approaches to problems, both basic and clinical in nature. Despite the responsibilities of organizing a new medical school, his research efforts were unabated: during his first twenty years at Rochester he published more than 125 papers, and was mentor to a variety of faculty, people in training, and students. His example clearly had a stimulating effect on the faculty he appointed, and set the expedition for research at Rochester into motion.

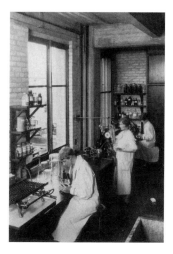

Dean Whipple's laboratory, 1926

The success of the research endeavor at Rochester was due both to the environment that Dr. Whipple created and the quality of individuals he appointed as his first faculty

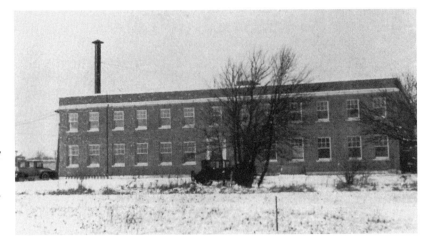

Research
laboratory
(Animal
House),
December,
1922

members. Most of his department chairs were young by today's standards, but they were already prominent in their research disciplines. Their selection of outstanding younger faculty expanded the research activities in the newly forming departments.

Importantly, Dr. Whipple established formal patterns of interaction among researchers in order to assure dissemination of knowledge. A research committee comprised of J.R. Murlin and Wallace Fenn led a regular interdepartmental science conference, which was attended by all faculty appointees. A medical society committee held regular meetings chaired by William S. McCann, chair of Medicine; these were attended by preclinical scientists as well as clinicians. A medical history club, chaired by George Corner of the Department of Anatomy, held regular meetings to discuss topics of interest to faculty and students. In addition, current developments in biomedicine around the world were discussed in these meetings.

During this seventy-five year period, literally tens of thousands of research papers have been produced by faculty and students of the School of Medicine and Dentistry. Many faculty have gone on to other institutions, often in leadership roles. It would be impossible to present more than a small number of selected instances of such research. The emphasis here is on major contributions, particularly those which have had a major influence on existing research fields or which were key to development in new directions. This

Dr. Wallace Fenn's hypobaric chamber for study of human respiratory physiology at altitude

140   PAUL L. LaCELLE

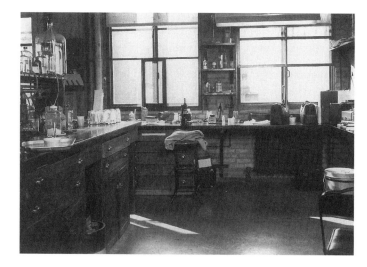

account does not include the contributions of individuals whose work is described by Gilbert Forbes in chapter three. The identification of recent research accomplishments has been restricted to novel contributions by senior faculty where work has been recognized widely. The research contributions are listed below by department and in chronological order.

Anatomy

George Corner, first faculty member appointed and chair of Anatomy, had research interests in the anatomy and physiology of the corpus luteum and its role in pregnancy. A medical student, Willard Allen, isolated progesterone, and crystalline progestin subsequently was characterized by Oskar Wintersteiner and Willard Allen. The next chair, Karl E. Mason, his colleagues, and Victor Emmel studied the role of vitamin E (tocopherol) on the lipids of muscle and fatty tissues in rats, emphasizing the antioxidant role of tocopherols. More recently Carl Knigge and colleagues pioneered the histocytochemical characterization of functions in the medial eminence of the hypothalamus. Robert Joynt and Alfred Weindl demonstrated that medial eminence-releasing factors are regulatory of pituitary function.

Subsequently, Manuel delCerro established techniques to transplant fetal retinal cells in the effort to treat blindness in animal models. Another important study was the first transplantation of monkey brain fetal cells into adult brain to test the hypothesis that brain renewal could be accomplished by such transplantation methods. A most recent emphasis in the department has been the work of Gary Paige on the dynamics of neural systems which effect balance control and orientation in space.

The department is currently titled Neurobiology and Anatomy, an appropriate recognition of its major research emphasis and teaching in neurobiology, as well as the ongoing commitment to teaching human anatomy.

Biochemistry

Walter Bloor, a chemist well known for his work on the fatty acids of plasma, established a research program in lipid metabolism. Bloor's graduate student, Warren Sperry, received a Ph.D. in the field of lipid metabolism in 1925; this was the first Ph.D. given by the University of Rochester. Together

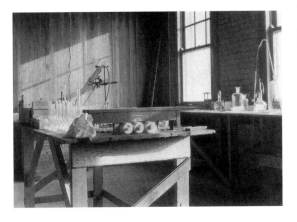

Walter Bloor's laboratory, 1925

they completed important work in cholesterol metabolism. Bloor and Robert Sinclair did some of the early work in phospholipid metabolism, using the newly available isotope deuterium. Harold Hodge, a physical chemist, did extensive work on the metabolism of both teeth and bones; he confirmed and extended earlier work on the positive effect of fluoride in preventing dental caries. Robert Burton, Alejandro Zaffaroni, and Henry Keutmann established chromatographic methods for characterization of steroids, particularly corticosteroids and related compounds.

Elmer Stotz characterized one of the cytochromes of the electron transport system; subsequently he and Guido Marinetti developed chromatographic techniques to study phospholipids and fatty acids. Using these new techniques, Marinetti studied key phosphoenzymes in liver and muscle. In 1952, Alexander Dounce published studies that predicted the nucleotide basis for the human

---

A Case of Perfect Preoccupation

Stories about absent-minded professors abound. One that has become legendary involves biochemist Alexander Dounce, one of the most prolific of Rochester's researchers—and a man who became oblivious to his environment when focused on his investigations.

Dounce was working in his lab with an assistant one day when his helper grew faint and collapsed in the doorway. The preoccupied professor stepped over her body, obtained a piece of equipment in a lab down the hall, and returned to his lab, once more stepping over the inert figure. Some seconds later, aware at last that something was missing from the scene, he noticed his helper sprawled in the doorway. "Here, here, what's this?" he is reported to have exclaimed, amazed by the scene's incongruity—and then, stepping over the assistant again, rushed to summon help.

Dounce's brilliance led him to propose the first model for a nucleotide genetic code template system for replication of nucleic acids. His paper on duplicating mechanisms for peptide chain and nucleic acid syntheses, published in Enzymologica *in 1952, predated Watson and Crick's discoveries by a year. (The final experiments in the confirmation of a model for replication necessitated that Watson and Crick employ radioactive material, material that Dounce refused to have in his laboratory.)*

---

142   PAUL L. LaCELLE

genetic code, in advance of the work of Watson and Crick in 1953. Dounce also established several new methods for isolating cell organelles, including nucleoli and plasma membranes. Leon Miller established the role of the liver in protein production and developed an in vitro liver perfusion system and techniques for studying individual plasma proteins.

James Wittliff and co-workers characterized steroid binding proteins in normal and tumor mammary gland tissue, work which contributed importantly to the development of therapeutic strategies for treating breast carcinoma. Russel Hilf established well-characterized animal models for breast tumors, particularly with respect to the enzyme distribution and patterns in malignant cells and the influence of hormones on the differentiation of tumor cells.

Fred Sherman became chair of the department in 1982. A member of the National Academy of Sciences, he has made exceptional contributions to the under-

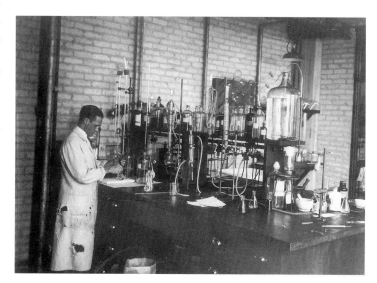

Biochemistry research laboratory, 1926

standing of biology and genetics of yeast, and for determining the mechanisms of cytochrome regulation, expression, and metabolism.

Donald Young identified precisely changes in cell protein synthesis induced by steroid hormones. He pioneered techniques for detecting such new protein, particularly the giant two dimensional electrophoretic gel which was key to his discoveries and has broad potential as a technique for gene identification. His most important accomplishment has been the isolation of the gene regulating production of cyclo oxygenase 2 (COX-2), a cause of inflammation; inhibitors of COX-2 are potent in treating disorders such as arthritis.

Robert Bambara, current chair, has used purified proteins to demonstrate and reconstitute the reactions required for synthesizing and joining nascent DNA segments during mammalian cell DNA replication. He also has clarified mechanisms by which estrogen induces expression of specific genes, and how the hormone bonds with receptor proteins in cell nuclei to influence the promoters of responsive genes. Alan Senior has characterized the synthesis of ATP in bacteria and mitochondria and has clarified the bases of multi-drug resistance in cancer cells.

William Bernhard has studied free radical processes by which ionizing radiation alters the structure of DNA, and has demonstrated the importance of base sequence and DNA hydration on the amount of damage. Christopher Lawrence has investigated the enzymatic mechanisms in bacteria, yeast, and human cells for replicating of DNA containing unrepaired damage. Since this is a source of mutations, understanding these mechanisms could lead to novel disease prevention strategies. Thomas Gunter and colleagues have examined metabolic aspects of calcium signaling and have discovered a novel mitochondrial efflux mechanism for sequestration of calcium.

Edward Puzas, director of the Musculoskeletal Research Center in Orthopaedics, has identified functional insulin-like growth factor receptors in isolated bone cells and a regulatory role for retinoic acid in the expression of bone morphogenetic protein in chondrocytes, key contributions to understanding bone development and dynamics. His group has shown that toxic agents, such as lead, may contribute to osteoporosis.

Environmental Medicine

The precursor to this department began in the mid-1960s with the establishment by Harold Hodge and Thomas Clarkson of a nationally designated Environmental Health Center, funded largely by the National Institute of Environmental Health Sciences, which provided support for a large program of associated research and for a related toxicology training program. The Center has had continuous support since its beginning, clear evidence of the exceptional quality of its faculty in research and education.

In 1992, the school established the Department of Environmental Medicine, with Thomas Clarkson as chair and members from several departments as faculty. Included in the new department's activities were activities in environmental science and a variety of clinical pulmonary studies directed by Richard Hyde and Mark Utell of the Department of Medicine.

Bernard Weiss and Victor Laties, both members of the original EHS Center, are pioneers in examining, in animal models, behavior related to addiction, especially secondary to nicotine and narcotics. Thomas Gasiewicz has done extensive studies of mechanisms whereby halogenated heterocyclic compounds, such as dioxin, cause toxic effects in animals. He has also demonstrated features of a gene-regulatory protein, the AhR receptor, to genes, interactions with DNA, and identification of cells such as thymus and embryonic tissues affected by these compounds.

Debra Cory-Slecta, current department chair, and her colleagues have used in vivo electrochemistry and autoradiographic methods to demonstrate the neurochemical localization of lead in brain structure and its role in behavioral deficits in animal models. Other studies by the group describe the effects of low lead levels on behavior in groups of children.

Microbiology

Stanhope Bayne-Jones, first chair of Microbiology, was interested in factors regulating bacterial growth. His successor, George Packer Berry, significantly advanced the understanding of virus transformation. Conrad Birkhaug and colleagues established the relation of streptococcus to scarlet fever, while Philip Jay and Ralph Voorhees studied the role of bacillus acidophilus in dental caries. William Bradford, a pediatrician known for his work on whooping cough, isolated bacillus parapertussis in children who had whooping cough. Henry Sherp performed important early studies in the biochemistry and immunology of meningococcus.

Herbert Morgan and Donald Hare characterized a psittacosis virus multiplication phenomenon; Morgan also examined viral transformation in tumor and embryogenic cells. Howard Slavin and George Packer Berry, later dean of the Harvard Medical School, carried out some of the early studies of herpes infection in a mouse model.

Barbara Iglewski, current chair of what is now the Department of Microbiology and Immunology, has performed important studies in Pseudomonas aeruginosa, characterizing a system of genes regulating proteases which cause host tissue damage. Edith Lord has developed tumor models to demonstrate the role of cytokines and the stimulation of cytolytic T cells. Richard Phipps has developed systems for characterizing the growth and regulation of fibroblasts and inflammation in the healing process and in fibrosis in lung; he also is examining his hypothesis that prostoglandines are not only immuno-inhibitory agents, but are regulatory for normal and malignant B lymphocytes.

Robert Marquis, a microbiologist and physiologist, has focused his studies on oral pathogenic bacteria, characterizing the oxygen metabolism and the organisms' strategies to counter acid and oxidative damage. Tim Mosmann, director of the Center for Vaccine Biology and Immunology, is examining immune regulation by T cell subsets of CD4+, which induce different types of functions useful in combating pathogens in autoimmune disease and allergy. He also studies differentiation of TH1 and TH2 cells under regulation of cytokines, and mechanisms of selective repression during pregnancy to suppress immune reactions against the fetus.

Oral Biology

When the School of Medicine and Dentistry was established in 1925, it was anticipated that undergraduate dental students also would be enrolled. However, since even the strongest dental schools in the country at that time required only two years of undergraduate training, Rochester did not attract students with three years of preparation and an undergraduate program in dentistry was not established.

In 1929 the Rockefeller Foundation provided grants to the University of Rochester and to Yale University for fellowship programs for research and training in dentistry. At Rochester, fellows were appointed to medical school departments, where they carried out their research. Following the Rockefeller Foundation grant, the Markle and Carnegie Foundations provided additional funding.

In 1952, John Hein became chair of the newly-formed Department of Dentistry of the university. He was succeeded in 1955 by Erling Johansen, a researcher known for his electron microscopic studies of apatite crystals in tooth structure. In 1957, the department's scope was broadened and it was renamed the Department of Dentistry and Dental Research. In 1972, a separate Department of Dental Research was established and a Department of Clinical Dentistry set up.

Basil Bibby, one of the first Rockefeller Foundation fellows in 1930, made important contributions in terms of his studies of dental plaque and the role of fluoride in preventing cavities. Harold Hodge of the Department of Biochemistry, another of the Rockefeller fellows in dentistry, performed classical analyses of the chemical structure of teeth. With Stafford Warren, he used x-ray techniques to examine tooth structure, and he extended the work on fluoride as a highly effective preventative of caries.

William Bowen, the next chair of the Department of Dental Research, greatly broadened the department in terms of faculty and research programs, attracting major increases in federal funding for research and graduate education. (Bowen's contributions are described in detail in chapter three.) This highly productive department was further expanded by Lawrence Tabak, and in 1998 it became the Center for Oral Biology of the University of Rochester Medical Center. Tabak has contributed major new insights into the biochemistry of salivary gland mucins and other cell-surface glycoproteins, which are

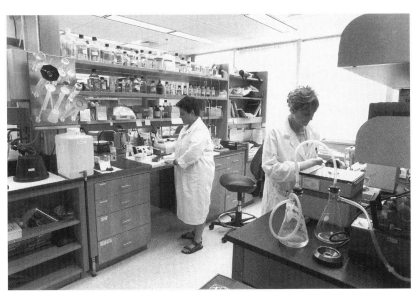

Laboratory in the Center for Oral Biology, in the Arthur Kornberg Medical Research Building; Anne Vacca Smith *(left), and* Kathleen Scott-Anne *(right)*

PAUL L. LaCELLE

important in cell-to-cell communication during development processes. He has discovered a family of enzymes, glycosyl transferases, that transfer N-acetylgalactosamine from sugar donor to peptides. Tabak's unique ability is exemplified by his talent in analyzing biochemical and structure-function studies with gene ablation to elucidate the importance of post-translational mucin modification in development biology.

Pathology

When Dean Whipple came to Rochester, the first completed element of the medical school building was a research building. This enabled him to continue the work he had underway at the University of California San Francisco. Thus, the first research in the new school took place in the Department of Pathology, which Dean Whipple chaired. A number of faculty investigators became interested in blood regeneration in anemic states, and their work was of utility in contributing to Dr. Whipple's studies. For example, Stafford Warren, who had been interested in the deleterious effects of radiation of various body tissues, contributed by his demonstration of x-ray–induced abnormalities in liver function.

Leon Miller subsequently established liver's role in producing many of the plasma proteins. Russell Holman and Earle Mahoney of Surgery demonstrated the positive effects of transfused plasma protein on metabolism; this early work stimulated much subsequent work in intravenous support of patients.

Utilizing the isotope iron 59 as a tracer, Paul Hahn and Whipple studied the role of iron in iron-deficient anemia; this work was made possible by instrumentation developed by William Bale of the Department of Radiology and by isotopes furnished from Ernest Lawrence's cyclotron at Berkeley. In 1935, a cyclotron was built at the University of Rochester and a number of isotopes, including sodium, potassium, and iron, became available for use in studies in the departments of Pathology and Physiology at the School of Medicine and Dentistry. Lee DuBridge, chair of Physics, required faculty members to handle and distribute the isotopes to the medical school for use in experimental protocols. This involvement

Dean Whipple—Up in Arms
The Medical School's involvement with the Manhattan District (the code name for work involved in making the first atomic bomb) began in February 1943 when, as the result of negotiations among the federal government, Dean Whipple, and University President Valentine, a top-secret research project was agreed on. The goal of the Rochester research was to determine the effect of radiation by uranium and other radioactive elements on humans. In addition, Rochester scientists were to assess the consequences of inhaling dust from isotopes containing ores and measure the toxicity of chemicals employed in processing the materials.

By September, a new building had been completed across Elmwood Avenue from the medical school. Faculty were at work and research apparatus was in place. So was a heavy military guard.

One evening, Dean Whipple strolled across the street to discuss a matter with a scientist. When the autocratic Whipple was challenged by a soldier with a gun, a military policeman who adamantly refused to permit the Dean's entry without requisite military credentials, Whipple returned to his office in a huff. Thus rebuffed, he never paid a second visit.

of faculty in River Campus-based departments with medical school faculty was extended even further during the war, when faculty from Physics, Chemistry, and Biology all worked with faculty in the School of Medicine and Dentistry.

Eric Schenck and A. El-Badawi characterized the autonomic innervation of arteries and of the genito-urinary system components. Jules Cohen and Schenck described the clinical and pathological features of human heart in chronic alcoholism.

J. Lowell Orbison, dean of the School of Medicine and Dentistry and director of the University of Rochester Medical Center, 1967–1980, extensively studied experimental malignant hypertension in the dog and examined factors which influenced it. In lathyrism (spastic paralysis) induced in rodents, Orbison and colleagues investigated impairment of the immune system and alteration of cartilage and elastic fiber development. In collaborative work with William Peck, then a medical student, estrogen and estrogen-like compounds were shown to reduce atherogenesis in cholesterol-fed cockerels.

Goetz Richter studied ferritin metabolism and its immunology in malignant disease processes, and Lowell Lapham, a neuropathologist, demonstrated the unique organization of cerebellar cortex in the development, organization, and maturation in the human fetus. Leon Wheeless, an engineer, worked with Stanley Patten (who succeeded Orbison as chair of Pathology) in developing automated equipment for cytopathology screening systems; this was particularly useful in studying cervical cells as prescreens for malignancy. More recently, Charles Sparks has examined the mechanisms of development of triglyceride-rich lipoprotein and apo B assembly, attempting to characterize a role for apo B in lipid transport and as a risk factor in coronary occlusion and in stroke.

Pharmacology

The Department of Pharmacology was established in 1958 with Harold Hodge as its first chair. Hodge's successor, Louis Lasagna, established a strong emphasis in clinical pharmacology. Subsequently, faculty from the Center for Brain Research were brought into the Department of Pharmacology, as well as into Physiology. Among these were Leo Abboud, who had investigated the characteristics and regulation of nicotinic receptors in brain, and Jean Bidlack, known for studies of the biochemistry of opioid receptors and molecular basis of neuropharmacology of opiates.

Robert Doty, recognized for pioneering work that demonstrated intercerebral communication in brain and who is a national leader in neuroscience, was appointed in Neurobiology and Anatomy.

Patricia Hinkle has examined the structure and function of pituitary receptors, particularly those important for thyrotropin-releasing hormone and the activation of G proteins and stimulation of phosphoinositide turnover with increase in cytoplasmic calcium and activation of protein kinase C.

Shey-Shing Sheu has examined receptor-mediated calcium dynamics in signaling processes in striatal neurons and in regulating contraction in cultured heart cells. Angelo Notides examined the estrogen receptor, particularly with respect to the physical chemistry of hormone receptor interactions.

Lawrence Raisz developed single-cell methods for assay of hormone effects on bone, particularly focusing on parathyroid hormone and thyrocalcitonin; he established the role of the latter as an inhibitor of bone resorption. Eugene Boyd and colleagues demonstrated the effect of convulsant drugs on electrical transmission through nuclei of the brain.

M. W. Anders, current chair of the department, has contributed to the understanding of biotransformation and the effects of toxic organic chemicals and their metabolites, and determined the bioactive and bioprotective pathways in cells. A particular interest has been the glutathione pathway for the bioactivation of nephrotoxic and nephrocarcinogenic halogenated alkenes, and also the metabolism of hydrochlorofluorocarbons.

Physiology

The Department of Physiology at the University of Rochester began in 1917 as the Department of Vital Economics, headed by John Murlin. When the medical school building was completed in 1925, Murlin and his staff moved to the School of Medicine and Dentistry; subsequently Vital Economics became part of the Department of Physiology. Wallace Fenn was appointed chair of Physiology; at age thirty-one, he was the youngest of the school's first chairs. Trained at Harvard University by Walter Cannon, Fenn had worked with Professor A.V. Hill in England and had established an important research field with his studies of oxygen consumption by nerve during stimulation. Fenn extended his work in muscle mechanics, and subsequently demonstrated for the first time the dynamics of potassium exchange in muscle during contraction.

Murlin continued his interest in the pancreas, studying pancreatic extracts. While examining carbohydrate metabolism in depancreatized animals, he recognized the existence of what later was described as insulin. In 1927, Murlin discovered another hormone, glucagon. Murlin's graduate student, Vincent DuVigneaud, elucidated the chemical structure of insulin and subsequently was awarded the Nobel Prize for isolation and synthesis of vasopressin and oxytocin. Later, Murlin and Charles Kochakian were the first to demonstrate the effect of androgens on protein and energy metabolism.

Edmund Nasset discovered a new intestinal enzyme, enterocrinin, which stimulated intestinal secretions. Newell Stannard first demonstrated quantitatively oxygen utilization in resting muscle. Harry Blair, a Princeton-trained physicist, established one of the first mathematical models to describe muscle mechanics.

Edward Adolph completed early studies of metabolism and distribution of water that became a basis for subsequent clinical manipulations of body fluids in various disorders. With the advent of World War II, Adolph extended his work in water metabolism to the body mechanisms important for water conservation; as war was anticipated in the North African Theatre, this work had timely applicability. At the same time, Hermann Rahn and Fenn extended their work in pulmonary function to examine the effects of hypoxia on high-altitude flight. Their analysis of the physiology of relative hypoxia was important not only for the aviators of World War II but subsequently as standards for NASA.

The advent of the availability of radioisotopes permitted examination of ion permeation in cells and tissues, and the Department of Physiology was one of the first in the country to make use of such isotopes. R. B. Dean, an associate of Dr. Fenn, demonstrated the movements of sodium across cell membranes by use of sodium 23 isotope. Dean coined the term "active transport," recognizing the energy requirement of such sodium movements. This work stimulated the initiation of studies worldwide to further characterize electrolyte movement in cells.

William Lotspeich succeeded Fenn as chair of Physiology; his work focused on the kidney's capacity to metabolize acid compounds using induced enzymes important to that metabolism. Julius Cohen demonstrated mechanisms whereby energy is conserved in the kidney by interconversion of a variety of substrate. Albert Craig, a pulmonary physiologist, investigated respiratory function during underwater swimming and demonstrated the potential for hypoxic loss of consciousness during such maneuvers.

Paul Horowitz, a muscle physiologist who trained with Professor

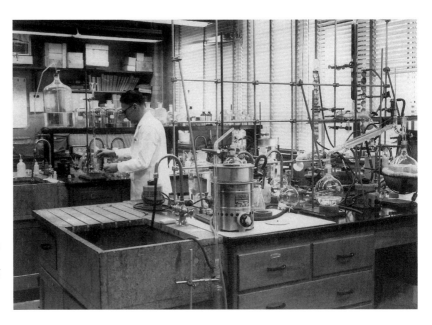

Research laboratory, 1956

PAUL L. LaCELLE

Hodgkin of Cambridge, succeeded Lotspeich as chair. His extensive studies of individual muscle fibers during active function and in the passive state contributed substantially to an understanding of muscle dynamics. His students and fellows have extended his novel work and have become prominent in the field of muscle physiology.

Carl Honig extended his interest in oxygen metabolism of cardiac muscle to collaborative studies with Thomas Gayeski in which oxygen utilization in individual cells was examined using novel microspectrophotometric methods developed by Gayeski. Honig later developed mathematical models to characterize oxygen flow from the hemoglobin of cells in the capillaries through tissue to myoglobin to active metabolism sites in muscle cells.

Ted Begenisich has examined the nature of ion channels in cardiac and neuronal cells from carcinoma and from squid axon. Trevor Shuttleworth has demonstrated the temporal relationship between calcium influxes in exocrine cells, and the intracellular calcium mobilization as a result of signaling pathways, which stimulate ion and fluid secretion. Camillo Peracchia has demonstrated a role for calcium and the compound connexin in gap junction and their role in cell-to-cell communication. Ingrid Sarelius has shown that contraction of single-muscle fibers under groups of capillaries initiates upstream arterial dilatation; this mechanism becomes a means to modulate the number of capillaries and enhance oxygen delivery. Peter Shrager has characterized the ion channels in myelinated axons during axonal development and in demyelinating disorders.

Richard Waugh, formerly of the Department of Biophysics, has interest in the viscoelastic properties essential for cell membrane integrity. He has developed novel techniques, such as pico-newton force transducer, to measure bending stiffness of model phospholipid membranes in normal states and when the membranes have been reconstructed from lipids and other structural elements. He has demonstrated the role of individual structural elements to the visco-elastic properties of such membranes. Waugh recently was appointed chair of the new Department of Biomedical Engineering at the University of Rochester.

Radiation Biology and Biophysics

In February 1943, the University of Rochester was asked by leaders of the U.S. Army's Manhattan District to become part of the activities leading up to the development of the atomic bomb. Rochester's role was to characterize the effects of radiation on various systems, to establish exposure parameters to protect workers preparing materials for atomic fission, and to develop instruments to define radiation in the workplace. Stafford Warren, chair of Radiology, was asked to direct the work at Rochester, since he had extensively studied the effects of x-radiation on human tissues. A facility was built in the summer of 1943 and a large number of faculty began studying inhalation of

The first mammogram, using radiological techniques refined at Rochester, was made in 1930 by Stafford Warren, first chair of the Department of Radiology. Not for another twenty or more years, however, would mammography become a widely-used diagnostic procedure.

Warren was one of the most successful researchers in the history of the School of Medicine and Dentistry, exploring ways to apply the use of radiology in diverse medical disciplines. He and colleagues in Surgery were among the first to employ dye-markers effectively, enabling him to examine diseased arteries using radiographic techniques.

particles in animals, toxic effects of chemicals used in uranium processing, and the effects of the isotopes themselves in animal models. Harold Hodge, a physical chemist from the Department of Biochemistry, led a division that examined the toxicology of the various agents. Hodge was involved in a broad range of studies, ranging from effects of fluoride in bone to toxicity of uranium; he subsequently produced a compendium on the pharmacology and toxicology of uranium compounds. With Marian Gleason and colleagues, Hodge published *Clinical Toxicology of Commercial Products;* this became the standard of information concerning commercial products of potential human toxicological import. In 1958, Hodge became the first chair of the Department of Pharmacology.

William and Margaret Neuman began work on localizing heavy elements in bone, particularly those isotopes important to the work of the Atomic Energy Project (as the Rochester portion of the Manhattan District was named). Subsequently, Neuman brought together a group of collaborators interested in the development, regulation, and metabolism of bone from the unique standpoint of the physical chemistry, as compared to conventional biochemical studies of calcium metabolism. He worked closely with dental researchers, in both research and teaching. Aser Rothstein, working with heavy metals, demonstrated that although heavy metal ions do not pass through a cell membrane, they may exert effects on the membrane's function, including regulation of glucose and ion transport. This established the key role of membrane-

---

Those are the breaks . . . that can influence a lab style!

Aser Rothstein, who co-chaired the Department of Radiation Biology and Biophysics in the '60s, became a leader in research graduate education at Rochester in the new department that developed during World War II, from the Atomic Energy Project. A chance accident early in his career, however, changed forever the way Rothstein conducted the research carried out in his own laboratory.

In studying yeast metabolism and utilization of potassium, the young scientist was required to use calibrated glass manometers, each attached to a closed flask, to determine the rate of oxygen utilization by a specific number of yeast cells. Each of the two-foot-long manometers required individual calibration—a long and tedious chore, since many of the delicate procedures were involved in the calibration process.

On one occasion, intent on securing the newly-calibrated manometers in an upright position, Rothstein stood them upright carefully in a partially opened lab bench drawer, using pressure from the drawer to hold them in place. At last, the laborious task was over. With a sigh of relief, the scientist turned away from the bench—and with an automatic gesture of completion, slammed the bench drawer shut. The sound of breaking glass manometers accompanied Rothstein's decision never, ever to do manual work in a laboratory again. (And, says his colleague Paul LaCelle, he never did.)

related enzymes in cell metabolism. Rothstein further used nonpenetrating compounds, including heavy metals, to dissect the various mechanisms for transport through cell membranes, studying yeast and blood cells.

In 1948 the Department of Radiation Biology was formed, its faculty including many—such as Hodge, Neuman, and Rothstein—who had been involved in the Atomic Energy Project. Henry Blair, formerly of the Department of Physiology and known for his mathematical characterization of the excitation process in muscle, was named the first chair of the new department. Subsequently, Neuman and Rothstein became leaders of the department, which in 1966 was renamed the Department of Radiation Biology and Biophysics.

William Bale, who had received his Ph.D. at Rochester in 1937 and who worked with Dr. George Whipple on the early utilization of iron 59 in the studies of anemia, also employed radioactive sodium as a means to trace metabolic processes. Bale used radioactive iodine tags on plasma proteins to localize radio isotopes immunologically to tumors, delivering radiation to malignant cells. Leon Miller, who also had worked with Dean Whipple, established techniques to perfuse animal livers, and by this technique established the liver as a site of protein synthesis. George Casarett contributed importantly to radiation biology by establishing that there is a threshold for low-dose radiation to induce pathological effects in tissues, a concept key to current understanding of induction of tumors.

Philip Chen and Taft Toribara developed a highly sensitive, widely used microanalytic method for phosphorous determination; their highly cited work

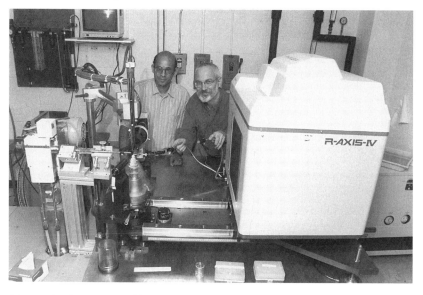

Macromolecular x-ray crystallography facility showing a high intensity x-ray source (left), crystal freezing device (center), and electronic image plate detector (right). The facility is directed by Professors Barry Goldstein *(right) and* Ravi Basavappa *(left).*

ACHIEVEMENTS IN THE BASIC BIOMEDICAL SCIENCES

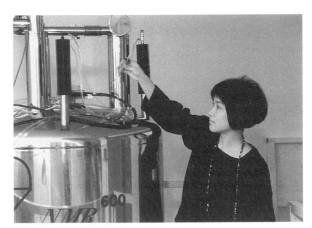

Nuclear magnetic resonance spectrometer for study of protein structure, 1998

was identified by *Analytical Chemistry* as one of the ten most important papers published 1950–1999. Gilbert Forbes with John Hursh established a whole-body scintillation counter to determine naturally occurring potassium 40 isotope in humans, thereby permitting estimates to be made of lean body mass and body fat. This pioneering facility, among the first of its kind in the country, is the last still functioning. Hursh and Alexander Dounce of the Department of Biochemistry pioneered biochemical assays to detect early effects of heavy metals on renal function, Dounce from the biochemistry standpoint, and Hursh from that of heavy metals. Thomas W. Clarkson, a postdoctoral fellow in the department in the 1950s, subsequently contributed to a broad range of research fields: transport across the gastrointestinal tract, renal function, and, importantly, to the epidemiology of alkyl mercury compounds in three major exposures to humans in Canada, Japan, and Iraq. These epidemiologic studies have been extended to the Seychelles Islands. They are pioneering classics in terms of experimental design and analysis. Robert Weed and co-workers, including Aser Rothstein, studied the ion transport in erythrocyte membranes and pioneered efforts to establish metabolic factors important to the visco-elastic properties of the membrane, as well as to the viscosity of whole blood.

George Kimmich developed a model for the sodium-dependent metabolic transport in epithelial cells from intestine, and Philip Knauf first used a nonpenetrating compound to characterize the transport of anions in cell membranes. Paul Morrow established theoretical and experimental models for the deposition of inhaled particles in humans and established one of the first environmental chambers in the United States for the careful study of human inhalation processes, including pathophysiology and clinical function. Gunter Oberdoerster has become a world leader in characterizing the effects of atmospheric particles, especially those from combustion, on inflammatory lung injury.

In 1996, the Department of Biophysics, successor to the Department of Radiation Biology and Biophysics, was disbanded and faculty assigned to other departments within the School of Medicine and Dentistry.

PAUL L. LaCelle

Arthur Kornberg Research Awards

Since 1997, the University of Rochester School of Medicine and Dentistry has conferred Arthur Kornberg Research Awards on outstanding senior faculty, on mid-career faculty in recognition of exceptional research contributions, and on young faculty who have demonstrated exceptional promise for significant work. The awards honor Nobel laureate Arthur Kornberg, M.D., a member of the School of Medicine and Dentistry Class of 1941, and now Professor of Biochemistry, Stanford University.

The following basic science faculty are Arthur Kornberg Research Award recipients:

- Robert A. Banibara, Ph.D., *Professor and Chair, Biochemistry and Biophysics*
- William H. Bowen, B.D.S., Ph.D., *Professor, Center for Oral Biology*
- Thomas W. Clarkson, Ph.D., *Professor, Environmental Medicine*
- Jeffrey D. Hayes, Ph.D., *Assistant Professor, Biochemistry*
- Patricia M. Hinkle, Ph.D., *Professor, Pharmacology and Physiology*
- Barbara H. Iglewski, Ph.D., *Professor and Chair, Microbiology and Immunology*
- Gary D. Paige, M.D., Ph.D., *Professor and Chair, Neurobiology and Anatomy*
- Richard P. Phipps, Ph.D., *Professor, Cancer Center, Microbiology Immunology*
- Fred Sherman, Ph.D., *Professor, Biochemistry and Biophysics*

In addition the following faculty from clinical departments are Arthur Kornberg Research Award recipients:

- Robert Ader, Ph.D., *Professor, Psychiatry*
- Leon G. Epstein, M.D., *Professor, Pediatrics, Neurology*
- Howard J. Federoff, M.D., Ph.D., *Professor Neurology, Director, Center for Aging and Development*
- Gilbert B. Forbes, M.D., *Professor, Pediatrics*
- Arthur J. Moss, M.D., *Professor, Medicine (Cardiology)*

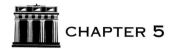 CHAPTER 5

Edward G. Miner Library: Print, Pillars, People, and Passwords

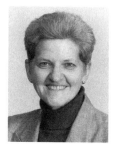

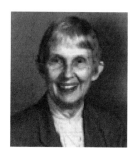

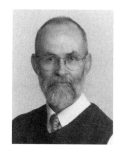

JULIA F.
SOLLENBERGER,
M.L.S.

LUCRETIA W.
McCLURE, M.A.

CHRISTOPHER
HOOLIHAN,
M.L.S.

In 1926, when George W. Corner, the medical school's Library committee chairman, sent his first report on the state of the Library to Edward G. Miner, chair of the University Trustees' Library Committee, he addressed one primary theme—the status of the collections. After describing in some detail the books and journals that had been brought together for use by the physicians and scholars of this new medical school, Corner finally mentioned that "the University Librarian . . . feels that the progress of the Library would be greatly helped if we had in charge of it a trained medical bibliographer. . . . The committee is of the opinion that such a librarian, if he can be found, will be necessary at some time in the future, whenever the library gets beyond the stage of a tool for daily work and begins to be a scholarly enterprise."

Seventy-five years later the Library is still a "tool for daily work," but it is now surely a "scholarly enterprise" as well. Located at the heart of the Medical Center complex, it holds a unique place in the institution—it is a shared resource, an agent of scholarly communication, a technology center, a focal point for learning and teaching, and for many, a place of welcome refuge on a busy day. The Library is also a group of talented information professionals with creative ideas and a track record of significant accomplishments. Many of the tools they use have moved from print to electronic, from static to dynamic. The Library is more than just a place to house print volumes—the "pillars" and the print. To the print and the pillars have been added people, and passwords.

The Library's early mission—to support teaching, research and patient care with recorded knowledge—remains its core purpose. The Library works with all affiliates of the Medical Center, including the faculty, staff, and students of Strong Memorial Hospital, the School of Nursing, and Eastman Dental Center, as well as the School of Medicine and Dentistry. The following mission is stated in the *Edward G. Miner Library Three Year Plan, March 1999*:

> To promote excellence in education, research, and patient care at the University of Rochester Medical Center and among its affiliates, the Edward G. Miner Library acquires, develops, manages, and delivers information resources and provides instruction and assistance in their use.

The Edward G. Miner Library does not have the largest collections of any medical library in the country, nor does it have the finest architecture, or most technology-rich innovations. The Library is recognized, however, for high-quality service; for collections of historical materials and rare books that rank among the best in the nation; for attractive use of vintage architectural details; for excellence in teaching of information management skills; for collaboration with community colleagues; for making wise decisions based upon solid data; and finally, for leadership in the profession of medical librarianship. While set in the context of an historical narrative, this chapter will emphasize these significant accomplishments.

Lucretia W. McClure *(photograph on previous page), sixth director of the Edward G. Miner Library, served the Library in a variety of positions from 1964 until her retirement in 1993. She came into the field when libraries functioned with manual operations, when being up-to-date and automated meant having photocopiers and electric typewriters.*

During her tenure the move from a manual environment to one of high technology occurred. The Miner Library had strong collections and an experienced and knowledgeable staff in the 1960s, making it well positioned to take advantage of the opportunities offered by automation.

Developments that occurred during these years included:

- *online database searching*
- *online cataloging system*
- Chester, *the University-wide online catalog*
- *online automatic routing for interlibrary loan*
- *learning center with public computing*

The major renovation and expansion that was completed in 1987 contributed to the Library's ability to provide computers for both staff and users, accommodate the continuing growth of the History of Medicine Section, and provide good study space. The next generation of technology will bring further changes and advances, and no doubt, some surprises.

The First Fifty Years

The beginning of the Edward G. Miner Library and its early growth is documented in "Crossroads: The Story of the Medical Library" in the anniversary volume *To Each His Farthest Star* (pp.145–161). The Library was designed to serve all segments of the Medical Center and the first requisite was to establish a collection of books and journals in medicine and science that would support educational, research, and clinical programs. From the opening in 1925 when there were some 17,000 volumes in place to 1975 when the count rose to 136,000, including a fine historical collection, the Library served as a center for learning and knowledge, a vital part of the work of the Medical Center.

But size of collections alone does not tell the story of a library. Changes were taking place in libraries with the advent of automation. In 1974, the Miner Library was the first medical library in New York State to install OCLC, an online computer system for cataloging books and journals. The Library was also one of the original members of the SUNY Biomedical Communication Network that offered computer searching of *Index Medicus.* The BCN was the first interactive online database in medicine, and Miner was one of nine libraries to introduce this service in 1968. It was nothing short of a revolution: the ability to retrieve citations from the medical literature using a combination of subjects. It was just the beginning of a sea change in library service.

From this time forward the Library continued to follow three avenues: select, catalog, and make available the best books, journals, and other resources; expand the use of computers in library applications as new technologies emerged; and maintain the high standard of services provided by the knowledgeable and enthusiastic staff. The Library provided an array of services: circulation of materials, reference assistance, database searching, photocopying, and interlibrary loan for all faculty, staff, and students in the Medical Center. In addition, the Library served health professionals in the medical community as well as the University of Rochester community. The Library participated in a number of national and regional organizations and consortia.

All of these contributed to the strength of the Miner Library, a strength that was necessary to meet the needs and changes that were ahead. New technologies, staff with new kinds of skills, new services, and budget constraints were all to come in the years ahead, making an interesting quarter century, from 1975–2000.

RESOURCES AND SERVICES:
FROM PRINT TO ELECTRONIC

The trend of the past twenty-five years in regard to medical library resources and services is, indeed, PRINT to ELECTRONIC. In 1975 the print version of *Index Medicus,* the premier index in the biomedical sciences, was still a major resource for those searching for articles of interest on a particular medical topic. As of January 2000, the Library no longer receives the print version of *Index Medicus; Medline,* its greatly expanded electronic equivalent, is now freely searchable via the Internet and is the ubiquitous source of biomedical information worldwide.

Online catalogs have now replaced the card catalog. A growing number of full-text journal articles and reference books are available at the desktops of faculty and students. The range of electronic equivalents and enhancements to print is great indeed. New multimedia formats (streaming video, audio, digital images, and interactive web-based instructional materials) support the information needs of health professionals and students.

Print Collections and "Traditional" Services

The years from 1975 to the present have seen changes in both the acquisition of materials and how they are used. From its beginning in 1925, when 239 journal titles were on the shelves, until the present, with 1,671 print and 366 electronic titles available, the number of journals acquired has not been a steady upward growth. Many factors have forced libraries to study their collections in terms of use and value and make difficult decisions because of budget constraints.

With the launching of Sputnik in 1957, the nation acknowledged its failure to be first in space with a great influx of money into science and medicine. Responding to an enormous growth in the number of scientists and the rapid increase in the number of publications, libraries bought more materials. Funding from both the government and the institutions fostered this growth. The Miner Library benefited from two grants provided through the Medical Library Assistance Act.

By the mid-1970s the economic scene had changed. High inflation had devastating effects upon libraries, as did the increasing cost of periodicals. A study by the Ebsco Subscription Services showed that in 1992 the cost of 2,352 titles listed in *Index Medicus* cost $660,772, an increase of 58% over the cost of the same titles in 1988. By 1993, journals in an academic library, that had cost $656,217 in 1989, cost $1,012,699. Many libraries were forced to cut journal expenditures by hundreds of thousands of dollars. The Miner Library began annual reviews of its journal collection. Journals in foreign languages, those of peripheral subject content, and those with little use were targeted for cancellation. Since 1994 the Miner Library has been tracking journal use through a quarterly reshelving count. Using this utilization data, as well as citation analysis, the Library and the faculty have worked together to make the difficult decisions necessitated by financial constraints. During the period of 1994–97 over 300 titles were cancelled.

Librarians have found creative ways to provide both print and electronic resources since the financial "crunch" began. Many book budgets were cut to support journals. Major reference tools, available online, were discontinued in print form. Cooperative buying with the libraries on River Campus, of particularly expensive journals and databases, has helped.

Many libraries turned to interlibrary borrowing to provide access to journal articles they did not own. Miner Library is an active member of the Rochester Regional Library Council, an agency that encourages sharing of resources in the five-county area surrounding Rochester. The use of automated interlibrary loan services such as DOCLINE and OCLC (an international online catalog with library holdings and an interlibrary loan module) makes access to hundreds of libraries possible. The photocopier, fax machine, and Internet have transformed the library-to-library document sharing service. In addition to borrowing items for Miner Library users, the Library has also been a major lender. In 1974/75, the Library filled 9,336 requests but borrowed only 2,808 items from other libraries. In 1998/99 the Library loaned 10,500 items and borrowed 8,136.

Libraries must adapt to changes in medicine and science, to the evolving developments of the Medical Center. The Miner Library has not simply collected and held titles to build numbers. The Library responded to new areas in brain research, molecular biology, and nuclear medicine, as well as the addition of a doctoral program in nursing. The Library will continue to adapt to new programs in teaching and in new areas of research. Providing the best journals, books, databases, etc., in all formats, will continue to be the standard.

Managing the Collection with Automation

Since the arrival of computers in the 1960s, change in library practice has been rapid and often dazzling. Until that time, libraries had functioned in a manual mode, cataloging for internal use only, typing and mailing interlibrary loan requests, and preparing bibliographies by reading the literature. This time-consuming work brought rewards to the librarians; they became knowledgeable about medical literature and experts in using the bibliographies and abstracts. Just when the burgeoning medical literature seemed ready to engulf the library, the computer came along and library applications soon followed.

Miner Library quickly adopted automated services to help manage the collections and began cataloging online with the OCLC system in 1974. Automated cataloging provided catalog records in machine-readable form, a necessary step for building an online catalog. For the first time, it was possible to see records of libraries across the nation and beyond.

The next move toward an online catalog came in 1984 when the University of Rochester began developing a university-wide catalog with Geac

Computer International. With some two million records in the university libraries, the Geac System had to accommodate not only a large collection, but one of great variety and on four different campuses. For example, the Miner Library uses the National Library of Medicine classification scheme for books; the other libraries use the Library of Congress. An enormous staff effort was required in preparing for the online catalog.

While the Miner Library records from after 1974 were in machine-readable form, the records from earlier years had to be converted. The Library was fortunate to receive several New York State grants through the Rochester Regional Library Council for conversion of these records. By 1987 some 800,000 records from all of the libraries were available in "Chester," the university's first online catalog. Plans were underway to utilize the Geac system for an acquisitions module and automated circulation began in 1988.

By 1992, with all its records in Chester, the Library closed the card catalog. The dismantling of the card catalog in 1994 signaled the end of an era; automated services had become the standard.

Though the Geac System served the university libraries for well over a decade, the need for greater capabilities and state-of-the-art systems architecture required the university libraries to seek a replacement. In the fall and winter of 1996/97 the libraries implemented Voyager, a new client-server system with both a Web and Windows-based online catalog, as well as a serials management module. The University of Rochester was the first large research library to implement Voyager, and it soon became clear that enhancements were needed, especially in the acquisitions/serials module. The Library worked with the company to define requirements and test enhancements. Contributions made by UR libraries staff helped bring Voyager to the forefront of integrated library systems by the late 1990s.

Interlibrary Loan: Sharing Collections

Electronic applications improved many of the services provided by the Library. With the online catalog, the collections of all University of Rochester libraries could be searched without trudging across to another campus. In addition, OCLC made the holdings of thousands of other libraries known, giving the Library many avenues for borrowing and lending books.

In the mid-1960s, the Miner Library had a practice, thought very sophisticated at the time, of automatically forwarding interlibrary loan requests. When a request from the Library was sent, by mail, to another library, several additional mailing labels were enclosed so that the request could be forwarded until it was filled. This would be considered clumsy today, but it is exactly the model of the many automatic routing systems in practice now. For example, OCLC developed an interlibrary lending module with automatic forwarding. The National Library of Medicine created DOCLINE, an online routing system for medical libraries in 1987.

JULIA F. SOLLENBERGER, LUCRETIA W. MCCLURE, CHRISTOPHER HOOLIHAN

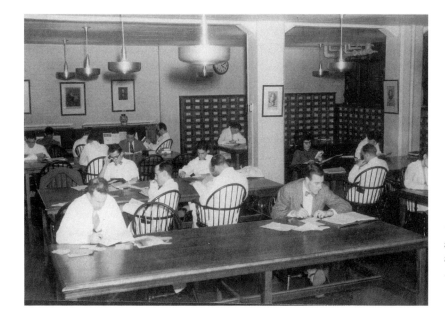

"Readers"
using print
resources,
1950

Reference and Database Search Services

Perhaps the most compelling change in library service came with the development of the computer database. Searching the literature was an important function for both librarians and users. The staff spent much time instructing users in ways to search the indexes, as well as pointing out the differences between a subject source and a cited-reference source.

Librarians often chose to be reference librarians in order to have the opportunity to read the rich and interesting literature while compiling bibliographies. That this is no longer essential is one of the casualties of automation. When the SUNY Biomedical Communication Network (BCN) came online in October 1968, it was the end of the library as we had known it—the BCN changed the way libraries served users and the way librarians practiced their art.

The BCN was the first interactive, online database for the field of medicine. At first, the system was cumbersome and slow. There were only a limited number of *Index Medicus* citations to search, and no instruction manuals for librarians. But as one of the original nine libraries to come online with the BCN, the Miner Library staff was ready to participate. To be able to enter a combination of subjects and let the machine do the searching was nothing short of astonishing. In the manual world, compiling a dozen bibliographies a month by reading the articles to determine relevance was an achievement. With the computer, one could produce twelve a day and more.

The BCN was created by Irwin Pizer, librarian at the SUNY Upstate Medical Library. His plan was to develop a complete reference service. The database would include *Index Medicus,* indexed chapters of books, and an

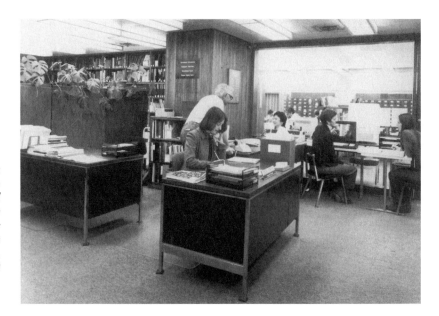

interlibrary loan module for acquiring copies not owned by the Library. (The last two items have been achieved in other ways.) His design also allowed for searching by the library's users, long before end-user searching became the mode it is today. Faculty and students at URMC were invited to reserve time to do a literature search. While many individuals enjoyed the experience, it became evident that librarians could do it better and faster, and the practice was ended.

The database grew, and many other indexes, such as *Psychological Abstracts* and *Biological Abstracts* were added. The Library staff joined BCN user groups, participated in training sessions at regional and national meetings, and developed training manuals to help teach users. Being experts in database searching gave a new dimension to the role of the librarian. The Library continued to provide online search services through various successor systems to the BCN.

All of these computer applications contributed to a new kind of library, one that could be accessed from outside of its walls.

Self-Service Searching

In 1984 the Library procured its first personal computer, to be used for interlibrary loan transactions and database searching. Prior to this time literature searching was accomplished on "dumb" terminals connected through phone lines and by acoustic couplers to remote mainframes; interlibrary loan was done on a TWX teletype terminal. Printer speeds ranged from ten to a whopping thirty characters per second! With the advent of personal computers, online literature searching could be performed by the users themselves.

Faculty, staff, and students began to have PC's on their desks, and some wanted the convenience and speed of searching *Medline* and other databases themselves.

The role of reference librarians, long considered the major link between the user's need for information and the information itself, was changing. By the mid-'80s, users became more sophisticated in their information requirements and PCs were used for personal information retrieval and management. In response to this shift, the Information Services librarians at Miner began, in 1985, to integrate more user education and end user search support into their programs and services. In 1984/85, BRS Colleague, an end-user version of the search interface that Miner's reference librarians were using for mediated searching, was made available to individual subscribers by the vendor and eventually through a library-managed account. The BRS Colleague Group Account began with 13 members in April 1986 and swelled to 79 in 1989/90. In 1986/87 the first training of end-users took place; Miner librarians taught 14 medical students to do their own bibliographic searching, at a designated workstation in the Library; that year they completed 70 searches, using twenty-one hours of online time. Late in 1987 the Library also began to teach searching using PaperChase, a menu-driven version of *Medline* that offered half-price online access for medical students, residents, and fellows.

In 1987, all searchers, librarians, and end users were paying for database access by the minute, with some discounts applied for library-administered group billing. End users always knew the clock was ticking! Miner Library developed end-user search training to teach users to become efficient and effective searchers and to keep the cost of searching to a minimum. In the spring of 1988 a critical event occurred that transformed literature searching. Instead of searching via phone lines and paying for online time, databases could be purchased by subscription and mounted locally. A segment of the database was stored on a compact disk and accessed through a CD-ROM drive, with search software contained on the hard disk of the workstation. With the Library paying one subscription price, library users had unlimited access to the CD-ROM database on several in-library workstations equipped to provide direct access to *Medline*.

Directed by Julia Sollenberger, head of Information and Access Services, and Kathryn Nesbit, reference librarian, the Library in 1988/89 participated in a three-month evaluation project sponsored by the National Library of Medicine. Miner was chosen as one of nineteen libraries across the country to receive the hardware and software necessary to run one of the *Medline* CD-ROM products. Users could sign up to search the system at no charge. The overwhelmingly positive response provided justification for the Library to order Compact Med-Base, a CD-ROM *Medline* system which would lead the user through the search process step-by-step and map free text terms to Medical Subject Headings; this was the very first iteration of the Ovid search system, which is still in use at Miner Library in 2000.

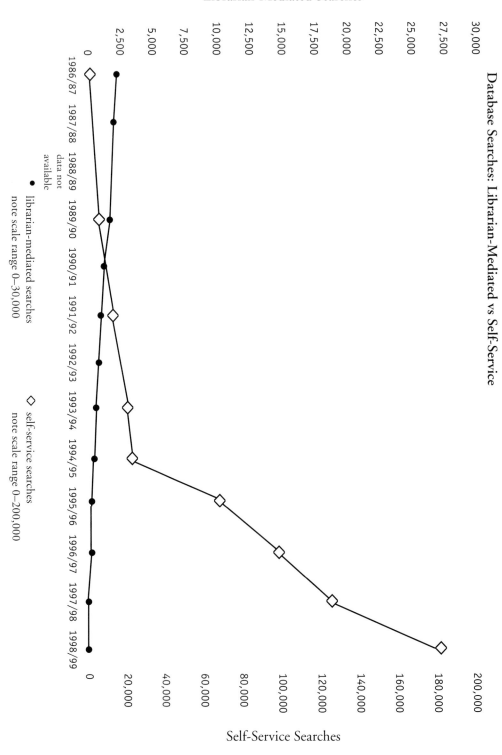

Database Searches: Librarian-Mediated vs Self-Service

Librarian-Mediated Searches

Self-Service Searches

- data not available

● librarian-mediated searches
  note scale range 0–30,000

◇ self-service searches
  note scale range 0–200,000

In 1989 three CD-ROM workstations were available for *Medline* searching in the Library, and an estimated 225 self-service searches were performed by end-users each month. The number of librarian-mediated searches declined sharply. In 1989/90 reference librarians performed 36% fewer computer literature searches than the previous year, while the number of self-service searching sessions doubled. This explosion in self-service searching can be traced to the ubiquitous nature of personal computers. The explosion was fueled by the appearance of local and wide-area networks in the late '80s and early '90s. In 1990 after-hours remote access to CD-ROM *Medline* workstations became available over telephone data lines. In 1991, a network version of the CD-ROM *Medline* product, then in use at Miner, was installed. The "Miner Network" provided multiuser in-library access and limited twenty-four hour remote access to four biomedical literature databases.

The next few years marked an increase in self-service searching, both in the Library and from remote locations. The number of self-service searches grew from 8,750 in 1990/91 to 18,356 in 1994/95. In that year the Internet was just coming into view; "gopher" and "Mosaic" were creeping into the vocabularies of the computer literate. By 1995/96, however, the world was beginning to change. Netscape had become a freely-available web browser and many in the workplace and at home were accessing information via the Internet. In 1996, the "Miner Network" was replaced with a Unix-based system that provided faster response time, improved remote searching, greater availability of a graphical user interface, and, most important of all, a Web Gateway. Searches could be done with an Internet connection and a web browser, without the need to download and configure a software client for the user's local PC. End-user searching grew more than three-fold in one year and has been growing by leaps and bounds ever since. In 1998/99 there were 167,410 computer literature searches performed on more than twenty different databases on the Ovid system alone.

The Internet and the Web: First a Tool, then a Service

The Internet has indeed changed the course of information access and management. For the first time in 1992/93 Miner Library staff members had access to the Internet from their desktop workstations. In the 1993/94 annual report a stated goal of the Reference/Information Services Department was to "enhance reference staff's knowledge of the Internet and begin to use appropriate Internet resources in providing reference assistance to patrons." Figures in the Library's 1996/97 annual report show a one-year increase of 29% in the use of the Internet for answering reference questions, and a 19% decline in reference librarians' use of print material.

The web also became a tool for providing information about the Library to clients. In 1994 the first Miner Library home page was built by Director

Valerie Florance on a server in the Department of Environmental Medicine. Early users of the web shared their expertise and their hardware and software, and in the Medical Center they worked together to create a partial web presence for various aspects of the institution.

An Internet Services department in the Library was established in 1995 and web development was expanded. Miner Library staff were known to be knowledgeable and helpful, and web development projects began to trickle in. A web "front door" for the whole Medical Center was created, and in 1996 the Library purchased a web server to be the "official" home of the Medical Center's web presence.

Now individual departmental web authors could request accounts on the server and work with Library staff to create web pages. During 1996/97, fifty-seven web projects were added to the URMC site. Projects ranged from single page announcements of upcoming seminars to multi-page developments representing a whole new departmental presence. The Library also began to explore new opportunities for using web capabilities in School of Medicine and School of Nursing courses. "Course pages" for one School of Nursing course and two School of Medicine courses were developed.

Since 1997 the role of the Edward G. Miner Library has evolved to be the primary provider of education and research-related web services and systems for the Medical Center. The Library's Head of Web Services is the URMC Webmaster, who is responsible for both the technology and the development services provided for non-clinical activities. In the summer of 1999, Library staff redesigned the web site and published the URMC Web Standards and Guidelines. This was the first step toward a unified web presence for the Medical Center.

The Library is represented on the Strong Health Web Steering Committee, working with consultants to build a strong web presence for clinical activities and programs. In addition, Miner staff has a leadership role in developing and providing web and computer-based instructional materials for students. Increased interactivity and multimedia formats are developing in the education arena, as well as in research and patient care.

Full-text Resources: The Digital Library

The move to full-text electronic resources began with access to a limited number of full-text journals on BRS Colleague in the late '80s. Use was low, interest small, and online cost high. In 1992/93 the Library offered single, in-library workstation access to the full-text equivalent of the textbook *Scientific American Medicine* on CD-ROM. During the next two years Miner's Computing and Network Services staff developed several ever-improving methods for networking a growing number of CD-ROM-based full-text electronic resources. The Library also offered the *New England Journal of Medicine* as the first full-text journal to be linked directly from a *Medline* citation; an entire

Julia F. Sollenberger, Lucretia W. McClure, Christopher Hoolihan

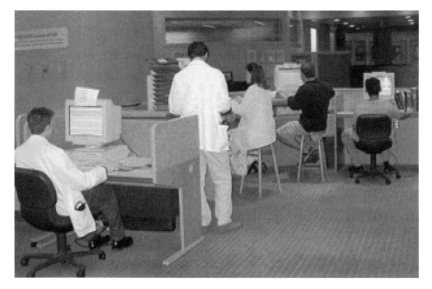

In the year 2000, students, faculty, and staff search for information in the Digital Library and on the Internet

article was just a click away from the online reference during the database searching process.

In November 1996 the Library began to provide quick and easy remote access to Miner's growing collection of electronic resources. A web-based menu offered integrated access to all its databases, as well as full-text resources (on CD-ROM or on the Internet), from desktop computers within the Medical Center or from home or office. The Library had entered into a two-year agreement with the Department of Anesthesiology to share access to a new technology product (Citrix Winframe) that would open a Windows application from a user's web browser, even from a remote location. This integrated menu was dubbed the "Miner Digital Library" and was recognized nationwide as the first application of Winframe technology in a medical library environment.

The Miner Digital Library has been transformed several times in its short five year existence. The initial version included nine online book resources as well as the Ovid databases; there are now more than 350 full-text journals, 30 databases, and 50 online reference books. The interface was updated in 1999. In the year 2000 the Library is offering a new version that can be customized by individuals to become "my digital library."

INFORMATION MANAGEMENT EDUCATION: FOSTERING UNDERSTANDING AND INDEPENDENCE

From the earliest days, librarians have helped users to become independent learners. Traditional "bibliographic instruction" started with a library book truck laden with carefully chosen reference books, wheeled into a classroom and presented in a show-and-tell format. Learners became familiar (if not by title, then by sight) with the materials considered to be key resources for answering their questions. The orientation tour—a walk through the Library with a knowledgeable guide—was, and still is, a core method of instruction.

Health professionals throughout the years have had, however, increasingly more knowledge to assimilate. Tools to access the literature have become diverse and technology-based, and the "lifelong learner" now needs a whole cadre of skills in information seeking and evaluation. Information management education has evolved to be a primary role for librarians.

Self-service searching marked the beginning of a sea change in library-based instruction. In 1985 the Library offered its first "course" to fourteen medical and graduate students—"Computer Searching: Finding Information the Easy Way." With funds from New York State's Hospital Library Service Program, Julia Sollenberger, head of Information and Access Services, and Kathryn Nesbit, reference librarian, collaborated with Bernie Todd Smith, director of the Werner Health Sciences Library at Rochester General Hospital, to develop a curriculum that could be adapted to different user groups. The twenty-hour elective was conducted in a hands-on mode that reinforced each specific retrieval skill. The curriculum was sold in notebook format to medical librarians across the country and used as a model for similar training programs. Nuggets of the original curriculum are still used to train health professionals to retrieve information on *Medline.*

From 1986 to 1989 the course was shortened to a nine-hour evening class offered to practicing health professionals as well as students. Physicians and nurses trained in the intricacies of MeSH (Medical Subject Headings) and the indexing process became the initial members of the Library's BRS Colleague End User Search Service group account.

Over the next few years the *Medline* training course became shorter, as the sophistication of the search software increased. Automatic mapping of the users' keywords to the terms used by indexers was the single enhancement that most reduced the end users' need for in-depth knowledge of the controlled vocabulary. Command language searching gave way to the graphical user interface with step-by-step prompts for user input. As search systems improved, the need for in-depth training was reduced; by 1992 the *Medline* class had become a one-hour demonstration. With the leadership of Valerie Florance, library director from 1993–1998, the education program at Miner returned to its former hands-on format. Seeing is NOT the same as doing; the quality of searches could suffer if no search exercises were completed in class.

The Library's education program expanded significantly with the advent of the Internet. From Gopher and Lynx classes in 1994 to courses like Internet Basics, Internet Searching, HTML, Molecular Biology Resources, and Electronic Drug Resources in the year 2000, the Library has remained the single best source of instruction in information management for Medical Center students, faculty, and staff.

All reference librarians now participate in the Library's teaching programs. Regularly scheduled courses, as well as "custom" classes targeted to a particular audience, are offered for all affiliates of the Medical Center. Educating our clientele has become one of the highest priorities of the Library; we know that skill in acquiring and using knowledge is a key to success in any health professional's career.

Instruction in the Curriculum

The Library's role in teaching information management skills to students as part of the formal curriculum has changed significantly. For years a "bibliographic instruction" session was provided to students at the invitation of particular faculty members. Beginning in 1985 the Library offered the *Medline* searching course as an elective to medical students. From 1987 to the early '90s library staff participated in the "Introduction to Medical Informatics" course given to all third year medical students. A lecture on the principles of searching *Medline* using PaperChase, a menu-driven search system, was followed by a supervised individual hands-on practice session. In the School of Nursing graduate students taking the Research courses received instruction in information retrieval, with an emphasis on searching the CINAHL nursing database.

In 1995 a hands-on training session covering *Medline* and the student email system was offered during orientation for first year medical students. As part of the physiology course, a computer-based competency requirement was implemented for first year students, with a mandatory, graded homework exercise on searching *Medline*. The following year an exercise requiring the use of Internet resources was assigned to all second year pathology students. The idea of "information competencies" was taking hold, and the teaching of information retrieval skills was becoming more pervasive in the curricula of both the School of Medicine and the School of Nursing. Its inclusion in the curriculum, however, was still dependent upon individual faculty members' willingness and desire to include it.

The new Double Helix curriculum in the School of Medicine has recently changed all that. Launching the new problem-based curriculum is the "Mastering Medical Information" course (first taught in August and September 1999). All of the one-hundred first year students take the course, designed by a team of librarians and medical faculty to integrate the topics of biostatistics, epidemiology, evidence-based medicine, and medical informatics. Learning objectives include: retrieving information from databases and the world-wide-web using effective search strategies; filtering information for quality and relevance; and finding evidence-based answers to clinical questions.

Eight hands-on informatics labs, each directed by pairs of library staff members, provide a skill-building environment that is reinforced with homework exercises and a take-home exam. To prove their competency, students

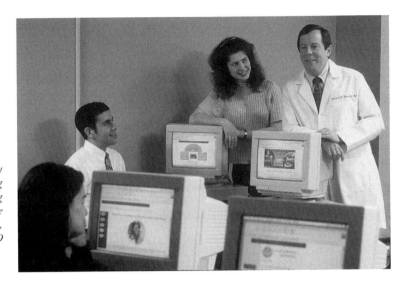

must demonstrate a minimum level of skill in developing an effective *Medline* search strategy. This initial exposure to information management skills is reinforced in two additional exercises during the first year, and at least one during the second year of medical school. By exposing students to information skills both early and often, we encourage students to become lifelong learners.

The Library's full participation in developing the Mastering Medical Information course as the first course in the undergraduate curriculum is unique in medical education. It serves as a model of collaboration and emphasizes that student mastery of information management skills and evidence-based medicine principles is critical to success in a problem-based learning environment.

In the School of Nursing, necessary information competencies for master's students have been identified and included in the objectives of particular courses. The inclusion of these objectives is an integral part of the course content, consistent from year to year and from instructor to instructor.

TECHNOLOGY AND THE INTEGRATED INFORMATION ENVIRONMENT

Public and Instructional Computing

For more than thirty years the Library has been using technology to manage its collection and to provide knowledge resources to its users. In the mid-1990s the Library also began to provide technological services. The newly-created Learning Center (see renovation section, p. 174) provided computer workstations for students, faculty, and staff so that they can access the Library's resources, as well as utilize a myriad of "personal productivity" software—for word processing, data analysis, and graphics creation and manipulation. In 1988 the Learning Center housed fewer than twenty workstations; average monthly use of the facility was less than 200. Ten years later use of the Learning Center's forty PC and Macintosh computers had climbed to 1,200 per month.

The Library expanded its technology services in 1997 when the Division of Medical Informatics decided to shift its focus to research and development, rather than provision of services. The Library took on the following responsibilities: the student email service; maintenance and upkeep of medical student computing labs (including computers in the new problem-based-learning rooms); support of computer-assisted instructional software; and collaborative development, with faculty, of web-based and multimedia educational modules. Students have come to rely on the Library's Information Systems staff, including student assistants at the Learning Center Help Desk, for a wide variety of technical assistance.

Integration of Information Systems and Services at the Medical Center

In the past half decade the Edward G. Miner Library has taken its place as a technology leader at the Medical Center. Library staff have been at the forefront as integration of information systems and enhanced communication about technology-related projects have benefited all faculty, staff, and students. Valerie Florance served as co-principal investigator for a two-year IAIMS (Integrated Advanced Information Management Systems) planning grant, awarded to the Medical Center by the National Library of Medicine in September of 1994. The Library created an IAIMS project office, which became the center for this institution-wide effort.

The IAIMS planning grant created an opportunity to develop a plan for an all-inclusive, integrated information environment that advanced the clinical, research, administrative, and educational missions of the Medical Center. Planning committee reports were written and synthesized, and a master plan evolved. Recommendations ranged from enhancing the network infrastructure, to teaching information competencies in the curricula, to developing policies on information security, confidentiality, ownership, and access. The stage was set for becoming a technology-rich institution that uses information when and where it is needed, in the format required, to facilitate work and study. The Library was, and still is, a leader in this integrated information environment.

In 1997 Miner Library joined all Rochester-area hospitals and the Eastman Dental Center Library in a project called MIRACLEnet (Medical Information Retrievable At Computers Located Everywhere). With Julia Sollenberger leading the effort, libraries pooled their resources, increased their buying power, and moved forward through an increasingly competitive healthcare environment to facilitate access to knowledge-based information for all. Miner Library continues to serve as host institution for the systems and services that are provided through this collaborative project.

FACILITIES AND RENOVATION

When the new School of Medicine and Dentistry and Strong Memorial Hospital were planned, the founding dean, George Hoyt Whipple, M.D., recognized that the Library should serve the entire facility and he placed it in the center of the building. The original Library was 11,095 sq.ft., designed to hold some 100,000 volumes. The space was doubled to 26,607 sq.ft. in an expansion completed in 1962, with room to hold a collection that would

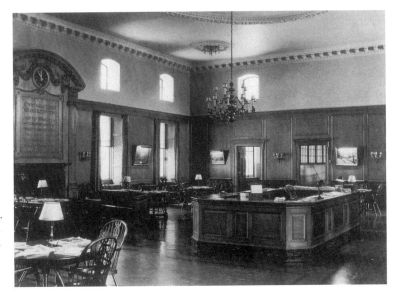

Original lobby of Strong Memorial Hospital, 1926

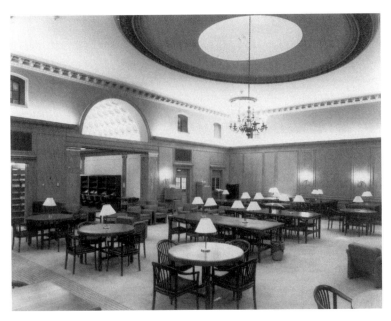

Renovated lobby becomes Library Reading Room, 1987

JULIA F. SOLLENBERGER, LUCRETIA W. MCCLURE, CHRISTOPHER HOOLIHAN

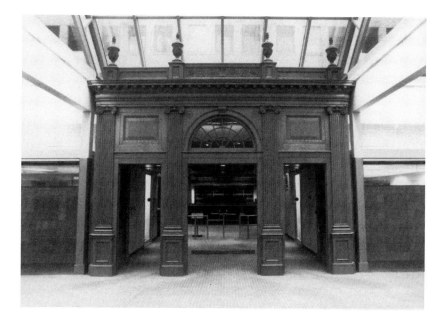

Original hospital entrance portal now graces Library entrance

grow over the next ten years. By the mid-1980s, the Library was in critical need of additional space. While the Library ranked in the top quarter of medical school libraries in terms of volumes and services, it ranked 89th of 132 medical libraries in terms of space.

The Medical Center administration acknowledged that providing adequate space for the Library was a high priority, and planning began under the leadership of Lucretia McClure, Library director. The only unused area adjacent to the Library was the lobby of the original hospital, left vacant when the new Strong Memorial Hospital was built in 1975, and the only beautiful room approved by Dr. Whipple for the hospital. Its oak paneling, handsomely carved wood portals, and molded ceiling had welcomed patients and their families for nearly fifty years. What a fine reading room it would make!

In 1985 the university and Dean Robert J. Joynt approved the $3.1 million plan designed by the Rochester firm, Kaelber, Meyer, Miller and Ungar. Funds were secured through loans from the New York State Dormitory Authority and from donors, including alumni and faculty, local and national foundations, and a number of long-time university supporters. Construction began in March 1986 and was completed in May 1987. The renovation brought the Library to nearly 39,000 sq.ft. The new space provided a quiet, elegant reading room and study area with seats for one hundred readers; a new stack area with independent study carrels; a Learning Center and microcomputer room; an archives room; good office space and working areas for the staff; and an improved environment with new heating/air conditioning/ventilation systems. Formal dedication of the new Library was held October 6, 1987.

In the thirteen years since the renovation, several smaller facility enhancements have taken place. Two computer classrooms have been outfitted for hands-on instruction. Changes in our computing environment required adaptations in the physical facilities that now house and support the new technology, and in 1998 the Learning Center was redesigned and renovated.

OUTREACH: BEYOND OUR WALLS

Changes in health care and in health education in the last decade have extended the reach of the Medical Center beyond the physical facility. The Library serves affiliated community practices, as well as the institutions that comprise Strong Health and the Upstate Health Partners. Document delivery is provided, on a fee basis, to two rural hospitals, Jones Memorial and St. James Mercy, as well as Highland Hospital and the Visiting Nurse Service.

In 1997 the Eastman Dental Center (EDC) was affiliated with the University of Rochester to become one of the entities of the Medical Center. The EDC's Basil G. Bibby Library became a branch of the Miner Library in 1998. With the retirement of June Glaser, director of the Bibby Library, Christine DeGolyer was hired to become the medicine and dentistry outreach librarian. DeGolyer is also project coordinator for a two-year contract awarded to the Miner Library by the National Network of Libraries of Medicine to provide training and other information services to the professionals who work in the public health departments of Monroe and surrounding counties.

HISTORICAL COLLECTIONS AND SERVICES

In a 1926 report on the Library prepared by George Corner for Edward G. Miner, chair of the University Trustees' Library Committee, Corner described the acquisition of classic texts in the history of medicine. "The field is very large," he wrote, "the books expensive, and much bibliographic skill is required if mistakes are to be avoided. Opinions differ as to the extent to which it is advisable to put money into books, which cannot be considered essential to the modern worker. The Committee has felt it a duty to plan at least a modest collection of historical books sufficient to illustrate teaching in the history of medicine." No one in Rochester was better qualified to direct the formation of such a collection. A 1913 graduate of Johns Hopkins School of Medicine, Corner had absorbed the sense of historical tradition epitomized at Hopkins by the figure of William Osler, and had spent the year prior to the opening of the School of Medicine in London working on a history of early medieval anatomy.

Although several hundred books had already been acquired for the historical collection, Corner realized that he would need resources from outside the university to acquire the "thousands of volumes" that he felt would constitute a good medical historical collection. Through his friendship with the elderly Edward Wright Mulligan, chief of Surgery at Rochester General Hospital and George Eastman's personal physician, the Library received gifts of $5,000 per annum in 1926, 1927, and 1928 to acquire rare medical books. Mulligan's gift gave Corner access to a fund that would be the equivalent of $147,000 today. Between 1925 and 1939, Corner purchased some 1,200 classic titles in the history of medicine, laying the foundations of what currently constitutes one of the finest rare medical book collections in the nation. In 1939, Corner left to become chair of the Department of Embryology at the Carnegie Institute, and with his departure there was no one on the faculty with the interest, expertise or funding to continue development of an historical collection. As a result, additions to the rare book collection were few and sporadic, and it was largely neglected over the next twenty-five years.

In 1964, another fund was established in the Medical Library for the purchase of rare books. The establishment of the Walter Wile Hamburger Memorial Fund signaled a revival of interest in the history of medicine at the School of Medicine and Dentistry. In 1965, the Library Committee, chaired by Librarian Stanley Truelson, recommended to the school's advisory board the appointment of "a faculty member possessing considerable enthusiasm and ability in teaching medical history." The committee also recommended funding for the continued acquisition of rare books and for a salaried history of medicine librarian to organize and develop the collection. In October 1965, the first History of Medicine Librarian was appointed to the professional staff.

Although a formal academic program in medical history never materialized, gifts of sizeable historical collections were made to the Miner Library by the Rochester Academy of Medicine (1969), from the library of Henry Foster (1821–1891) by the Clifton Springs Hospital (1970), from the orthopedics collection of R. Plato Schwartz, M.D. (1973), several hundred 19th century titles were donated from the library of Edward C. Atwater, M.D. (1976), as well as the working library of Rochester physician Edward Munn, M.D. (1801–1847). New funding mechanisms supported the historical collections, most notably an endowment from the estate of Thomas Lamont, Edward G. Miner's son-in-law (1972).

Throughout the 1980s, the historical collections continued to grow. A major stimulus to the development of the historical collections came with the renovation of the Miner Library in 1987. The History of Medicine Section acquired two new areas: a large room adjacent to the History of Medicine office that provided ample storage for housing archival collections; and a room equipped with mobile shelving that enabled us to transfer more than 300 18th- and 19th-century periodicals from the open stacks to the historical collections. A formal archives program was initiated that focused on the acquisition of faculty manuscript collections. Over the next thirteen years, the faculty manuscript collection would expand to twenty-five collections, including the papers of George Hoyt Whipple, Wallace O. Fenn, Edward Adolph, John Romano, George Engel, Loretta Ford, and other important figures.

Inventories of these collections were added to the History of Medicine Section's website, enabling scholars worldwide to survey our manuscript holdings at the most detailed level. Automation also affected the use of our rare book collections. Since the early 1980s, machine-readable records (MARC) have been created for each rare book added to the collection using the OCLC database. Scholars and bibliographers worldwide can now access our collections either on the OCLC database, its WorldCat web version, or on the University of Rochester's online public catalog accessible on the Internet. Using a more traditional format, *An Annotated Catalog of the Miner Yellow Fever Collection* was published in 1990, a collection that began as a gift of forty-one titles by Edward G. Miner in 1927. In the decade following the catalog's publication, the yellow fever collection grew by another hundred titles.

Throughout the 1990s, hundreds of titles were acquired for the rare book collections, through gifts and purchases. The largest single gift ever made to the historical collections was received in 1996. Edward C. Atwater, M.D., donated some 1,200 18th- and 19th-century books, pamphlets, and broadsides from his personal collection of American popular medicine. Between 1996 and 2000, this collection grew by nearly another thousand titles, the result of Dr. Atwater's continued generosity and through purchases made by the Library. Because the Atwater Collection is so thoroughly representative of the health reform movements that gripped 19th-century America, a two-volume annotated catalog of the Atwater Collection is being compiled, with the first volume scheduled for publication late in 2001.

Today the Miner Library's rare book holdings number some 15,000 volumes. The collection represents all disciplines and periods in western medical history, but is particularly strong in early printed anatomy, obstetrics & gynecology, yellow fever, cholera, orthopedics, dentistry, 19th century American medical imprints, and American popular medicine.

A recent major acquisition occurred with the transfer of 300 18th-through early 20th-century titles on dentistry from the Basil Bibby Library of the Eastman Dental Center. The History of Medicine Section also maintains a supporting collection of some 5,000 circulating and reference titles on the history of the biomedical sciences.

Coinciding with the growth of the History of Medicine Section's facilities and collections over the last fifteen years of the 20th century has been a substantial increase in the use of materials and services. Patronage nearly doubled between 1985 and 2000, indicating the scope, quality, and uniqueness of our rare book and manuscript holdings and their value to scholars within the university and across the eastern United States and Canada.

LEADERSHIP AND COLLABORATION

The Edward G. Miner Library is a medium-sized medical library, but its reach extends far beyond the walls, and the staff is recognized for its leadership, both within the Medical Center and in the profession. Until the 1960s, the Library was closely tied to the Rush Rhees Library and in some avenues, such as selection of materials, depended upon the members of the Library Committee. Stanley Truelson became the first medical librarian to report directly to an administrator within the Medical Center, rather than to the university Librarian. Each director has contributed to the development and achievements of the Library. In addition, they have provided leadership on university committees, in national, regional, and local organizations, and through publishing and speaking.

Over the years individual directors have served at the highest levels of the Medical Library Association (MLA) and have received national honors and awards. Lucretia McClure, director of the Miner Library from 1979 to 1993, served as president of the MLA and also received the Marcia Noyes Award, the highest award bestowed by that professional association. Valerie Florance served as editor of the Annual Statistics of Medical Libraries in the United States and Canada, the premier source of benchmarking data for academic medical libraries. Julia Sollenberger served on the Board of Directors of the MLA and received the Estelle Brodman Award for Academic Medical Librarian of the Year. The leaders of the Miner Library have indeed been notable leaders within their profession.

The Library as an institution has been a strong contributing member of a number of organizations, including the Regional Medical Library, housed at the New York Academy of Medicine, and now the National Network of Libraries of Medicine. Library directors have served on the RML Advisory Committees and offered services to support the work of this arm of the National Library of Medicine. The directors and many of the staff serve on committees and boards of the Rochester Regional Library Council (RRLC). One of the Council groups is the Hospital Library Services Program that fosters cooperation among the hospital libraries, and supports the circuit librarian program and the MIRACLEnet shared database project.

The Miner Library was a participant in the Rochester Study, a research project supported by the RRLC and the MLA. The research involved a survey of some 448 physicians in the Rochester area concerning the impact of library services on clinical decision making. The results of the study had a significant impact on the medical library community. The published report, indicating that physicians rate information provided by the library higher than that provided by other sources, has been widely read and cited.

The librarians of Miner have been active in a number of library-related organizations. Many are members of the Medical Library Association and its regional group, the Upstate New York and Ontario Chapter of the Medical Library Association. The Library has also been represented by staff in numerous other organizations such as the American Association for the History of Medicine, the Association of Academic Health Sciences

Libraries, the International Federation of Library Associations, and the American Medical Informatics Association.

YES, IT HAS ALL COME TRUE!

The work of any library is complex with its links to the cyber world as well as its traditional in-house printed resources. This chapter has pointed to the major changes and achievements that have occurred throughout Miner Library's existence, as well as providing a window to the future. Lucretia McClure, in the Library's annual report for 1984/85, predicted the state of the Library in the year 2000:

> Fifteen years from now, in the year 2000, today's Medical Center students returning for reunions will find a library, looking perhaps much the same, but with many changes in the way to use its facilities. The card catalog will be gone, replaced by an online catalog. . . . Individual items can be searched for by the traditional author, title or subject and also by keyword, . . . or by any combination of these elements. The catalog will tell which of the University Libraries owns a particular item, whether it is checked out and whether the latest issue of a journal has been received.
>
> If a book or article is not owned by the library, it will be obtained almost instantly by long distance facsimile transmission. All the indexes and abstracts will be available online as will the full text of many articles.
>
> There will still be books and journals, of course . . . [but] . . . we will be working in electronic libraries before the end of this century. What we will also see is the need for librarians to take the lead in teaching library users about the sources of information and, once located, how to sift the information for the most relevant data, how to evaluate what is read and above all, how to become intelligent and discriminating users of the wealth of information in the biomedical sciences.

The Internet has accelerated the pace and we have arrived at an even higher plane in our information-seeking sphere. Yes, it has all come true!

 Directors of the Edward G. Miner Library
George W. Corner, M.D., *1924*
Mildred Walter, *1929*
Stanley D. Truelson, *1963*
Willis Bridegam, *1966*
Henry L. Lemkau, *1970*
Lucretia W. McClure, *1979*
Valerie Florance, *1993*
Julia F. Sollenberger, *1998*

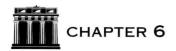 CHAPTER 6

Achievements in Clinical Care, Research, and Service

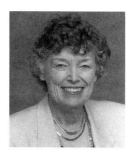 RUTH A. LAWRENCE, M.D.

Since its earliest days, the Medical Center has been home to skilled and innovative faculty dedicated to advancing clinical care through research, teaching, and practice. In this chapter, some of the many highlights of that distinguished seventy-five year history are recalled.

ANESTHESIOLOGY

A leader in developing new understandings about pain and how to control it, the Department of Anesthesiology at Rochester developed one of the country's first pain clinics during the 1980s and '90s. That clinic, a landmark achievement for the region, represented the latest in a series of advances that began in the old Division of Anesthesia, which until 1969 was part of the Department of Surgery.

The development of anesthesiology as a separate specialty began in the 1930s and '40s, although at that time most of the service was provided by nurse anesthetists. By the '50s, the field was being recognized generally by Departments of Medicine and Surgery for its potential contributions in applied pharmacology and respiratory physiology. Aware that departments spe-

cializing in anesthesiology
were being developed at Massachusetts General Hospital,
at the Mayo Clinic, and at the
University of Iowa, faculty
here joined the movement.

Robert Sweet became
head of the division in 1950.
He was succeeded by Nicholas
Greene who left to go to Yale
later in the decade, taking
with him most of his recruits;
Greene eventually published
a textbook on spinal anesthesia and contributed significantly to the anesthesia literature. With Greene's departure,
D. Vernon Thomas was named
head of the division and served
in that capacity until 1959.

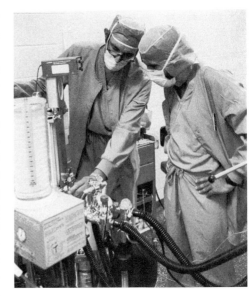

Seymour J. Sandler, M.D., *Associate Professor of
Anesthesiology, instructs a resident on the use of an
anesthesia gas machine*

Allistair Gillies, a member of the department in 1954 and 1955, had left to
follow Greene to Yale; he returned to Rochester and was named chair when
the division was elevated to departmental status in 1969.

The department's major teaching efforts included a residency and fellowship program in clinical anesthesia. The residency program was started in
1953. The first resident was Robert M. Lawrence, who had been a surgical
house officer before being called to Korea where he served in the original
MASH unit. Lawrence clearly recognized the critical role played by anesthesiologists in the care of the injured.

Department faculty participated in the pharmacology/toxicology pro-

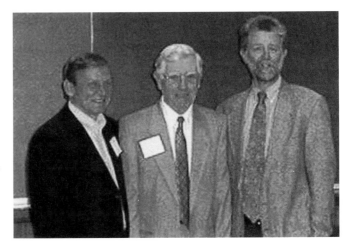

Chairs of Anesthesiology,
Ronald A. Grabel, M.D.
(1983–92), Alastair J. Gillies,
M.D. *(1969–83), and*
Denham S. Ward, M.D.
(1992–present)

RUTH A. LAWRENCE

gram for second year medical students, conducted in the dog laboratories and focused on the use of general anesthetics to relieve pain. The faculty also taught fourth year students, half of whom usually chose the anesthesia clerkship elective.

The department conducted both basic laboratory and clinical research. Among many notable works and publications were those of Jose Calimlim, whose multiple drug studies in blinded, placebo-controlled trials often involved the postoperative control of pain. Frank J. Colgan performed many of the initial evaluations of high-frequency ventilation. In 1982, he developed a prototypical device to determine the degree of gas exchange with this modality; his device was a forerunner of the present-day jet ventilator. Robert G. Merin conducted extensive studies in the laboratory and in the operating room on the effects of halothane anesthesia. In addition to measuring the effects on myocardial hemodynamics, Merin also studied glucose metabolism in concert with halothane anesthesia, known to have an effect on the liver; many of his other studies focused on the cardiac toxicity of inhaled anesthetics.

COMMUNITY AND PREVENTIVE MEDICINE

The Medical Center Department of Community and Preventive Medicine, established in 1958, evolved from an informal interdisciplinary course led by Albert D. Kaiser, a respected community pediatrician and health officer. Robert L. Berg, a Harvard trained internist, was appointed to the endowed chair named for Dr. Kaiser.

Following Berg's retirement, Charles Phelps, an economist from RAND and director of the University Public Policy Program, was appointed chair in 1989. When Phelps became university provost, Thomas A. Pearson, a cardiovascular epidemiologist who trained at Johns Hopkins, was appointed chair in 1997.

The department's broad mission over the years, to promote teaching and research in population health and health services, has evolved from an initial focus on comprehensive personal health services to encompass epidemiology, social and behavioral science, and health services research. Senior faculty and their areas of academic focus, with national and international recognition, have included Ernest Saward, a lifelong leader in developing the health maintenance organization concept; James Zimmer, a gerontologist with an extensive portfolio of research on health services for older people, in collaboration with Berg and others; Stephen Kunitz, a medical sociologist and author of several books dealing with his longstanding research on health problems of traditional societies, including the Navahos and Australian aborigines; William Barker, an internist-epidemiologist, with a broad interest in health promotion for older persons, including leadership of the Monroe County "McFlu" project, prototype for the influenza vaccine amendment to

Medicare; Theodore Brown, a medical historian, with a principle interest in 20th century American medicine, including development of the biopsycho-social model at the University of Rochester and elsewhere; Sarah Trafton, applied policy analyst and consultant, with many leadership roles in Rochester health-care forums; Alvin Mushlin, Jack Zwazinger, and Dana Mukamel, all with strong interest in health services research, emphasizing econometric dimensions, including cost effectiveness analysis, medical decision-making, and quality of care measurement.

As for educational programs, the department has long provided required core medical school courses in community medicine in the first year and epidemiology in the second year. This material is now combined in a single six-week course, Mastering Medical Information, taught at the beginning of the medical school's new Double Helix curriculum.

A master of public health program, initiated in the 1970s for general training in epidemiology and health services, was expanded in the late 1990s to offer a clinician investigator track.

In the 1990s under the leadership of Phelps, Mushlin, Zwazinger, and Mukamel, the department established both a postdoctoral and Ph.D. program emphasizing health services research. At the national level, both Saward and Phelps were appointed members of the Institute of Medicine, and Berg and Barker were elected president of the Association of Teachers of Preventive Medicine.

EMERGENCY MEDICINE

The Medical Center's new and enhanced emphasis on emergency care is clearly evident in the new two-story wing now under construction near the Elmwood Avenue entrance to Strong Memorial Hospital. Strong's role as the

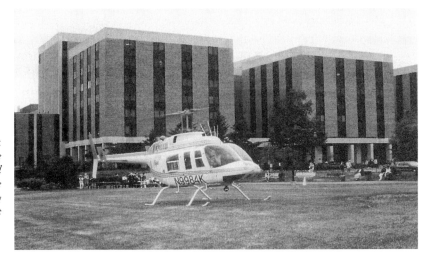

Mercy Flight landing on the helicopter pad near the Emergency Department

RUTH A. LAWRENCE

region's Level I trauma center places it at the hub of an expanding—and improving—network of emergency care. Mercy Flight helicopters fly ill and injured patients from outlying counties to the Medical Center; a new roof-top heliport, adjacent to the Emergency department, will ensure that these patients arrive with even greater efficiency into the hands of the appropriate ED team.

After many years of providing outstanding services to the community and a superb clerkship experience to senior medical students, Emergency Medicine was recognized as a full department in 1992. A year later Sandra Schneider was recruited from Pittsburgh to become its first chair. A residency and fellowship program was developed and specialty areas have emerged, including Pediatrics, Sports Medicine, and Clinical Toxicology.

Major areas of clinical research have been greatly augmented by a unique program which employs "enrollers"—specially trained interviewers who identify Emergency department patients who are appropriate candidates for various research protocols. With the approval of patient and/or family, patients are enrolled in the appropriate protocol promptly, even as treatment is underway. As a result of this grant-funded program, therapeutic studies can be carried out in an intense environment where clinical research traditionally has been extremely difficult.

The department also takes an active role in improving pre-hospital stabilization, working in partnership with the Emergency Medical System.

FAMILY MEDICINE

The Department of Family Medicine was established as an academic unit in 1979. Initially an arm of the Department of Community and Preventive Medicine, Family Medicine achieved full departmental status in 1988.

At its beginnings in 1970, under the leadership of Eugene Farley, Family Medicine's agenda was to create a high quality residency program. When established, the residency was one of the first three such programs sponsored by an academic, research-intensive institution in this country, and it quickly became nationally recognized and attractive to many high quality applicants from many medical schools. Its first patient care base was the practice of David E. Reed, a member of Rochester's class of 1957. Trained in Internal Medicine, Reed was attracted to Family Medicine and his practice served as the clinical base for residency education in the new program.

There have been two major themes of scholarly investigation by faculty in the department. The first grew out of a landmark study, published in 1972–73; it described the range of 100,000 clinical encounters in the practices of family physicians in Virginia. This study was the basis for a national wave of interest in family medicine related to the classification of health problems in primary care. Here in Rochester, Jack Froom and Larry Culpepper, who had been recruited to the Family Medicine Unit by Farley, crafted the "International Classification of Health Problems in Primary Care." This came to serve as the defining database for education and population research in family medicine nationwide and had a wide-ranging impact on population-based research in primary care.

The second theme grew out of the work of Jack Medalie, an internist turned family practitioner, who performed early studies in Israel on the family context in which cardiovascular disease develops in individual patients. One of his findings was that the presence of a pet in the family was cardioprotective. His studies and others led investigators here, notably Thomas Campbell and Susan McDaniel, to conceptualize the field of Family Systems Medicine. Their work grew out of the broader interest in biopsychosocial medicine here at Rochester and resulted in much collaborative work between the Family Medicine faculty working in this area and the faculty in Psychiatry with similar interests. All of these works dealing with the impact of the family on health have had international significance.

In more recent years, Kevin Fiscella and Peter Franks have been studying disparities in health care, using national databases, focused on the impact of social and demographic variables on the care received by various segments of the population. This work has been facilitated by the deep involvement of the department in the care of disadvantaged patients, in its main practice and at the Westside Health Center where efforts are focused.

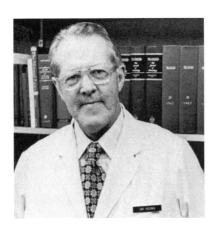

Lawrence E. Young, M.D., *Charles A. Dewey Professor of Medicine and Chair of Internal Medicine, 1957–1973*

DEPARTMENT OF MEDICINE

The early faculty in Medicine were first of all generalists, as was the case for other clinical departments. Although some had special areas of clinical and research interest—like McCann in respiratory physiology and disease and Slavin in the infectious diseases—these more focused interests were in addition to the faculty's primary responsibility to serve as general clinical internists and teachers of internal medicine. The breadth of knowledge and experience that these early faculty brought to the care of their patients and to teaching, and which informed their approach to research was critically important to the nature and substance of their accomplishments in the early years of the school.

Beginning in the 1950s, and especially in the 1960s, federal funding for research and training expanded greatly. As a result, there were dramatic advances in the subspecialties of medicine. This growth stimulated the development of subspecialty units and the recruitment of substantial numbers of highly specialized faculty. Especially during Lawrence Young's tenure as chair, from 1957–1973, the department grew dramatically. Several nationally distinguished leaders in the subspecialties and in General Internal Medicine were recruited and built units whose scholarly achievements became nationally recognized.

Cardiology

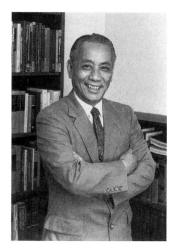

Paul N. Yu, M.D., *Professor of Medicine (1963–1982) and head of the Cardiology Unit, Department of Medicine*

Cardiology is one of the most clinically active units within the Department of Medicine and has a strong history of advancing care for patients with heart disease. Under the leadership of Paul N. Yu, the Cardiopulmonary Unit in its early activities enlarged the diagnostic scope of the then-new 12-lead scalar ECG and contributed to the development and clinical application of treadmill-based exercise stress testing. One of the early participants in this work, Robert Bruce went on to develop a nationally accepted standardized protocol for exercise testing.

During its first fifteen years, the cardiac catheterization laboratory was the focus of a combined clinical and research effort related largely to the study of pulmonary circulatory dynamics and pathophysiology in patients with a variety of heart and pulmonary diseases. Regulatory mechanisms were studied

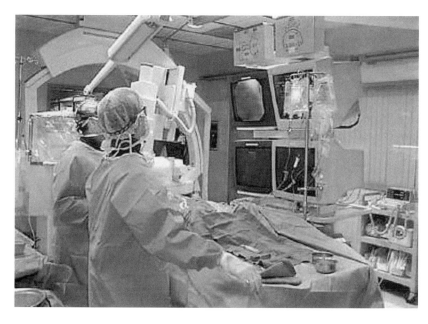

Cardiac Catheterization Laboratory, modern era

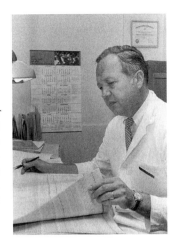

Bernard F. Schreiner Jr., M.D., *Professor of Medicine, and head of the Cardiac Catheterization Laboratory, 1960s–1980s*

in a large cohort of patients with valvular heart disease in preparation for surgery. The effects of exercise, hypoxia, and various pharmacologic interventions were studied in numerous patients to assess pulmonary vascular regulatory mechanisms, both active and passive, as well as the associated interstitial pathophysiology. Techniques to measure pulmonary blood volume and extra-vascular lung water were developed to facilitate these investigations, which brought about a better understanding of the central role of the pulmonary circulation in patients with heart failure, especially those with rheumatic mitral valve disease. The cardiology laboratory was among the first to use transseptal left atrial puncture in the evaluation of left heart dynamics. Bernard Schreiner, director of the laboratory, and Gerald Murphy, were important contributors to this work.

In the late 1960s, Pravin Shah and David Kramer, working with radiologist Raymond Gramiak, made a major contribution to the understanding of intracardiac hemodynamic events in patients with hypertrophic obstructive cardiomyopathy with the echocardiographic recognition of abnormal systolic anterior movement of the anterior mitral valve leaflet (SAM) as a major factor responsible for the intraventricular pressure gradients characteristic of this entity. The finding has stood the test of time and remains a central diagnostic echocardiographic feature of obstructive cardiomyopathy.

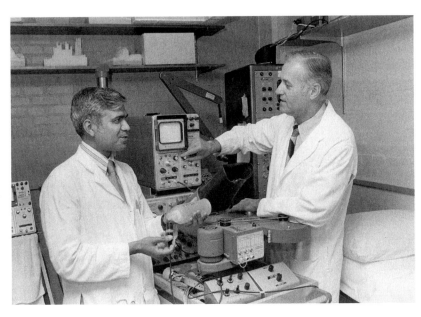

Pravin M. Shah, M.D., *Professor of Medicine, and* Raymond Gramiak, M.D., *Professor of Radiology, with an original cardiac echo machine*

RUTH A. LAWRENCE

During the early years of the development of Rochester Cardiology, Paul Yu, at first single-handedly, provided his consultative expertise to a large in- and out-patient-based clinical practice that served large numbers of patients not only in Rochester but also throughout a large segment of New York's Southern Tier. His efforts provided the solid foundation upon which has been built the comprehensive general and special cardiology consultative services of the current era.

The Cardiology Unit was one of ten units nationwide selected by the National Institutes of Health to develop a specialized Myocardial Infarction (MI) Research Unit. The unit in Rochester was physiologically and clinically oriented and contributed to the recognition of factors important during the pre–hospital phase of acute MI, as well as the rapid advance of bedside invasive hemodynamic assessment of patients during acute infarction. This small cadre of units contributed enormously to the understanding of early events in acute myocardial infarction, leading to the current highly sophisticated intensive cardiac care units such as our own at Strong Memorial Hospital.

The work of Arthur Moss has extended these early studies. His work over the past twenty years has led to better understanding of the natural history of ischemic heart disease, as well as the impact of various preventive, rehabilitative, and pharmacologic therapies. He has also made major contributions to the understanding of the Long Q-T Interval Syndrome and its management.

Faculty in the affiliated hospitals have made significant contributions to a variety of multicenter national trials. Working at the Genesee Hospital, Serge Barold made substantial early contributions to our understanding of a variety of cardiac electrophysiologic problems and the use of implantable pacemakers.

In more recent times, William Hood and his colleagues made major contributions, as participants in multicenter studies, to the modern-day management of congestive heart failure, using angiotensin converting enzyme inhibitors. With the coming to Rochester of Bradford Berk, as chief of Cardiology in 1998, the unit's basic research program became very much enriched, focusing on Berk's work in vascular biology.

Endocrinology

Endocrinology did not become a formal unit of the Department of Medicine until the late 1950s. Even before then, however, Rochester faculty were making major contributions in this field. In the 1930s, Rochester was one of the few institutions nationally to have a hospital ward devoted to clinical investigation. This unit, guided by Samuel Bassett, was a forerunner of modern clinical research centers. In the 1940s and 1950s, Henry Keutman and his colleagues applied measurement of urinary steroid excretion to the understanding of endocrine, metabolic, and renal diseases. Christine

Waterhouse and her colleague Leonard Fenninger, made ground-breaking observations leading to a better understanding of malignancy-related cachexia. Waterhouse also studied electrolyte metabolism in heart failure, metabolism of bone, and changes in lipoprotein phosphatides in various disease states. Her professional interest and expertise spanned the fields of nephrology and endocrinology and set an early standard in the field for the careful assessment of clinical laboratory observations.

In 1962, the Endocrinology Unit was established as a separate entity after Seymour Reichlin arrived from Washington University in St. Louis. His recruitment to Rochester initiated a long period of outstanding clinical research achievement. Reichlin saw the importance of brain-endocrine connections, stimulated by his Ph.D. work in London, where he studied pituitary control of the thyroid. His views of hypothalamic-pituitary-endocrine physiology, summarized in his landmark paper, which appeared in the *New England Journal of Medicine,* had a major impact on thinking in this field.

No less significant was the work in that same era (the 1960s and early 1970s) conducted by Lawrence Raisz and William Peck, who made important contributions to the study of bone cell function. Peck's achievement of isolating bone cells for study *in vitro* enabled a host of observations regarding hormonal influences on bone physiology.

When Peck left for St. Louis in 1976, Dean Lockwood became head of Endocrinology. He and his colleagues, John Amatruda, and Nicholas Livingstone concerned themselves with pathophysiologic mechanisms in diabetes; in particular, they contributed greatly to our understanding of interactions between insulin and its receptors and the cellular actions of those receptors.

Lawrence Jacobs' work represented an effort to unravel the molecular events surrounding exocytotic mechanisms. Stephen Welle has made highly significant observations on muscle protein homeostasis, especially in the elderly, while Paul Woolf's work helped illuminate neuro-humoral responses to brain injury. John Gerich, current director of the Clinical Research Center, has been a leader in the field of intermediary metabolism; one of his seminal contributions was the identification of the kidney as a gluconeogenic organ.

Gastroenterology

The Gastroenterology Unit was formally established in 1957, with Harry Segal as the first unit head, although he and others had been consulting in gastroenterology for some time before that. The unit's academic activities were based at both the Genesee Hospital (TGH) and Strong. When Segal became Chief of Medicine at TGH, Michael Turner was recruited from England to serve as unit head, and Turner then brought Frederick Klipstein from Columbia and Gerald Bevan from England who served as the core faculty for the unit at its inception.

Segal was primarily an outstanding clinical internist and teacher, but one of his contributions was the development of the "tubeless gastric analysis." Turner's work focused on studies of bile salt metabolism, on which he and Bevan collaborated. Klipstein, in 1970, became the director of the Tropical Medicine Malabsorption Unit, a cooperative undertaking of the Universities of Rochester and Puerto Rico. The most notable achievements of this unit were the following: (1) identification in 1973 that showed that certain enterotoxigenic bacteria were the cause of Tropical Sprue among Puerto Ricans, and in 1975 similar findings among Haitians through studies conducted at the Albert Schweitzer Hospital in collaboration with Helen Short of our Microbiology Department; (2) demonstration through clinical studies in Puerto Rico, the Dominican Republic and Haiti that subclinical malabsorption contributed to nutritional deficiencies that were widespread in the populations of these countries; (3) development in the early 1980s, in collaboration with Richard Houghten at the Scripps Clinical Research Foundation, of a synthetic toxoid vaccine for the prevention of the acute diarrhea caused by enterotoxigenic strains of *e. coli*. A report of this important work appeared on the front page of the *New York Times Science Section.*

In more recent years, William Chey has conducted important studies of various GI hormones, and their functional role in normal GI function and various disease states. This work was conducted initially in Chey's laboratories at TGH, and more recently in the Konar Center at Strong.

General Medicine

Coincident with the maturation of the unique Rochester health-care system in the early 1970s, the General Medicine Unit (GMU) was founded under the leadership of Paul Griner. The major focus of the unit was in the area of Health Services Research, especially rigorous evaluation of hospitalization utilization. Some of the studies were seminal in introducing the concept of clinical pathways and guidelines. One of the first research fellowship programs in General Medicine in the country was established by Griner and Alvin Mushlin, who subsequently became the head of the GMU. Mushlin has contributed key studies in the use of higher technology diagnostic procedures. The unit is currently under the direction of William J. Hall and continues its broad research interests in health improvement strategies, especially among minority populations in the Rochester area.

Geriatrics

A long tradition of geriatrics at the URSMD began with the pioneering work of T. Franklin Williams in the 1970s. Under his direction, Monroe Community Hospital became one of the first teaching nursing homes in the country, while one of the first geriatric assessment clinics was established at Monroe Community Hospital. A geriatrics fellowship program has been in existence since that time and has produced some of the current leaders of academic geriatrics in the country, including Knight Steel, Mark Williams, and Mary Tinetti. At present, the Geriatrics division's activities are organized under the Division of Geriatrics headed by William J. Hall.

A major research focus of the division is the Rochester Claude C. Pepper Older Americans Independence Center, one of the first such comprehensive research centers funded nationally by the National Institutes of Health. The center has encouraged and developed broad interdisciplinary research programs in aging aimed at maintaining and improving function in older persons, including studies in muscle metabolism (Steven Welle), therapy in Alzheimer's disease (Pierre Tariot), and urinary incontinence (Thelma Wells). At present the center is focusing on the immunologic and vascular effects of respiratory infection in older adults. Monroe Community Hospital (Paul Katz, director) continues to provide an important educational focus in geriatrics, including the Finger Lakes Geriatrics Education Center. The Geriatrics division has been recognized nationally for its leadership role in developing novel educational strategies. Recognition has included a designation as a Geriatrics Center of Excellence by the John A. Hartford Foundation.

Hematology-Oncology

The Hematology-Oncology Unit has a long and distinguished history at the University of Rochester, having been established in the 1920s by William S. McCann, first chair of the Department of Medicine.

Even a brief look at the work of a number of distinguished faculty in hematology reveals a tradition of innovative research and clinical advances. In

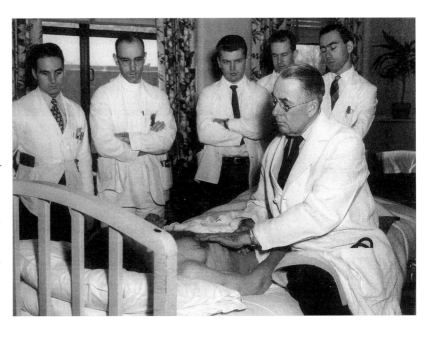

William S. McCann, M.D., *first Chair of Medicine, 1926–1956, demonstrating physical examination techniques to medical students*

RUTH A. LAWRENCE

1928, Lemuel W. Diggs began teaching the first course in hematology at the Medical School. The author of the widely used *Atlas of Morphology of Human Blood Cells,* Diggs established the first blood bank in the United States, following his departure from Rochester. He also established the first Sickle Cell Center in the country, where the natural history of patients with sickle cell hemoglobinopathies could be studied.

John S. Lawrence performed landmark studies on hematological disorders in animals, including studies of infectious feline agranulocytosis. Under Lawrence's tutoring, William Valentine studied the puzzling case of an Italian youth whose hemoglobin level was normal, but whose red cell count was very high. In 1944, Valentine published a report describing this case and others selected from a large population of Italian immigrants in Rochester, and proposed naming the condition thalassemia major (or its variant, thalassemia minor). Valentine began a distinguished career, becoming well known for studies of red cell enzymopathies, radiation effects on hematopoiesis, and for the initial description of leukocyte alkaline phosphatase.

In 1948, Lawrence E. Young became the second head of the unit. He pursued research in immunohematology and studies of hereditary spherocytosis. Young and Charles Yuile, in the Department of Pathology, performed landmark studies on dog blood groups and abnormalities occurring after transfusion of incompatible blood in animals. Scott Swisher, head of the Hematology Unit from 1957 to 1967, became a world-renowned expert on hematologic morphology. Also, a large collection of dog blood typing sera assembled by Swisher in Rochester gave rise to the world's first dog blood group reference laboratory.

Robert Weed, who became head of the Hematology Unit in 1967, was the first to apply fundamentals of membrane physiology, derived from studies in yeast cells, to the study of red cell structure and function. His studies with phase microscopy and electron microscopy contributed greatly to our understanding of human red cells. Weed was a pioneer in applying scanning electron microscopy to studies of red cells. Together with Paul LaCelle, he established and directed the Clinical Investigator Training Program at Rochester, an innovative program that gave academic clinicians a foundation in the basic sciences.

Victor Marder and Marshall Lichtman became co-chiefs of the Hematology-Oncology Unit in 1977 and directed the unit until 1990. Lichtman studied hematopoiesis and leukemogenesis and Marder performed numerous landmark studies on vascular biology, the biology of fibrinogen, and endothelial cell function, resulting in an international reputation in hemostasis and thrombosis. Lichtman and George Segel in Pediatrics did seminal studies in defining the activity of the L-system amino acid transporter in normal and malignant lymphocytes.

In recent years, a significant clinical advance led by the Hematology Unit was the establishing of the Bone Marrow Transplant (BMT) Program at

Strong Memorial Hospital, at the urging of Lichtman and through the strenuous efforts of Jacob Rowe. The BMT Program recruited as director John DiPersio (who now holds a major leadership position at Washington University). Rowe, DiPersio, Camille Abboud, and later Jane Liesveld were instrumental in establishing this clinical, educational, and research program, the first of its type in Upstate New York. The program is noted for its studies of cytokine biology and its application to transplantation, as well as for aggressive pioneering work in matched unrelated donor transplantation.

In late 1995, Joseph Rosenblatt joined the Hematology-Oncology Unit. Rosenblatt was noted for his studies of the biology of HTLV-II, closely related to the HTLV-I virus, a cause of leukemia and neurological disease in man. While at UCLA, he had cloned an HTLV-II provirus used to develop screening assays both in the United States and Europe. Rosenblatt is also known for studies of RNA regulation in HTLV-I/II, by the Tax and Rex genes, unusual regulatory genes which served as models for understanding similar regulation of complex retroviruses such as HIV-I. Together with Pia Challita-Eid, Rosenblatt has recently focused on novel immune therapy approaches to cancer, and has developed the first antibody fusion proteins, which merge antibody function with a chemokine or a T-cell costimulatory ligand for purposes of eliciting immune response to human tumors. This synthesis of genetic engineering and immunology provides a new approach to eradication of residual disease.

Faith Young, who recently joined the unit from Tufts University, is a recognized authority on lymphoid development. Together with her mentor, Fred Alt at MIT, Young pioneered a unique model in RAG/blastocyst mice, particularly useful for understanding lymphoid differentiation, that is now being applied to studies of lymphomagenesis.

At Rochester General Hospital, Pradyumna Phatak, in collaboration with Charles Phelps (now University Provost), conducted the first systematic cost-effectiveness analysis of screening for hereditary hemochromatosis. Based on this analysis, the unit conducted the largest United States primary care screening study for hemochromatosis between 1993 and 1996. The center at RGH currently cares for 230 hemochromatosis patients and is one of the largest of its kind in the country. Phatak is internationally recognized for his expertise in this arena. Work by Peter Kouides has established von Willebrand's disease as a relatively common cause of menorrhagia. His work led the Mary M. Cooley Hemophilia Center to be one of four national sites for von Willebrand's research chosen for funding by the Centers for Disease Control and Prevention.

Infectious Diseases

In the early years of the school there was no unit in the Department of Medicine devoted to the study and care of patients with infectious diseases. Through the 1930s and 1940s Howard Slavin served in this capacity; much of his work dealt with varicella zoster, but he had broad clinical interest in other infectious diseases.

In the late 1950s John Vaughan was recruited to head a combined Immunology/Infectious Diseases Unit. During the late '60s, Vaughan's unit achieved several accomplishments. Ward Bullock conducted studies of the pathophysiology of leprosy and its treatment with Dapsone. Carl Norden developed a rabbit model for osteomyelitis that he continued to work on after he left Rochester. Norden's findings became applied widely across the nation in studies of the pathogenesis and treatment of that disorder.

Vaughan was also charged with recruiting the director for a separate Infectious Diseases Unit. With the arrival of Gordon Douglas in 1970, a series of major studies involving respiratory viruses was undertaken. Robert Betts and then John Treanor joined Douglas in these studies, with collaboration from Caroline Hall in the Department of Pediatrics. Early studies of influenza vaccines, starting with an inactivated virus and the study of the immune response thereto, ultimately led to studies of attenuated influenza vaccines that may have become the standard for the modern era. Seminal studies with anti-influenza antivirals were conducted by Treanor and Betts and for respiratory syncytial virus (RSV) by Hall. Norbert Roberts conducted important studies of cellular defense mechanisms against RSV.

Michael Brandriss and Jacob Schlesinger, working at Rochester General Hospital, developed the first monoclonal antibodies against yellow fever and mapped yellow fever epitopes. Their antibodies were used to construct sensitive immunoassays for rapid, early diagnosis. Schlesinger and Brandriss also demonstrated that a non-structural glycoprotein (NS1) induced protective immunity, a concept that underlies current lines of research on flavivirus vaccine development. In more recent years, Ann Falsey and Edward Walsh conducted important studies of the epidemiology of respiratory syncytial virus, especially in the elderly.

In parallel here at Strong, Richard Reichman carried out studies of herpes simplex infection and, with his colleagues Bonnez and Rose, have studied papillomavirus pathophysiology and the role of that agent in neoplasia; they are now moving towards a vaccine. Roy Steigbigel conducted studies of animal modes of infection as well as the function of white blood cells in various diseases; he was the author of one of the "most often cited" papers for the NBT test for the assessment of white blood cells in sepsis. Betts and Roberts demonstrated that antibiotic overuse bred resistance and that removal of a specific antibiotic (gentamicin) from the formulary led to disappearance of resistance. Betts was one of the first investigators to demonstrate the transfer of CMV during renal transplantation; this phenomenon has been confirmed for other organs including liver and heart.

The involvement of the unit in various vaccine trials, dating back to the early influenza trials spearheaded by Gordon Douglas, set the tone for research in the unit. In recent years, substantial federal research support enabled faculty to conduct various vaccine studies. These include HIV vaccine candidates, the value of live attenuated influenza vaccine, the use of vaccine in the prevention of varicella zoster, and the role of conjugated pneumococcal vaccine and pertussis vaccine in adults. Rafael Dolin, who succeeded Douglas as head of the Infectious Diseases Unit, along with Betts, Bonnez, Tom Evans, Paul Graman, Mike Keefer, Reichman, Roberts, and Treanor, have been involved in this work. Graman's role has been to define hospital-associated viral transmission.

Reichman has coordinated the various treatment trials in HIV-infected patients. He works closely with Susan Cohn, Evans, Amneris Luque, Keefer, and Peter Mariuz. Cohn has also defined features of rural AIDS. Margie Urban has spearheaded studies to lead to better control of sexually transmitted diseases in the urban poor. Most recently, Lisa Demeter has become recognized nationally for her studies in the development of viral resistance and its molecular characterization.

The unit has perhaps been most widely recognized for delineating the epidemiology, pathogenesis, diagnosis, prevention, and treatment of respiratory viral illness. This has embraced the studies of influenza and RSV in both the very young and the very old, as well as those in between. This has been a collaborative effort, both at Strong and at Rochester General, including faculty in both Medicine and Pediatrics.

Pulmonary and Critical Care

The founding of the Pulmonary and Critical Care Unit dates back to the 1930s. Nolan Kaltreider, former chief resident in Medicine, developed gas dilution techniques to measure total capacity of the lungs and their subdivisions. Working with William McCann, first chair of the Department of Medicine, Kaltreider made the original observations of alterations in lung volumes with pulmonary emphysema, pulmonary fibrosis, and other pulmonary diseases. Kaltreider and McCann also pioneered a method to measure blood volume by isotope dilution and made some of the initial measurements in patients with congestive heart failure.

In the 1960s, Lawrence E. Young, then chair of the department, asked Dickinson Richards, Nobel laureate at Columbia University, to review the structure of the chest lab and cardiopulmonary division headed by cardiologist Paul Yu. Richards urged the creation of an independent Pulmonary division, and in 1968 Kaltreider was appointed the first chief of the newly founded Pulmonary Unit.

A year later, Richard W. Hyde was recruited from the University of Pennsylvania to be the unit's first full-time faculty member. He brought to Rochester unique expertise in pulmonary physiology; he measured pulmonary blood flow and lung tissue volume by having study participants rebreathe soluble and insoluble gases in health and disease. William J. Hall, Hyde's first fellow in Pulmonary Disease, joined Hyde on the faculty. Hall's research established the relationship of respiratory viral infection in the pathogenesis of asthma. At the same time, Hyde and Hall fostered the development of a strong clinical program that by the year 2000 has twelve full-time faculty.

In the late 1980s and early 1990s, the Pulmonary Unit at RGH conducted several studies describing the outcome, after life-support care of respiratory failure, in patients of advanced age. The unit also wrote the first description of the process and outcome of withdrawal of life-support care in a community hospital.

Pulmonary, Critical Care, and Occupational Medicine divisions now are coordinated by Mark J. Utell, whose own research examines the role of environmental pollutants in pulmonary disease.

Renal Disease

The Renal Disease Unit was developed in July 1965 and headed by John R. Jaenike, who was joined in 1967 by Richard B. Freeman. The most significant clinical research in the Renal Unit was the development of micropuncture studies of acute renal failure and studies of renal function in obstructive neuropathy, as well as long-term clinical studies of patients with glomerulonephritis and hereditary renal disorders. Through a training grant, more than fifteen nephrology fellows have been trained.

In the 1980s, Richard Sterns conducted several clinical studies addressing the treatment of hyponatremia, which gained the Nephrology Unit at RGH international recognition in this controversial area. These clinical studies have been amplified by animal models developed with Donald Kamm and Stephen Silver which expanded our understanding of the effect of fluid and electrolyte disturbances on the brain.

Rheumatology / Immunology

In the years before an Arthritis Unit was formally established, Ralph Jacox carried the primary responsibility for seeing patients with rheumatic disorders. While his main interests were in the infectious diseases, Jacox quickly became widely known and highly respected as a rheumatologist. It was therefore quite natural that Lawrence Young appointed him the first head of the Arthritis Unit, when the Department of Medicine was undergoing formal organization along subspecialty lines. Jacox's main efforts were devoted to clinical service and teaching, and he established the first immunology diagnostic laboratory in the hospital, focused on performance of the "latex fixation test" in patients with a wide variety of clinical conditions. He developed a high quality post-residency training program in clinical arthritis and served on the national panel of rheumatologists who crafted a set of standard diagnostic criteria and a system of classification for rheumatoid arthritis.

A year after the Arthritis Unit was established, John Vaughan was recruited as the first head of a combined Immunology-Allergy Unit. While the unit was administratively separate from the Arthritis Unit, the two were highly interrelated operationally and functioned collaboratively, a tribute to the generosity of spirit and collegiality of the two unit heads. Vaughan's major research contributions, recognized nationally, were his studies of rheumatoid factor and the antinuclear antibodies; he demonstrated that there were a variety of antinuclear antibodies individually associated with various disease states. A prolific clinical scholar with broad interest in rheumatological and other immunological disorders, Vaughan published extensively and was an important mentor to the several top-quality young faculty who joined the unit during his tenure.

When Vaughan left for San Diego in 1970, John Leddy became head of the unit, which formally merged with the Arthritis Unit in 1985. Leddy, working with Stephen Rosenfeld, observed and reported the first descriptions of genetic deficiencies in the Complement system. Their running of the clinical immunology diagnostic laboratory enabled them to make seminal observations of Complement deficiencies and relate the laboratory findings to clinical presentations. They studied in detail the functional consequences of specific Complement deficiencies, as related to host defense mechanisms and the process of inflammation. They confirmed and amplified their observations by isolating and purifying the various components of Complement, then adding them back to subjects who were deficient, reversing the clinicopathologic state.

In more recent years, Clark Anderson (with his Fellow John Looney) conducted ground-breaking studies in which they identified and characterized the molecular structure of two of the three Fc receptors for IgG in man. These receptors play critical roles in leukocyte function in host defense/inflammation, and the work has been recognized world-wide as a major contribution.

George Abraham has conducted important research on monoclonal rheumatoid factor and cryoglobulins. With Douglas Turner (Professor of Chemistry in the College), Abraham has done signally important research on the biophysics of cryoglobulin formation.

NEUROLOGY

The Department of Neurology at Rochester is well known internationally as a leader in advancing the understanding and treatment of neurological disorders including Parkinson's disease, Huntington's disease, Tourette's syndrome, periodic paralysis, and stroke.

In the early years of the medical school, Paul Garvey was one of the outstanding clinicians and teachers. Trained in neurology at the University of Michigan, Garvey was recruited by William S. McCann in 1929 into the

Department of Medicine, which later included Neurology as one of its divisions. Garvey retired in 1963, but continued to teach and consult. Forbes Norris headed the division until 1966. At that time, the other faculty members were Richard Satran, David Goldblatt, and David Marsh.

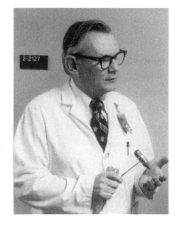

Robert J. Joynt, M.D., Ph.D., *Chief of Neurology and first Chair of the Department of Neurology*

In 1966, the Department of Neurology was established under the leadership of Robert J. Joynt. Joynt, a graduate of Iowa, had additional training at Royal Victoria Hospital in Montreal and was a Fulbright scholar in Cambridge. He then returned to Iowa in neurology until his appointment at Rochester. In addition to teaching and the laboratory study of the role of the hypothalamus in water metabolism, his clinical research included clinical trials in the treatment of strokes with surgery and specific medications.

Robert C. Griggs became chair when Joynt became dean of the medical school in 1984. Griggs and his colleagues had begun work on periodic paralysis, establishing a successful treatment in 1967, cloning the genes in 1994–1996, and finally confirming the effectiveness of the treatment in a randomized trial.

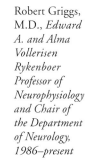

Robert Griggs, M.D., *Edward A. and Alma Vollerisen Rykenboer Professor of Neurophysiology and Chair of the Department of Neurology, 1986–present*

The work of Ira Shoulson on Parkinson's disease has resulted in several abstracts, papers, and public reports. He led a multicenter trial on the efficacy of deprenyl in delaying the signs of Parkinson's disease and was part of the team that located the gene responsible for Huntington's disease. He established the Experimental Therapeutics Unit with the departments of Pharmacology and Neurology where he continues his research in the experimental therapies of neurologic disorders. Shoulson and Griggs run a unique NIH-funded training program in experimental therapeutics of neurologic disease.

Roger Kurlan has dedicated his clinical research to the study of Tourette's syndrome. He has established that the syndrome is far more common than originally thought and may affect as many as 20 percent of children in special school programs. He is currently working on new therapies for the disorder.

Proximal myotonic myopathy has been identified by Richard T. Moxley III and Charles Thornton as a new disease. One of the most common adult muscular dystrophies, its symptoms, progression, and cause continue to be studied by Moxley and Thornton.

The department has also been prominent in medical journalism. Joynt served as editor of *Archives of Neurology* from 1982–1997 and was founding editor of *Seminars in Neurology* in 1981, with Goldblatt taking over the editorship in 1984. Griggs is editor of *Neurology* (1997–present).

OBSTETRICS-GYNECOLOGY

Among the most distinctive contributions of the Department of Obstetrics and Gynecology was the promotion in the 1950s of a kinder, gentler approach to the process of childbirth. This patient-centered innovation helped spur the development of the birth center/rooming-in concepts now so common throughout the country. Reproductive technology has also made strides here, with the department achieving a notable success rate in assisted pregnancies and managing the only sperm bank north of New York City.

In the early years, Rochester provided the nation with an unusual model among American medical schools by combining both specialties—obstetrics and gynecology—in one department. The first chair, Canadian-born Karl M. Wilson was one of the initial contingent recruited by Dean George Whipple from Johns Hopkins. Another Canadian, Robert Ritchie was brought from McGill to oversee Gynecology. Other early faculty included Willard Allen, Henry Darner, Richard TeLinde, and Ward Ekas. Ekas developed the department's outpatient unit and an innovative home delivery service.

Wilson organized a community program of cytologic screening for gynecologic cancer that began with 4,000 specimens the first year and quickly expanded to over 100,000 per year. This screening has been successful in identifying the disease early and has almost eliminated delayed diagnosis of advanced cervical cancer.

Both Wilson and Allen earned national reputations for their research. Wilson is best remembered for his 1945 paper which detailed the "Rochester ovum," a human ovum of sixteen days development; nine years later, he described an eleven day old pre-villous ovum. Allen, working with Rochester anatomist George Corner established a bioassay in 1928–29 that enabled them to isolate progesterone from sows' ovaries.

Wilson was a strong supporter of Rochester's new Department of Psychiatry and encouraged his residents to take a fellowship in the Medical-Psychiatric Liaison Unit. One of the first to do this was John Donovan, who later gained national prominence for his curriculum design and teaching philosophy and for his innovative work on the menopausal syndrome. The Division of Psycho-Social Obstetrics and Gynecology was established under the leadership of Anthony Labrum and later David Baram, with a special focus on PMS and on psychosexual dysfunctions.

Donald Kariher studied the Rh factor in pregnancy; the phrase "hemolytic anemia of pregnancy" was coined in his laboratory. Later, he and Tom Smith invented a new device for circumcising newborns that became widely used throughout the country.

William Jackson and Tom Smith established and promoted the use of cervical cytology in Rochester as a screening tool for cervical cancer. George Trombetta, a resident, later pioneered work in Rochester using colposcopy as a diagnostic tool to detect early-stage cancers in the lower reproductive tract. With Ruth Schwartz, he was instrumental in teaching and promoting colposcopy locally and nationally. Later, he championed laser therapy for cervical and vulvar lesions.

The department's second chair, Curtis Lund, came to Rochester with an interest in anemia. He became a leader in all the discipline's national societies and served on the American Board of Obstetrics and Gynecology. He published some provocative cinefluorography studies of bladder function in women with urinary incontinence. Of special importance were Lund's efforts to promote research; nearly all the many residents who took a year-out experience working in the laboratory later entered academic medicine.

Lund promoted the concept of having mothers and infants room together and he encouraged fathers and families to take part in perinatal education and care.

Henry Thiede, one of Lund's first appointees, worked with Herbert Morgan, chair of Microbiology, and Lund to establish a tissue culture laboratory. By making monolayer cultures of human early placental trophoblasts, they were able to describe the abnormal chromosomal karyotypes of human spontaneous abortions. Later, they demonstrated viable cells and their karyotypes in amnionic fluid of near-term pregnancies. An outgrowth of this work was the First Rochester Trophoblast Conference in 1961, which now attracts 200–300 international scientists for each meeting.

During the 1970s, Richard K. Miller established the placental perfusion laboratory which has served as a model for similar laboratories elsewhere. Miller, who helped propel Rochester's trophoblast research into the international spotlight, has developed an innovative consultation service for physicians and patients—one of two in New York State and only forty in the nation—that targets the effects of environmental/drug exposure on the perinatal environment.

Mortimer Rosen, working with neurologist Richard Satran, developed a transvaginal fetal scalp lead that could record brain distress before it became apparent in fetal heart tracings. (Rosen later became chair of OB/GYN at Columbia University.)

When Thiede became the department's third chair in 1974, he introduced three subspecialties: Maternal/Fetal Medicine, Gynecologic Oncology, and Reproductive Endocrinology and Infertility. Under the leadership of Vivian Lewis, Grace Centola, Eberhard K. Muechler, and John H. Mattox, the art and science of assisted pregnancy have made dramatic strides.

James Woods, director of the Maternal-Fetal Medicine division, leads the management of high-risk obstetrical patients in multiple sites in Rochester and surrounding communities. His regional high-risk consultation service is demonstrating a significant reduction in morbidity for participating mothers and infants.

Extramural diagnostic services (including ultrasound and Doppler) have been greatly expanded under the direction of Jacques Abramowicz, while genetic determination services are offered through the Reproductive Genetics Unit (initiated and directed by D. Neil Saller). Woods developed a fax-based educational program now used by 500 hospitals nationwide, and led his division in supporting the development of Strong Memorial Hospital's construction of the first labor-delivery-postpartum recovery unit in Rochester.

Under the leadership of the department's fourth chair, David Guzick, clinical and research advances continue. For example, work on autism by Patricia Rodier has uncovered evidence associating autism with embryonic insult and, perhaps more importantly, genetic defects with early embryonic expression.

OPHTHALMOLOGY

In 1929, Ophthalmology in Rochester began as a division of the Department of Surgery. Albert Snell, Sr., who can be called the "father of the Ophthalmology Department" in Rochester, was asked to organize the Division of Ophthalmology in the newly built Strong Memorial Hospital. Snell was named the first lecturer of Ophthalmology. He became an international leader in industrial ophthalmology, specifically in the area of eye injury compensation, and he was a pioneer in the screening of school children's eyes.

As a commitment to future growth, the institutional leadership recruited John Gipner from the Mayo Clinic to bring to Rochester the tradition of ophthalmology that he had helped to establish in Minnesota. Arriving in 1931, Gipner served as the first chair of the Division of Ophthalmology. He started the residency program and trained twenty-seven residents during his tenure. He also actively promoted the involvement of community physicians in the activities of the division.

Following Gipner's retirement in 1961, Albert Snell, Jr., served as chair. In 1952, Snell, along with Rosario Guglielmino, created the first Eye Bank in the country. In 1974, under Snell's auspices, the Ophthalmology division was moved into the outpatient building. He successfully carried on the strong traditions of community leadership and excellence in ophthalmology established by Gipner.

In 1978, Henry Metz became chair, and the status of the division was changed to the Department of Ophthalmology. With a renewed dedication to basic science research, the Ophthalmology Research wing was completed in 1985. Metz initiated the expansion of the residency program to include three new residents yearly for a total of nine residents. In 1993, Metz stepped down as chair, although he remains a part-time faculty member.

In 1993, Steven Ching was appointed interim chair. Ching has distinguished himself as a teacher, scholar, and cornea specialist, and has maintained an unwavering commitment to resident education. He served as interim chair until February 1994 when George Bresnick was appointed chair.

Bresnick's areas of clinical specialty were retina and electrodiagnostics. In addition, he had an interest in public policy, public health, and health services research. He created a strong vision for the department as a national center for health services and a model for delivery of care to underserved populations.

In 1998, Barrett Katz became interim chair upon Bresnick's retirement. Katz was instrumental in orchestrating the department's participation in an international project entitled Idealized Design of a Clinical Office Practice (IDCOP). The effort of this project was to design, test, and disseminate major improvements in the office-based practice of health care.

In July 1999, Katz left the department for other pursuits, and with his departure Steven Ching again assumed the position of interim chair. Ching has embraced the department's vision for quality improvement through the IDCOP project and continues to strive for excellence in ophthalmology.

Ching envisions considerable growth for the department in providing eye care services to the community, as well as increased productivity in clinical and basic research linked to collaborations with industry.

The department has begun a refractive surgery research and clinical care program with Bausch & Lomb and the Center for Visual Sciences that will enable state-of-the-art laser refractive surgery to be done in this community. Rochester will be one of the national clinical testing and development sites for laser therapies, optical instruments and ophthalmic devices, and a clinical research site for Bausch & Lomb. As faculty grows, it is anticipated that other B&L trials in pharmaceuticals and ophthalmic devices will be directed to this department.

In addition, Ching hopes to add faculty expertise in refractive surgery, neuro-ophthalmology, ocular molecular genetics, retina, inflammations and autoimmune diseases of the eye, and pediatric ophthalmology.

Ching and Ronald Plotnik specialize in diseases of the anterior segment of the eye, cornea transplantation and infectious diseases of the eye. John Burchfield specializes in diagnosing and treating patients with glaucoma, the leading cause of irreversible blindness. Donald Grover specializes in the management of retinal vascular diseases, including diabetic retinopathy, age-related macular degeneration, and other vascular abnormalities of the retina and choroid.

Basic research in the past year has focused on visual processing in the primate (human and non-human) and feline visual system. David Calkins' lab is particularly interested in the perceptual role of certain cell classes (K type) and certain neurochemical systems (especially glutamate) in the retino-cortical pathways of macaques. Robert Emerson uses computational methods to study the determinants of the motion responses of cortical cells in cat visual cortex. William Merigan studies how the unique response properties of neurons in the ventral (color and form) pathway in macaques and humans give rise to the perception of complex images. Krystel Huxlin studies the mechanisms of reorganization after cortical injury in cats. Gail Seigel studies Batten's disease, apoptosis, and retinal cell behavior.

ORTHOPAEDICS

Orthopaedics was initially a division of Surgery and as a division was led by R. Plato Schwartz from 1926 to 1957, Professor Robert Duthie from 1958 to 1966, and Louis Goldstein from 1969 to 1974. In 1974 Orthopaedics became a department in the Medical Center under the leadership of the chair, C. McCollister Evarts from 1974 to 1986. Since 1986 the department has been guided by Richard Burton, the current Wehle Professor of Orthopaedics. Frederick Zuck has twice served as acting chair.

The department has been a pioneer in many areas of orthopaedics. During the first fifty years, the major clinical activities of national reknown were foot and ankle (Schwartz), arthritis (Duthie), and children and adults with spine deformities (Goldstein).

Since becoming a department, Orthopaedics has grown exponentially in its clinical activities as well as educational and research productivity. Under Evart's leadership, the department was seeing approximately 20,000 patients a year by 1985 and performing 1,200 major surgical procedures. By 1999–2000, the outpatient clinical volumes grew to 70,000 patient visits per year, with over 5,000 surgical procedures. Much of this increase in clinical activities was facilitated by the philanthropy of Donald and Mary Clark whose generous contributions made possible construction of the Clark Musculoskeletal Unit. Because of this exponential growth, the department has now outgrown the Clark Unit and a new musculoskeletal institute building is in the offing, with construction scheduled to begin in the year 2000.

When Orthopaedics became a department, a fundamental policy decision was made by Evarts that clinical activities should be organized around areas of expertise. In 1974, these areas of expertise were spine surgery, led by Chan and Goldstein; adult reconstruction surgery, led by Evarts; and hand surgery, led by Burton. In 1976, sports medicine was added, led by Kenneth DeHaven. Initially these areas of the department were called sections, and by 1986 there were eight full time faculty members in these four sections.

Over the past decade many new full time faculty were recruited with many new areas of expertise, resulting in an organizational system of ten divisions in the department and a total of twenty-five full time faculty. These divisions and their current leaders include: Adult Reconstructive Joint Surgery, Allen Boyd; Foot and Ankle Surgery, Judith Baumhauer; General Orthopaedics, John Marquardt; Hand and Upper Extremity, Richard Miller; Musculoskeletal Oncology, Randy Rosier; Musculoskeletal Trauma, John Gorczyca; Pediatric Orthopaedics, Kenneth Jackman; Research, Edward Puzas; Sports Medicine, Kenneth DeHaven; and Spine Surgery, Paul Rubery.

Many accomplishments of the orthopaedic faculty merit specific emphasis. When Professor Duthie left the University of Rochester Medical Center it was to assume the position as the Trueta Professor and Chair of Orthopaedics at Oxford University in England. McCollister Evarts served as president of the American Board of Orthopaedic Surgery, President of the American Orthopaedic Association, and Chair of the Orthopaedic Residency Review Committee. He recently retired as vice president for Health Affairs and dean at the Penn State Medical Center at Hershey. Richard Burton served as a director of the American Board of Orthopaedic Surgery for ten years and as president of the American Society for Surgery of the Hand, 1992–1993. Kenneth DeHaven served as president of the American Academy of Orthopaedic Surgeons in 1996–97. Randy Rosier is currently a director of the American Board of Orthopaedic Surgery. Both Rosier and Regis O'Keefe have served on NIH study sections. Judith Baumhauer is a Council Member of the American Orthopaedic Foot and Ankle Society, and Edward Puzas is in line to become president of the Orthopaedic Research Society.

The American Board of Orthopaedic Surgery will thus have had thirty years of consecutive representation from the Orthopaedics department at the University of Rochester (Evarts, Burton, and Rosier for ten years each in sequence), a unique accomplishment not duplicated by any other university in this country.

Between 1926 and 1986, the department was well recognized for clinical research. R. Plato Schwartz was well known for his clinical research in gate and foot mechanics. Louis A. Goldstein was internationally known for his pioneering work in the non-operative and operative treatment of idiopathic scoliosis and was elected President of the Scoliosis Research Society.

C. McCollister Evarts achieved international recognition for his role in the development of total joint reconstructive surgery for the hip and knee and for his landmark research projects on the prophylaxis of deep venous thrombosis in orthopaedic patients, in collaboration with the Division of Hematology in the Department of Medicine. Kenneth DeHaven became an international leader and pioneer in arthroscopic knee surgery and the surgical repair of meniscal injuries; he also did pioneering work in arthrofibrosis of the knee and in various techniques for reconstruction of the anterior cruciate ligament of the knee.

Richard Burton developed a nationally recognized fellowship in hand surgery and an international reputation for his work in the treatment of patients afflicted with arthritis of the hand and wrist. In the late 1970s he developed a surgical procedure for osteoarthritis at the base of the thumb, one of the most common joints afflicted with arthritis and one causing great patient disability. Because of excellent clinical results with long-term follow-up, this operation is now the gold standard operation for thumb arthritis against which all others are now being compared.

Since 1986, the department has become particularly well known for research in cellular and molecular biology of cartilage and bone disorders. The main foci have been cartilage maturation and degradation, osteoarthritis, the mechanism of growth plate function, osteoporosis, and in the cellular and molecular biology of cancer metastasis. The most recent research involves various gene therapies for musculoskeletal disorders and pharmacologic mechanisms to prevent periprosthetic loosening. These pioneering research projects have been under the leadership of Rosier, Puzas, and O'Keefe. In 1986 the department had no extramural funding; in 2000, the department ranks second in the United States for NIH funded research at over $2 million per year.

The Department of Orthopaedics has been well recognized for its educational efforts. The number of residents in the program has gradually increased and by 1988 the department had ACGME approval for five resident slots per year, with 400 candidates applying each year for the positions. In 1992 the American Orthopaedic Association awarded a special certificate to our residency "in recognition of outstanding support of scholarly endeavor and fellowship among orthopaedic surgical residents."

The first decade of the new millennium has been declared the Bone and Joint Decade by the United Nations and by many countries throughout the world. The Department of Orthopaedics at the University of Rochester Medical Center stands poised on the cusp of this decade with one of the finest orthopaedic departments in the country. This strong position is based on its cutting edge research in basic bone cell and molecular biology of bone and cartilage, its broad clinical expertise in all areas of the musculoskeletal system, and its commitment to the highest quality of resident and medical student education.

OTOLARYNGOLOGY

When George Whipple made the decision as the dean of Rochester's new medical school to develop an Otolaryngology service, he looked once again to Johns Hopkins to hand pick the chairman for that position. His selection was Clyde Heatly, a young otolaryngologist in training at that institution. Before coming to Rochester, Heatly spent a year in Europe working with experts in Germany and Vienna studying the newest techniques in the fields of otology and laryngology. He arrived in Rochester in 1928 to begin the development of the division and a residency program. Heatly and Stewart Nash developed a large following in the community, with the result that many graduates remained in the community to practice.

During the thirty-four years that Heatly was chair, the division grew and developed a respect for the specialty which, along with Ophthalmology,

RUTH A. LAWRENCE

formed a combined Board—the first in the country to establish a certifying exam. During the 1940s the advent of antibiotics and their dramatic effect on the primary diseases and complications of head and neck infection, brought the specialty to its knees. During the 1950s a group of young physicians used new technology to improve the treatment of head and neck cancer, using microsurgical techniques to restore hearing after otologic surgery and to develop new treatments for managing sinus disease. One of these leaders, a resident graduate of the University of Rochester, Thomas C. Yarrington became chair of the Department of Otolaryngology at the University of Nebraska, and later at the Virginia Mason Clinic in Seattle.

Heatly stepped down in 1962 after thirty-four years of leadership, and John P. Frazer became the new chair. Frazer developed the clinical and residency program as the first full-time chair of Otolaryngology. To accomplish this task he had the continued assistance of Gertrude Bales and the Rochester Otolaryngology Group (ROG), a large private practice whose partners had a strong interest in assisting in residency training. The physicians in that practice were George Trainor, Donald Raines, Skip Frame, Robert Gulick, and Jules Musinger. Several years later, one of the graduates, John Norante, completed a head and neck fellowship at the University of Iowa and joined the faculty as the first fellowship-trained subspecialist, setting the precedent for future recruitments. Six residents now see patients in the various teaching hospitals in Rochester: Strong Memorial, the Genesee, and Rochester General.

During the 1970s the program grew as several additional otolaryngologists became involved with the training program including Paul Harrington, Arthur S. Hengerer, and resident program graduates Peter Mulbury, James Hadley, and Les Bergash, all with the ROG.

In 1980 Frazer stepped down as chair and on Jan 1, 1981 Hengerer was appointed the third chair of the Division of Otolaryngology. Charles C. Parkins, a graduate of the University of Rochester was recruited from Syracuse University to develop the research program; he brought the first NIH grant to the division. Because of the large hearing-impaired population and the interest in deafness in Rochester, Parkins' interest in nerve deafness and cochlear function made him a natural to lead the division's research. A new state of the art laboratory was constructed and Parkins' efforts had immediate impact for the division, for resident education, and for exposure to a research rotation. Faculty growth continued with Paul Dutcher, M.D., a former resident, returning after a neurotology fellowship with the House Ear Group in Los Angeles, bringing clinical skills to augment the basic otology research.

With the expansion into plastic and reconstructive surgery, resident exposure and training was required. The program successfully recruited Vito Quatela, a Rochester undergraduate and resident from Northwestern University who had completed a fellowship in facial plastic surgery with several national experts. His clinical and research efforts influenced many residents to enter this subspecialty area. Within the next few years, the growth of the division encouraged the program to request and receive a change in the program structure. The program changed from two years of general surgery and three years of otolaryngology to one and four years respectively. The number of residents was also increased to a total of eight.

In 1989 another significant step occurred when Robert Frisina, Ph.D., was appointed director of otolaryngology research. The division established a joint venture with the Rochester Institute of Technology's National Technical Institute for the Deaf to create a research effort that proved extremely successful and which became the Rochester International Center for Hearing and Speech Research (RICHS). This program resulted in research funding from a number of private foundations and a large program grant from the NIA to study hearing loss in aging. The result of these efforts has been the infusion of approximately $10 million of research funds in this decade. This multi-specialty, multi-institutional project promoted collaborative efforts and generated many scientific presentations and papers. All residents now spend a four-month research rotation, three resident research awards have been granted, to David Sherris for cartilage growth factor effects and to Chase Miller and Yvette Vinson for immunology research.

In the 1990s additional clinical faculty were added to the division: John Wayman, a neurotologist with fellowship training at the Michigan Ear Institute, and John Coniglio, with head and neck fellowship training at Vanderbilt University; both were graduates of the Rochester residency. During the '90s the residency program received national recognition and entering residents continued to show exceptional talent. Over the past fifteen years half the residents have elected to spend a year in fellowship training; of this group, seventeen have gone on to enter full-time academic positions at prestigious residencies around the country.

As we enter the new millennium, two additional faculty have been recruited to replace Quatela and Coniglio who have left the full-time staff. Saurin Popat from the University of Toronto is now the fellowship-trained head and neck surgeon for the division. Timothy Doerr has been recruited from Wayne State and the University of Michigan, to become the plastic and reconstructive surgeon. We view the new decade as a great challenge and believe we are prepared to meet the rapidly changing health-care environment in which we find ourselves.

PEDIATRICS

The Department of Pediatrics, now the second largest department at the School of Medicine and Dentistry in terms of budget and numbers of faculty, has a strong history of clinical achievements. Several research-based innovations developed at Rochester over the years have had a national impact,

RUTH A. LAWRENCE

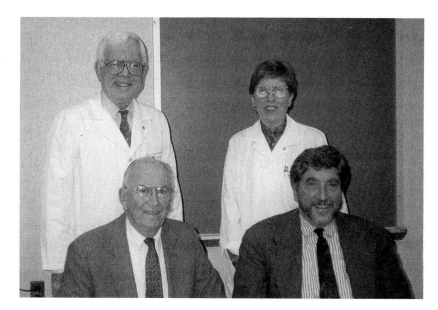

reshaping areas of pediatric care and the way treatment is delivered. At least one of these innovations—the development of a vaccine against Haemophilus b influenza—has saved the lives of thousands of children worldwide.

Pediatrics at the University of Rochester has had a national presence from its earliest days. Irvine McQuarrie, a member of the original small faculty, was a member of the first White House Conference on Child Health, convened in 1928, and the author of the committee's first report to the public. The present chair, Elizabeth R. McAnarney, currently is president of the Association of Medical School Pediatrics Chairs.

From the school's beginning in 1925, pediatric research and clinical care have been equally valued. The department's first chair, the scholarly Samuel W. Clausen, worked on evaporative water exchanges in children and on Vitamin A metabolism (the latter research conducted with Augusta McCoord, a pediatric chemist known to generations of students and residents).

Generally speaking, the major and most significant clinical achievements over the department's seventy-five year history have been in the areas of pediatric infectious disease, neonatal care, and health-care delivery to the region's medically underserved children

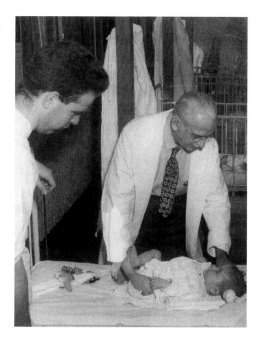

Samuel W. Clausen, M.D., *first Chair of Pediatrics, 1926–1952, examining a child on the infant ward (E-4)*

and adolescents. The advances in infectious disease include pioneering efforts to understand and treat pertussis, pneumococcal disease, and—in one of the major medical advances of the late 20th century—the development of the H flu vaccine that has reduced death and debilitation from the disease by 98 percent. (For a more complete telling of the H flu vaccine story, please see page 116.)

Many of these clinical advances have resulted from the unusually strong bond that has developed between the Department of Pediatrics and Rochester's pediatric clinicians, virtually all of whom have appointments as faculty at the School of Medicine and Dentistry. This long history of research partnerships between academicians and clinicians has improved treatments for several common infectious diseases.

William L. Bradford, the department's second chair, became nationally known for his work in pertussis and parapertussis (he reported the discovery of the latter simultaneously with a laboratory in Michigan). Bradford's work with children with whooping cough revealed that improved diagnostic results for the disease could be achieved by swabbing behind the child's nasal passages where bacteria often lurked, so well hidden they often escaped notice

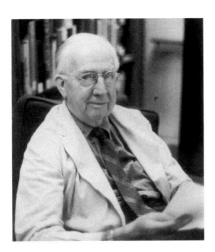

William L. Bradford, M.D., *second Chair of Pediatrics, 1952–1964*

when the traditional throat sample was harvested. The post-nasal "Bradford swab" became widely used throughout the mid-years of the century. His work comparing the efficacy of various antibiotics against parapertussis resulted in chapters on the disease and its treatment written by Bradford for several textbooks.

If there were an international "helping hand" award related to the Nobel Prize for clinical achievement, Bradford should certainly be considered as a candidate. Having observed that pertussis colonies did not grow well on culture plates coated with a particular fungus, he shared his specimens with his British colleague, Alexander Fleming. Fleming, of course, was later credited with being the first to isolate penicillin and to recognize its bacterial-inhibiting properties, a clinical advance of the first order.

Across the nation, the numbers of needless tonsillectomies and appendectomies were reduced as the result of the work done during the 1930s by Albert David Kaiser, health officer of the city of Rochester and a member of the Department of Pediatrics. After ten years observing several thousand children, Kaiser published *Tonsils—In or Out?* and began what was to become a great national debate that markedly reduced the frequency of unnecessary surgeries to remove tonsils and adenoids.

RUTH A. LAWRENCE

The department's longtime focus on infectious disease treatment and prevention parallels the issue's national importance. Burtis B. Breese and Frank A. Disney returned to Rochester after serving in World War II and formed a pediatric partnership that re-ignited their interest in streptococcal disease. They began the first office-based study of streptococcus, examining the epidemiology of the disease and the value of various therapeutic approaches. Based on their wide experience, they realized that an exact diagnosis of streptococcus by culture was essential; on house calls, each carried a little black bag equipped with materials for taking throat cultures and counting white cells. Their publications in this area spanned five decades, and they received jointly the first American Academy of Pediatrics Practitioner Award (in 1986) for their contributions to research in office practice.

Carolyn Breese Hall returned to Rochester after her residency to join the Division of Infectious Disease. Hall's study of respiratory syncytial virus led to trials of a vaccine for premature infants; she has also explored many therapeutic regimes for pediatric infections.

Clinical advances in the treatment of at-risk newborns are among the most notable achievements of the Department of Pediatrics. In 1959, Rochester neonatologists working with a team of anesthesiologists made medical history by being the first in America to place a newborn on a ventilator. The premature infant survived severe respiratory distress syndrome (RSD) at a time when the mortality rate from the condition was 90 percent.

Artificial ventilation, however, did not completely solve the problem of surfactant deficiency in prematurity. During the 1980s, under the leadership of Chair David H. Smith, the Division of Neonatology made a great advance in neonatal clinical care by developing a safe and highly effective exogenous treatment for RSD, the single greatest cause of neonatal mortality in the world's developed nations.

The team of Robert Notter and William Maniscalco, working with colleagues at the State University at Buffalo, initiated laboratory and animal work targeting surfactant, the lipid protein often deficient in the lungs of infants born prematurely. Between 1981–82, the two Upstate teams isolated and purified lipids from calves' lungs which proved effective in laboratory biophysical studies at Rochester and in treating premature surfactant-deficient lambs in Buffalo. In 1983, a decision was made to begin using the refined calf-lung extract to treat premature infants in the intensive care nurseries at both medical centers. At Rochester, the clinical application was directed by Donald Shapiro, who had been recruited from Yale to join the neonatology team. The innovative therapy met with great success. Since that time, calf-lung surfactant extract has become commercially available. Nationally marketed as Infasurf, the FDA-approved drug is produced using the methods and quality control procedures first defined by Notter.

In 1989, Dale Phelps became chief of Neonatology. Her research has resulted in successful prophylactic treatment of retinopathy in premature newborns, using laser therapy. Phelps is principal investigator for a large prospective multi-centered project, with a final analysis of results expected in this millennial year.

In the area of community health, a series of clinical advances was achieved during the 1960s when, under the leadership of Chair Robert J. Haggerty, Evan Charney, and others, a network of neighborhood pediatric clinics was established in urban and rural areas. Managed cooperatively by pediatrics faculty and neighborhood residents, the clinics not only provided important services to children and their families, but served as faculty research sites—becoming the source for medical and demographic data key to improving both health care and health-care delivery systems. These innovations became a national model for pediatric care among the underserved.

Work by Department of Pediatrics faculty with adolescents has resulted in still other clinical advances. Stanford Friedman, during his years in Rochester, developed what has since become the nationally-recognized subspecialty of Behavioral Pediatrics. Rochester's Adolescent Maternity Program (RAMP), developed and directed by Elizabeth McAnarney and Richard Kreipe produced research (by McAnarney) on adolescent mothering morbidity which indicated that—with proper medical care—the outcome of adolescent pregnancies could be as successful as those experienced by adult women. Kreipe developed a program (now interdisciplinary) that offers clinical help to adolescents with eating disorders.

Throughout Rochester's pediatric community—whether in the offices of the region's clinicians or in the state-of-the-art laboratories of the university's new Center for Vaccine Biology and Immunology—the quest for 21st-century cures and preventions continues.

PSYCHIATRY

The importance of the contributions made by Rochester's Department of Psychiatry to education, patient care, and research worldwide can scarcely be overestimated.

First and foremost among these contributions is the department's transformational influence on the school's teaching programs, work that reshaped medical education here and abroad. Through the work of John Romano, the department's founding chair, and his colleague George Engel, generations of physicians now take a holistic view of the patient. This humanistic orientation (then a new way of seeing the patient) has come to be called the biopsychosocial approach to care and is widely recognized as the hallmark of a Rochester-educated physician (see Chapter 1).

More recently, the development of the new field of psychoneuro-immunology by Robert Ader and his colleagues has put Rochester in the forefront of a movement that has documented scientifically what Romano, Engel, and their colleagues understood—importance of the mind-body connection in health and illness.

As was the case in most medical schools prior to World War II, Psychiatry at Rochester began as a unit within the Department of Medicine. It consisted originally of outpatient services provided in partnership with the Board of Education, the Society for the Prevention of Cruelty to Children, a criminal branch of the city court, and the Bureau of Public Welfare. The first in-patient service was provided in the old Municipal Hospital; the program, directed by Richard Jaenike, also was the source of some medical school teaching.

In 1945, a generous gift from Helen Woodward Rivas led to the establishment of a psychiatric clinic. That clinic in turn led to the founding of the Department of Psychiatry in 1946 and the recruitment of John Romano as professor and chair. Romano had studied under Soma Weiss at the Peter Bent Brigham Hospital in Boston. Weiss promoted a holistic view of psychiatry; he hired Romano to do rounds on the medical service as a psychiatrist. Romano's earlier experience with psychoanalysis at the Menninger Clinic and with Milton Rosenbaum at Cincinnati led him to believe that an analytic orientation was "an absolute necessity" for any department of psychiatry. As opposed to the neuropsychiatric model in place else-

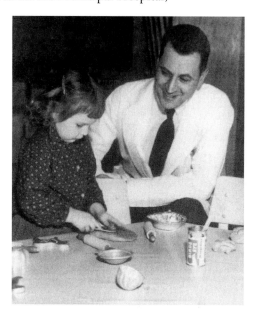

John Romano, M.D., *Chair of the Department of Psychiatry, 1946–71, observing a child at play*

Fridays in the car with John

A memorable experience for many third year medical students was the opportunity to spend time with the Department's charismatic founding chair, John Romano. Romano, a tall, often formidable man with an astonishing range of knowledge accompanied by great charm, enjoyed the time spent informally with students, as we see from this recollection:

> *Every Friday I would spend at Canandaigua [at the Veterans' Administration Hospital]. I would pick up four medical students or residents and drive them to my house to have coffee with my wife and son. . . . Then we would drive together to Canandaigua. I would have them taken on a tour of the whole place. At 10 a.m. they would come back and I would conduct teaching rounds. A patient would be presented to me. The nurses, social workers, nursing assistants, occupational therapists, psychologists, psychiatrists, physicians were there, as well as the dentist and clergyman. All persons relevantly concerned with the care of the patient would participate in the discussion. Then I would take these four students back with me, and we would take lunch at some little restaurant on the way home. This gave me an opportunity to know each student in the class.*

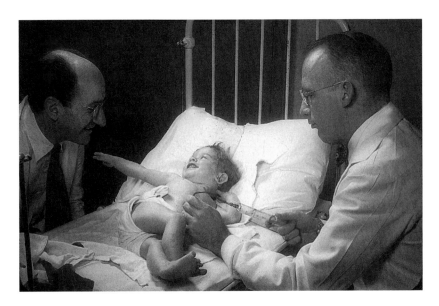

Franz Reichsman, Monica, *at age twenty months, while still hospitalized on E-4 in Pediatrics, and the "stranger"*

where during the 1940s, Romano oversaw the development of a more narrowly defined, but much more broadly oriented department.

At the same time, a new conceptual model was emerging. The scope of psychiatry was widening to include interactions with both biomedical and humanistic views. One of Romano's main objectives was to build greater rapport and communication between psychiatry and medicine. George Engel, an internist who also had been mentored by Soma Weiss, was recruited to Rochester by Romano to promote this broader orientation and to create a teaching program that would bridge both fields. In the course of instructing medical students, Engel and his colleagues wove aspects of psychiatry into the general curriculum. The establishment of the Medical-Psychiatric Liaison Unit created a visible link between psychiatry, medicine, pediatrics, and obstetrics and gynecology. In addition to Romano and Engel, key medical faculty included William Greene, Franz Reichsman, and Arthur Schmale. The biopsychosocial method remains the hallmark of a Rochester medical education.

In 1961, Engel took over the teaching of psychopathology to second year medical students and also rounded weekly with third year students; his work was crucial to the development of the general clerkship. With co-author and Rochester colleague William Morgan, he published *The Clinical Approach to the Patient,* the first text on physical diagnosis to recognize the importance of seeing each patient as a whole human being.

In a landmark essay in *Science* (1977) entitled "The Need for a New Medical Model: A Challenge for Biomedicine," Engel laid the foundation of the biopsychosocial model when he said, "The physician's basic professional

RUTH A. LAWRENCE

knowledge and skills must span the social, psychological and biological, for his decision and actions on the patient's behalf involve all three."

One of the great achievements of the new department was the construction of "the R-Wing" which opened in 1948. Gone were the drab facilities then common to "mental wards," replaced with rooms designed to resemble hotel accommodations; even the china was carefully selected to avoid an institutional look. Over the years R-Wing expanded; by 1957 it included five floors for patient care, research laboratories, and outpatient space. In 1969, R-Wing North was opened, to meet the increasing need for pediatric and adolescent accommodations and to support a family therapy program and a geriatric unit.

In 1971, Lyman Wynne replaced Romano as chair of the department. Former chief of the adult psychiatry branch of the National Institute of Mental Health, he is widely recognized internationally as an authority on schizophrenia and family and developmental psychology.

One of the department's scientists, Robert Ader is now known as "the father of Psychoneuroimmunology." After years of painstaking laboratory research, Ader was able to document in the laboratory that the immune and the central nervous systems operate as a functionally integrated defense system. At Rochester's Center for Psychoneuroimmunology, this work continues to develop under Ader's leadership.

Other distinctive research contributions of the department have been in the field of gero-psychiatry (Eric Caine and Pierre Tariot), including research on suicide in the elderly (Yeates Conwell), and more recently studies of sleep disorders (Donna Giles).

The restoration of mandatory internship training for residents in Psychiatry, accomplished through the influence of Romano and Wynne, was an important achievement. That requirement had been eliminated by the Board in Psychiatry, much to the distress of those who believed in broad, medically-oriented training for those entering the field.

Still another contribution was the department's influence in the development of the community mental health movement, a national effort that brought psychiatric and psychological care to the underserved and disadvantaged through the establishment of community mental health centers. This was an especially important contribution at a time when many patients were being discharged from mental hospitals into community settings. As a result, ambulatory mental health services were greatly expanded, and numbers of social workers, psychologists, and other health-care professionals joined the staffs of academic departments of Psychiatry.

Finally, the creation and expansion in Monroe County of a psychiatric register brought into a single database information on patients throughout the community who receive psychiatric care. The register continues to serve as an invaluable source of data for population-based research. A major subset resulted in a study of schizophrenic patients and their families.

RADIATION ONCOLOGY

After World War II, rapid strides in radiation physics technology and radiation biology research began to form the scientific basis for using radiation therapy to treat cancer. The physical separation of radiation therapy units from diagnostic radiology machines, a process that began in the early '50s, heralded the intellectual separation that would follow. At that time, only a few radiologists devoted themselves to treatment exclusively; since there were only kilovoltage units in Rochester, most radiologists practiced both diagnostic and therapeutic applications.

With the recruitment to Rochester in 1957 of Philip Rubin, many patients began being treated with radiation for either benign or malignant disease. Rubin had been chief of the Division of Radiation Therapy and Radioisotopes at the new Cancer Center at the National Institutes of Health. That center served as the model for a facility being planned at Rochester, a building devoted exclusively to radiation oncology and supervoltage equipment. Construction took place in a courtyard between Strong Memorial Hospital and the new animal facilities, and was completed in the early sixties.

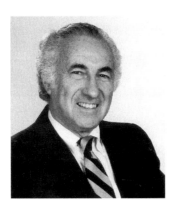

Philip Rubin, M.D., *Professor and Chair, Department of Radiation Oncology*

In the 1960s, the Department of Radiology, chaired by Louis Hempleman, consisted of three divisions: Diagnosis, Therapy, and Radiobiology. Hempleman's major contribution to oncologic practice was the detection of an increase in the incidence of second malignant tumors in thyroid cancer following thymic irradiation in newborns and the increase of breast cancer in patients irradiated for postpartum mastitis. As a result of these studies, the use of radiation treatment was restricted to oncologic diseases.

In 1961, a three-year residency program in radiation therapy and radioisotopes was established, funded by training grants from the National Cancer Institute (NCI). In 1965, Colin Poulter was recruited from London to become the program's clinical director. Faculty increased, as did the patient load. In the 1960s, the new facility included a 2 MV Van de Graaf accelerator, telecobalt and telecesium units, and a kilovoltage superficial x-ray machine.

A Radiobiology Unit was created under the direction of George Cassarett, an internationally recognized radiobiologist and radiation pathologist. His collaboration with Rubin led to the publication in 1968 of *Clinical Radiation Pathology;* the book became the basis for all late effects radiation research at our institution. In the mid-1970s, simple treatment planning computers evolved that facilitated the development of treatment plans for cancer therapy.

During the 1970s, the Medical Center planned and built a $6 million

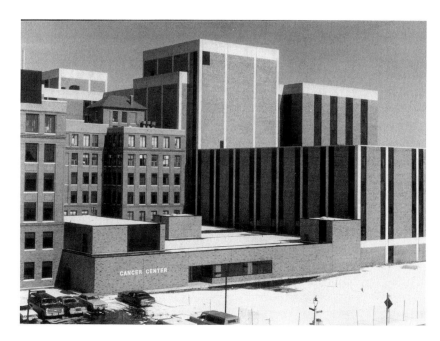

Cancer Center, and Robert Cooper was appointed director. The Division of Radiation Therapy and Radioisotopes (DRTR) became the Department of Radiation Oncology (DRO), with Medical, Surgical, Gynecological, Nursing, and Psychosocial Units. Radiation Oncology activity occupied major portions of this 25,000 square foot facility.

By 1980 Radiation Oncology consisted of five divisions devoted to clinical radiation oncology, radiobiology/pathology, medical physics, clinical investigations, and education. The new faculty promoted translational research and cooperative group clinical trials. The Division of Clinical Radiation Oncology increased its faculty to twenty-one, with appointments both in the DRO and the Cancer Center. Within the city of Rochester, all departments of radiation oncology were affiliated. Henry Keys was made clinical director and Bowen Keller became head of Radiation Physics. Linear accelerators were introduced and computerized treatment planning and simulation was begun. The NCI cooperative clinical trial effort in radiation research began in the late '70s with the formation of a national Radiation Therapy Oncology Group in which DRO investigators played a major role. In thirty years, the DRO has enrolled thousands of patients on studies and cooperated with other national cancer groups.

In the Division of Radiation Biology, a major accomplishment of the 1970s was receipt of an NCI grant to develop biological in vivo/in vitro models to simulate clinical problems and to provide a scientific basis for clinical Phase I, II, and III trials. Major research themes were tumor modeling and the use of in vitro spheroids, discovered by Rochester's Robert Sutherland and widely used to test new drugs, often in combination with irradiation.

The overall goal of the research program was to develop a scientific basis for combining radiation and chemotherapy to treat and control cancer. Over the years, the total research funding for this continuing project reached $50 million. With Sutherland's leadership, the Radiobiology Group expanded and additional faculty members and many post-doctoral fellows were recruited. Among those who joined the Rochester group and are still with the university are Edith Lord, Peter Keng, Bruce Fenton, and Jacquelyn Williams.

Perhaps most important to the field's rapid growth in the '80s was the increase in cancer patient curability and organ preservation. More than one hundred national training programs existed, and the DRO is among the first, having trained more than one hundred residents and fellows. Many of our faculty and trainees head major departments throughout the United States and Europe and have become outstanding leaders in the field of radiation oncology.

In the 1980s, Dietmar Siemann was appointed director of the Radiation Biology Division, followed by Peter Keng in the 1990s. Weekly research meetings, each on a different topic, were held, and a multidisciplinary approach to research was encouraged. During Siemann's and Keng's tenures, the research group was awarded twenty grants totaling over $10 million. Jacob Finklestein has led a conjoint program between the Department of Pediatrics and the DRO to develop predictive markers for radiation pneumonitis and fibrosis, most recently through plasma cytokines.

In the education arena, the *International Journal of Radiation Oncology, Biology, Physics* was edited and managed within the department for twenty years. The clinical oncology syllabus, *A Multidisciplinary Approach for Physicians and Students,* edited by Rubin, was first published in the 1960s. Now in its eighth edition, translated into five languages and sponsored by the American Cancer Society (ACS), the syllabus has reached most medical students here and abroad. Louis Constine, then associate chair, is an author and editor of *Pediatric Radiation Oncology;* now in its third edition, this is the bible for treating pediatric malignancies with radiation. Constine is renowned for his studies on pediatric malignancies and late-effects.

During the 1990s, many new biologic-technologic advances were made. The Medical Center developed a Bone Marrow Transplant Program in conjunction with the DRO, providing total body irradiation to prepare patients for the transplant. With Michael Schell directing the Physics section, the department was one of the first centers in upstate New York to treat patients using high-dose rate brachytherapy via interstitial and intracavitary implants. Schell's tenure has seen the introduction of stereotactic radiosurgery, real time prostate implantation, electronic portal imaging, and 3-D conformal treatment planning. The latter allows the linear accelerator to deliver treatment on target, excluding normal tissues. The clinical radiation oncology division had conjoint clinics and conferences with medical, pediatric, surgical, and gynecologic oncologists.

RUTH A. LAWRENCE

At the end of 1995, Rubin stepped down as chair after thirty-eight years, and Constine was named interim chair. A nationwide search culminated in the 1997 appointment of Paul Okunieff chief of Radiation Oncology at the NCI, as chair. Under his leadership, the department is expanding its research laboratories in molecular biology.

New faculty and research endeavors are adding strength to the department. A renaissance of interest in treating benign disease was pioneered here, starting with the inhibition of heterotopic bone formation using moderate doses of radiation in hip replacement patients. Jacquelyn Williams, in the laboratory, and Arvind Soni in the clinical setting, continue groundbreaking research into using radiation to control neointimal hyperplasia and vascular restenosis. Irradiating blood vessels following traumatic procedures to maintain patency has interested cardiologists and vascular surgeons and has revitalized radiation for benign disease. An international journal, *Cardiovascular Radiation Medicine,* was conceived in our department and heralds this new frontier.

A new shaped-beam Radiosurgery Center currently under construction will use this state-of-the-art therapy to control cancer, and give hope to patients with metastatic disease. These exciting activities will keep the Department of Radiation Oncology at the University of Rochester Medical Center at the forefront of research, and the institution in the spotlight.

RADIOLOGY

From Rochester's landmark studies during World War II on the effects of radiation to recent advances using contrast agents in imaging and techniques to improve small joint imaging, the Department of Radiology has made major contributions to the field.

Radiology has been present at the School of Medicine and Dentistry since its inception in 1925. Stafford L. Warren arrived with the first group of faculty recruited by George Whipple. Although he had no formal training in radiology, Warren developed the Department of Medical Photography.

In 1939, Radiology became a separate department. While Warren had published one of the first clinical demonstrations of film mammography in 1930, his major interests were in studying the biological effects of radiation. As a result of his early publications in these fields, Warren was selected to direct the Manhattan Project studies at the University of Rochester, carried out under the aegis of the Atomic Energy Commission. He was given a military position with the Manhattan Project and its study of the radiation effects of nuclear fallout.

Fully engaged with the top-secret project, Warren turned over the chair in 1947 to Andrew Dowdy, whose interests also were in radiobiology and radiation effects.

In 1948, George H. Ramsey was recruited to chair Radiology. During his twelve year tenure, he laid the framework for many modern aspects of clinical practice and training. These years saw the development by James Sibley Watson and Sydney Weinberg of cine radiography, a process of transferring fluoroscopic images to motion picture film.

On Ramsey's retirement, the chair was given to Louis H. Hempleman, Jr., director of the radiobiology program. Hempleman was well known for his studies of low-dose radiation and for demonstrating the deleterious effect of thymic irradiation in children and other radiation abuses. Since Hempleman was not a radiologist, the clinical programs were directed by Stanley Rogoff (diagnostic radiology), Raymond Gramiak (diagnostic ultrasound), and Philip Rubin (radiation therapy). Rogoff excelled in teaching, and in organizing the clinical practice and training program. Gramiak pioneered the use of contrast agents in ultrasound. He also developed collaborative relationships with Electrical Engineering, especially with Robert C. Waag, a leader in computer applications to ultrasound imaging.

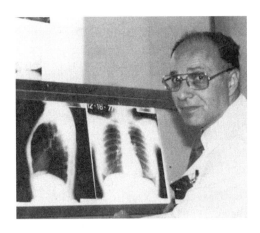

Stanley M. Rogoff, M.D., *Professor of Diagnostic Radiology and Chief of the Division of Diagnostic Radiology, 1965*

Hempleman retired in 1971 and Harry W. Fischer was brought from the University of Michigan to serve as the department's fifth chair. Fischer was most interested in departmental planning. He brought the European model of departmental design to this country and implemented these concepts for the radiology department of the new hospital, which opened in 1975. Many of these principles are still in place today. During his tenure, the first CT scanner (1977) and the first MRI scanner (1984) were installed. Fischer was also interested in contrast media development for radiological image enhancement. Under his direction, many research initiatives and clinical trials were completed, in particular those involving low osmolar contrast agents, then new, but commonly used today. Fischer and Francis Burgener, described early clinical techniques for intravenous cholangiography.

On Fischer's retirement in 1985, interim chair positions were held by John Thornbury, a prominent health outcomes researcher, and Robert O'Mara, the director of nuclear medicine; both men were international leaders in their fields. O'Mara subsequently served as permanent chair from 1988 to 1991. During the 1980s, imaging research continued within the department. Richard Katzberg and Per-Lennart Westesson developed techniques, including the use of MRI, to study temporomandibular joint pathology. Donald Plewes and John Wandtke refined techniques for digital chest radiography.

When O'Mara resigned to pursue full-time clinical practice, John

RUTH A. LAWRENCE

Wandtke became interim chair (1991 to 1993). In 1993, Arvin Robinson was recruited to lead the department. Recent clinical accomplishments include the development of special techniques for small joint MRI and the introduction of innovative interventional techniques in neuroradiology and angiography. The department has become consolidated within the hospital and fellowship training programs have expanded. Research has progressed in functional MRI, ultrasound tissue characterization, and volume tomographic CT scanning.

SURGERY AND ITS RELATED SPECIALTIES

An overview of the contributions made by Rochester surgeons must include their formative impact on the development of cardiac and vascular surgery nationwide; on plastic surgery; joint replacement; and the treatment of burn patients. The following includes many, but certainly not all, highlights from the department of Surgery's several divisions.

General Surgery

Rochester is distinguished for its work in gastrointestinal surgery, for first reporting a series of sclerosing cholangitis, introducing pitressin for bleeding of esophageal varices, and presenting the largest series of splenectomies performed for hematologic disease, including the largest series of myeloid metaplastic disease subjected to splenectomy.

The first primary lipoma of the liver and the largest personal series of hepatic resections were also reported by the department's fourth chair Seymour Schwartz, who also wrote the seminal volume on the liver. Schwartz also served as editor for the *Textbook of Surgery,* now in its seventh edition and the most widely-read text in the field.

The first chair of the Department of Surgery at the University of Rochester was John J. Morton (1924–1953), the surgeon credited with performing the first successful hemipelvectomy in the United States. Morton also reported the classic experience he and a team of investigators had recording the spontaneous regression of malignancies as they followed the medical consequences of the atomic bombing of Hiroshima.

National recognition of the value of managing biliary strictures using a Vitalium tube was explored and published by Herman Pearse. This was followed shortly by the work of Raymond Hinshaw in defining the 45 cm. requirement for a Roux limb to prevent reflux.

During its first three decades, the Department of Surgery included the Divisions of Orthopaedics (which became a department in 1974), Urology (which became a department in the 1969–1970 academic year), and Neurosurgery (which became a department in 1997). The Division of Plastic Surgery led by Robert McCormack contributed significantly to the treatment of burns and the early initiation of hand surgery. The Division of Pediatric Surgery was led by Robert White (1968–1979), who edited the first *Atlas of Pediatric Surgery*. He was joined by Thomas Putnam, M.D. (1966–1993) and later by Robert Emmens (1976). The current director is Walter Pegoli, Jr.

Over the years several dozen members of the faculty of the Department of Surgery have gone on to become department chairs at other universities and hospitals, including Vanderbilt, University of Chicago, New York Hospital, UCLA, Milwaukee, Beth Israel Deaconess, Harvard, Baylor, Cleveland Clinic, the National Children's Hospital in Washington, D.C., St. Christopher's, Temple, Tulane, University of Georgia, Vermont, and Hershey, to mention a few.

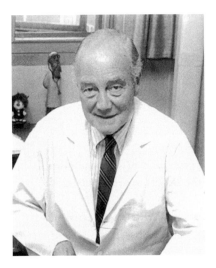

Earle B. Mahoney, M.D.,
Professor of Surgery, introduced cardiac surgery to Rochester in 1945, performed the first open heart procedure in 1955, and the first open heart procedure on cardiopulmonary bypass in 1958.

Adult Cardiac Surgery

Few surgical procedures for adult cardiac diseases were being performed anywhere between 1925 and 1950, except for occasional pericardiectomies. Bailey and Harkens performed the first successful closed operations for mitral stenosis in 1948, and by 1951 Earle Mahoney was performing mitral commissurotomies at Strong Memorial Hospital.

The period from 1950 to 1975 saw a progressive increase in the numbers of cardiac operations performed. Mahoney performed pericardiectomies and mitral and tricuspid commissurotomies. With Paul Yu, chief of Cardiology in the Department of Medicine, Mahoney reported pre- and postoperative studies of these patients in 1950, 1954, and 1956. A heart/lung machine was first used to successfully repair an atrial septal defect in 1953. In 1957, Mahoney, with the help of James DeWeese and Schwartz, first used a heart/lung machine during a surgical procedure at Rochester. Approximately twenty-five surgeries a year were performed during this time period, primarily to correct congenital cardiac defects. After extensive work in the dog laboratory in the 1960s, artificial valves became available as replacements for diseased aortic and mitral valves and the technology was perfected. By 1970, approximately 125 open-heart operations were being performed each year. By the year 2000, that number had grown to 750.

In 1967, DeWeese and Yu reported the first successful replacement of a carcinoid valvular defect. In 1970, DeWeese and Arthur Moss reported the first successful early repair of a ventricular septal rupture due to a myocardial infarction. DeWeese and Mahoney also reported one of the earliest series of successful repairs of traumatic ruptures of the aortic valve.

Interest in valve surgery continued, and in 1976 and 1988 long-term results of aortic valve replacements were reported. More recently, George Hicks, William Risher, and John Snider, have demonstrated the advantages of relocating the pulmonary valve to the aortic valve position (Ross Procedure) when treating aortic valve disease in many patients. Using contemporary techniques, this surgical team frequently is able to repair diseased mitral valves, avoiding valve replacement. Minimally invasive approaches for valve and coronary operations are becoming common.

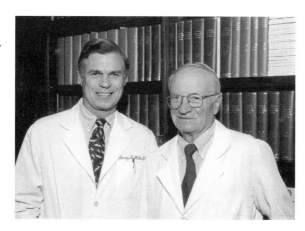

George L. Hicks, M.D., *and* James A. DeWeese, M.D., *leaders in cardio-vascular surgery*

A significant series documenting the successful use of venous grafts to bypass obstructed coronary arteries was reported in 1968 from Cleveland. The first such bypass was performed in Strong Memorial in December 1969 by DeWeese. As the success of this operation increased, the number of open-heart operations performed each year at Strong Memorial Hospital increased to more than 300 by 1975.

During the next decade, Scott Stewart and George Hicks joined the surgical faculty and the number of extracorporeal bypass surgeries performed jumped to 420. Hicks and others had learned that internal mammary arteries were superior to vein grafts as conduits for coronary bypass. In 1984, Hicks reported an improved technique for mobilizing the mammary artery for coronary bypass. Techniques for performing the replacement of thoracic aortic aneurysms were described by DeWeese in 1968. A series of successful operations to repair traumatically ruptured aortas and ascending aortic aneurysms were reported in 1979 and 1980. Risher, working with an endovascular surgical team led by Richard Green has been able to successfully introduce cloth-covered stents into the thoracic aorta through the femoral artery; this technique avoids major thoracic surgery during which the aorta is excised and replaced with a plastic graft.

Since the beginning of cardiac surgery at the university, there has been close cooperation among faculty in Cardiology, Radiology, and Anesthesiology (which became a department in 1969). Together they have developed and reported new or improved diagnostic techniques for selecting and managing patients undergoing cardiac surgery.

Congenital Cardiac Surgery

Earle Mahoney performed the first ligation of a patient's ductus arteriosus in Rochester and a repair of a coarctation. During the next twenty-five years, surgery to correct congenital heart disease became established under the direction of Mahoney and his colleague, James Manning, chief of the Pediatric Cardiology Division. DeWeese and Schwartz from Surgery and Chloe Alexson from Pediatric Cardiology worked closely to establish pediatric cardiac surgery.

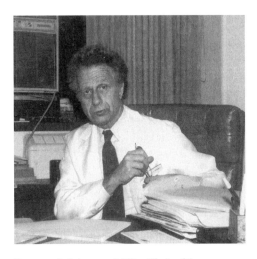

Seymour I. Schwartz, M.D., *Chair of Surgery, 1987–1999*

In 1957, they developed and initiated the use of extra-corporeal circulation while performing procedures to correct complicated congenital defects. In 1959 they reported one of the earliest successful open-heart operations to correct congenital heart defects using hypothermia, in collaboration with colleagues in Anesthesiology.

The team of Stewart, Manning, and Alexson followed the course of all the children who had had surgical corrections. In addition, Stewart modified and developed new approaches to the surgeries used with these children, many of whom had extremely complicated defects; twenty-one publications document his findings and results. Ten other publications report his work with cardiolo-

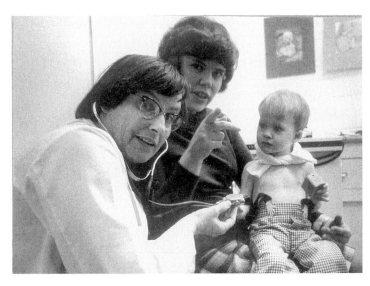

Chloe Alexson, M.D., *pediatric cardiologist, examining a child*

RUTH A. LAWRENCE

gists, radiologists, and anesthesiologists in developing and testing new techniques for the diagnosis, management, and follow-up of these patients.

Manning also developed an influential network of clinical ties to hospitals in northern New York. Through regular visits, during which he consulted with community pediatricians over problem cases involving children with heart disease, Manning brought specialty care to these outlying areas.

During the 1990s, an extracorporeal membrane oxygenation (ECMO) service was developed to support children with poor cardiac ventricular function before and/or after surgery to correct complicated heart defects. Working in conjunction with the neonatologists, ECMO is now also available for use with neonates and other children who have persistent pulmonary hypertension.

Thoracic Surgery

From the years 1926 to 1950, surgical procedures within the chest were rarely performed at Strong Memorial Hospital—except for thoracic sympathectomies first performed by the department's second chair, W. J. Merle Scott, to treat hypertension. Surgical treatment for pulmonary and esophageal diseases was added when George Emerson (the first general surgical resident to obtain additional training in thoracic surgery at Yale) returned to Rochester in 1948.

During the next twenty-five years (1950–1975), thoracic surgery became commonplace and members of the Rochester faculty contributed to the growth of the specialty. Emerson reported early successful treatments of chest wall deformities in children, and he continued to advance the surgical treatment of pulmonary tuberculosis and cancer of the lung and esophagus. In 1954, Mahoney, with Charles Sherman advanced the technique of using the right colon to reconstruct the esophagus.

From 1975 until 1987, Emerson and Clay Phillips reported their extensive experience with esophago-gastrectomy for carcinoma of the esophagus. Richard Feins returned to the university in 1987 and developed a strong non-cardiac clinical thoracic service, performing and advancing leading technology in several areas. These include minimally invasive thorascopic surgery for pulmonary, esophageal, and other intra-thoracic diseases, using techniques such as endoluminal laser ablation and the stenting of esophageal, tracheal and bronchial tumors or stenoses, and most recently, the use of photodynamic therapy for mesothelioma.

Neurosurgery

The major recent clinical advances in the field of neurosurgery at the University of Rochester include the development of a system of computerized surgical navigation for interactive image-guided neurosurgery employing implantable fiducial markers for treating brain tumors and Parkinson's disease. This has resulted in a marketable commercial product.

The development of artificial intelligence software for stereotactic radiosurgery for previously inoperable brain tumors has been equally successful.

From a historical view, many believe that neurosurgery at the University of Rochester began when Harvey Cushing came from Boston to Rochester in October of 1927 to preside at the first surgical clinic at Strong Memorial Hospital. Cushing spoke on the treatment of pituitary tumors, and many of his patients from the surrounding area were presented. Cushing had worked with George Whipple while they were both at Hopkins under the leadership of Osler.

In the early years, neurosurgery at Rochester was performed by John Morton, who had been one of Cushing's first house officers in general surgery at the Peter Bent Brigham Hospital in Boston. William P. VanWagenen joined the surgical staff to specialize in neurosurgery in 1928; he too had trained under Cushing. By 1930, VanWagenen was made an assistant professor of neurological surgery, the very first mention of the specialty in the medical school catalogue.

The Abner Perry Hard Fund was established to support a clinical research fellow in Neurosurgery in 1931; in 1935, Jean Rossier came from Switzerland as the first fellow. The training program in neurosurgery advanced briskly with as many as three people in training at any time. VanWagenen was a leader in the development of the specialty. His report of the successful removal of a pineal tumor and his careful ten-year follow-up review of brain tumor patients from 1924–1925 who had been operated on by Cushing was a landmark.

VanWagenen was the first neurosurgeon to section the corpus callosum in patients with intractable epilepsy and one of the first to perform lobotomies. Since that time, surgical treatment of epilepsy has been advanced and refined; it has been available as a clinical treatment at Strong Memorial Hospital since the 1980s.

Frank P. Smith, a 1941 graduate of the medical school, began his training under VanWagenen. Following a year of fellowship he returned to the faculty in 1949, and in 1954 he replaced VanWagenen as chief upon the former's retirement. Smith's major research was in surgery for pain, intra-arterial chemotherapy for brain tumors, and a variation of common carotid artery ligation of partial sparing of the external carotid artery in the treatment of cerebral aneurysms. In 1974, Smith moved his practice to California but maintained his great interest in Strong and in Rochester neurosurgery.

Joseph V. McDonald became chair in 1975. Shige Okawara had joined the faculty, and his major interest was in clinical research, which spanned ten years, involving endocrinologic and autonomic changes in patients with head injury, as well as the surgical management of severe open head injuries. Okawara began his studies on primate brain implants in association with the Department of Anatomy. McDonald, in the meantime, had developed a successful surgical approach to the heart's autonomic nerve supply in order to treat patients with the prolonged QT Syndrome, a cause of sudden death. Beginning in 1968 McDonald also organized and led the National Neurological Committee, which undertook the arduous but useful task of introducing into modern medical economics a study of cost containment.

Following McDonald's retirement, the department was led by Eugene George and briefly by Okawara and then by Paul Maurer, who had originally trained in Rochester and returned from an academic post at Walter Reed Hospital. Frank Smith, an Emeritus Professor, assisted the Division of Neurosurgery in becoming an independent department. Robert J. Maciunas was recruited to this new chair and became the third Frank P. Smith Professor of Neurosurgery. Maciunas' expertise is in the technological advancements within the field, including stereotactic and image guided surgery.

Plastic Surgery

The program in plastic surgery began in 1935, when Forrest Young was appointed first head of the division. A graduate of Stanford, Young had received surgical training at Rochester and then at Washington University before returning to Rochester to head the newly established unit. He quickly achieved national prominence as a pioneer in the then new field of plastic and reconstructive surgery. Young contributed one of the first papers on immediate excision of a third degree burn in a child, with grafting of the wound on the very day of injury. He became a regional and national leader in the care of children with cleft lip and palate, anomalies of the extremities, facial deformities, and genitourinary deformities.

Robert McCormack became the first plastic surgery resident at Strong Memorial in 1947, working under Forrest Young. Since then, over eighty residents have been trained in this specialty, and many have gone on to leadership positions and prominence nationally. When Young left, McCormack was recruited to return from the practice he had entered in Milwaukee; in 1950 he became head of the Division of Plastic Surgery. He was soon joined by Harold Bales, and then Lester Cramer, who respectively developed special expertise in the care of burns and in maxillo-facial reconstruction. Cramer was the lead investigator in an NIH-funded study of optimal approaches to the management of cleft lip and palate.

After McCollister Evarts arrived as head of Orthopaedics, the two units collaborated in the development of microsurgery of the hand. Plastic Surgery subsequently developed teaching linkages with units around the world, especially in Britain, Scandanavia, and Southeast Asia.

The unit developed special expertise in the care of patients with burns. Faculty physicians and Florence Jacoby, a nurse with special knowledge and skill in burn care, provided national leadership for developing new approaches to the care of patients with this often disfiguring and always painful clinical problem. The high regard in which they were held by their patients is recorded by one of the survivors of the 1963 Mohawk Airlines crash at the Rochester airport, Alan Breslau. He wrote of the superb care he had received and became an advocate and organizer of support groups, nationally and internationally, for patients who had suffered burns and for improvements in the quality of burn care. A distinctive research contribution of the unit was the development of techniques for the growth of skin cells in tissue culture. These studies were the forerunner of current efforts to grow such cells to be used for covering burned surfaces.

McCormack, who served with "unparalleled distinction" as head of the division for thirty-three years, felt himself fortunate to have as associates such outstanding surgeons and teachers as George Reading and Elethea Caldwell who achieved national recognition in their own right.

When McCormack retired in 1983, he was succeeded by Chris Wray, who came to Rochester from Barnes Hospital in St. Louis. More recently, Joseph Serletti has been directing the division.

During Wray's tenure, the department achieved national recognition and prominence because of the leading contributions of Joseph Serletti and his colleagues, in the area of reconstructive microsurgery.

Vascular Surgery

Vascular surgery came into its own as a specialty in the mid-twentieth century. The Society for Vascular Surgery was formed in 1947 as a result of the growing interest in surgical treatment of vascular disease. Rochester faculty surgeons were in the forefront of the field, and John Morton, W.J. Merle Scott, and Herman Pearse became founding members of the Society, based on their published experiences with experimental and clinical application of sympathectomies and popliteal vein ligations for treatment of arteriosclerosis obliterans and for the wrapping of aneurysms with cellophane.

The era of direct arterial reconstruction began in the 1950s. Aneurysms were resected and replaced with homografts or prosthetic grafts, and endarterectomies were performed for arteriosclerotic stenoses or occlusions of the aorta and peripheral vessels. Homografts, veins, and prosthetic grafts were used to bypass or replace occluded or stenotic arteries. These operations were being performed in Rochester by Merle Scott, Andrew Dale, James DeWeese, Seymour Schwartz, and their residents.

Charles Rob became chair of the Department of Surgery in 1961. He had had extensive experience with vascular surgery in England; with Eastcott, he had performed the first carotid artery reconstruction for carotid stenosis and transient ischaemic attacks. Because of the interests of Rob, DeWeese, and Allyn May at Strong Memorial, Wheelock Southgate at Genesee, John Lyon at Highland, and Joseph Geary at Rochester General, and others, general surgery residents became increasingly involved with and interested in vascular surgery. Many went on to more fully develop their skills in this area, and ultimately to perform vascular procedures in their own practices.

The growth in vascular surgery in Rochester and extensive clinical investigation in this field, beginning in the 1960s and 1970s, were largely the fruits of Rob's influence and that of James DeWeese, who soon became a national leader in the discipline. In addition to his work in adult cardiac surgery, DeWeese contributed to the development of a first-rate vascular surgery training program in Rochester and to improvements in vascular surgical treatments. His work was reported in a host of publications on a wide variety of vascular surgical problems. Especially noteworthy was his development of autogenous venous bypass grafts for occlusive peripheral arterial disease, his design of a vena caval clip to prevent recurrent pulmonary embolism, and—with James Adams—his study of primary deep vein thrombosis in the upper extremity.

DeWeese also played a leadership role nationally and was a key player in the development, under the aegis of the American Board of Surgery, of standards for "Certification for Special Competence in Vascular Surgery." Later—after years of negotiation—a plan was developed and approved for separate accreditation of vascular surgery by the ACGME, and DeWeese was deeply involved in these developments as well.

In 1976, Richard Green joined the faculty in Vascular Surgery; he has been extraordinarily productive as a scholar in this field, with experimental and clinical contributions extending across a wide spectrum. Especially noteworthy have been his contributions to the experimental and clinical use of antiplatelet agents to prevent intimal hyperplasia and atherosclerotic occlusion in native vessels and at anastomoses after surgery. He and his colleagues Kenneth Ouriel, John Ricotta, and others have explored the use of thrombolytics to treat graft occlusion. They have conducted studies of the predictors of success after treatment of carotid disease for non-hemispheric symptoms, and more recently—with colleagues in the Department of Radiology—they have developed advances in the endovascular treatment of aneurysms.

In 1997, the Vascular Surgery Section, under the leadership of Green and with the involvement of Ouriel, Cynthia Shortell, and Karl Illig, became a Vascular Center which also included three interventional radiologists—David Waldman, Oscar Gutierrez, and Roy Sumida. The section became a formal division of the Department of Surgery in 1998.

There have been nineteen graduates of the vascular residency. Twelve have gone on to academic appointments, either full time or clinical, and seven are in private practice. Kenneth Ouriel has become chief of Vascular Surgery at the Cleveland Clinic.

UROLOGY

Major advances of the Department of Urology can be summarized by reviewing the work in the field of fertility and the field of prostate cancer research. These also represent major interdepartmental collaborations.

The pioneering work in fertility of the department's first chair, Abraham T. K. Cockett and Ronald Urry has been continued by Robert Davis and Grace Centola. Their efforts are providing andrology and male reproductive services for the entire Rochester region, including consultations, semen analyses, microsurgical vasal and epididymal surgery, electroejaculation, and semen banking. These efforts are very closely coordinated with the university's programs targeting female infertility and in-vitro fertilization.

The role of neuroendocrine cells in cancer of the prostate was originated by Cockett and P. A. di Sant'Agnese. Their work identified the phenomenon of neuroendocrine (NE) differentiation of prostate adenocarcinoma and documented its prognostic significance. This work has been markedly expanded by Guan Wu and Sten Gershagen, who helped identify many of the mediators produced by these NE cells. They are now investigating how, through paracrine and juxtacrine mechanisms, these substances can promote the survival of prostate cancer cells in the androgen-deprived state, and particularly how NE-differentiated cells promote the initiation and progression of osseous metastases. The latter studies are being carried out with members of the Departments of Orthopaedics and Pathology.

Elucidating mechanisms of prostate cancer's escape from androgen deprivation has been the work of Chawnshang Chang, George Hoyt Whipple Professor of Pathology, Urology, Oncology and Biochemistry, in collaboration with Edward H. Messing, M.D., current chair of Urology. Chang and Messing have explained how estrogens, anti-androgens, and normally very weak adrenal androgens can induce the expression of androgen response genes in prostate cancer cells via the androgen receptor and androgen receptor cofactors.

The PIPER genetic algorithm, developed by Yan Yu of the Department of Radiotherapy and its implementation by Yu and Messing have enabled the University of Rochester Medical Center to establish the Finger Lakes' first program for prostate brachytherapy. This unique radiotherapy implant planning system has greatly enhanced the accuracy of treatment planning and the guidance of radioactive seed insertion into the prostate. The computer program uses artificial intelligence to go through 10^{16} iterations to identify optimal seed placement, maximizing radiation to the prostate and minimizing doses to neighboring tissues and the urethra. By being able to perform this treatment planning "real time" in the operating room, Yu and Messing and colleagues, Michael Schell, Ralph Brassacchio (Radiation Therapy), Deborah Rubens, and John Strang (Radiology), have made it possible to achieve optimal dosing in every patient undergoing this treatment.

The use of FLOW cytometry, image analysis, chromosome 9, 9p21 and 9q22 FISH in the detection, monitoring, and prognosis of bladder cancer, initially pioneered by Leon Wheeless (Pathology and Urology) and Irwin Frank, has made important research and clinical contributions through large clinical trials and clinical care.

Pediatric Urology

Ronald Rabinowitz brought specialty urologic care to pediatric patients in the Southern Tier, Finger Lakes, Adirondacks, and Rochester in 1976. Shortly thereafter, he introduced ambulatory pediatric surgery, initially with outpatient orchidopexy. Remaining at the forefront of advocating shorter hospital stays, he also popularized outpatient catheterless hypospadias repair. With the arrival of William Hulbert in 1989, new reconstructive and neuro-urologic services were offered. Clinical and laboratory research regarding testicular torsion, its effect on subsequent fertility, including the value of the cremasteric reflex and the use of color doppler ultrasonography was initiated. Rabinowitz and Hulbert also clarified the optimum timing of penile nerve block for post-operative analgesia in hypospadias repair.

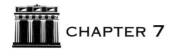

CHAPTER 7

The School of Nursing: Integrating Practice, Research, and Education

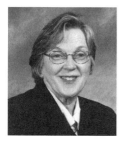
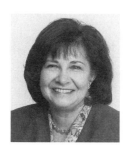
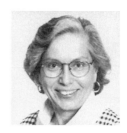

HARRIET J.
KITZMAN, R.N.,
PH.D.

BETHEL A.
POWERS, R.N.,
PH.D.

MADELINE H.
SCHMITT, R.N.,
PH.D., F.A.A.N.

Nursing at the University of Rochester, while holding firm to the high standards set by the School of Nursing's first superintendent, Helen Wood, has evolved in ways that are responsive to the needs and values of other university units (particularly those in the medical center), as well as to society's changing needs. Through research, clinical innovations, and preparation of leaders, nurses here have significantly shaped their discipline and enriched its contributions to health care.

Nursing has evolved over nearly a century, against a national and international backdrop of sociocultural, political, economic, educational, and medical forces. During the history of nursing at Rochester, nursing nationally came to be seen as a profession wherein nurses were accountable for their own practice, a practice governed by scientific knowledge as well as by art and ethics. Preparation for nursing practice changed from an apprenticeship-like training in hospitals to a professional education in colleges and university schools of nursing. Prior to the 1970s, nursing research was conducted by nurses who were well inspired to discover and document but were ill equipped in the methods to analyze the complex phenomena of clinical nursing. Now nurse

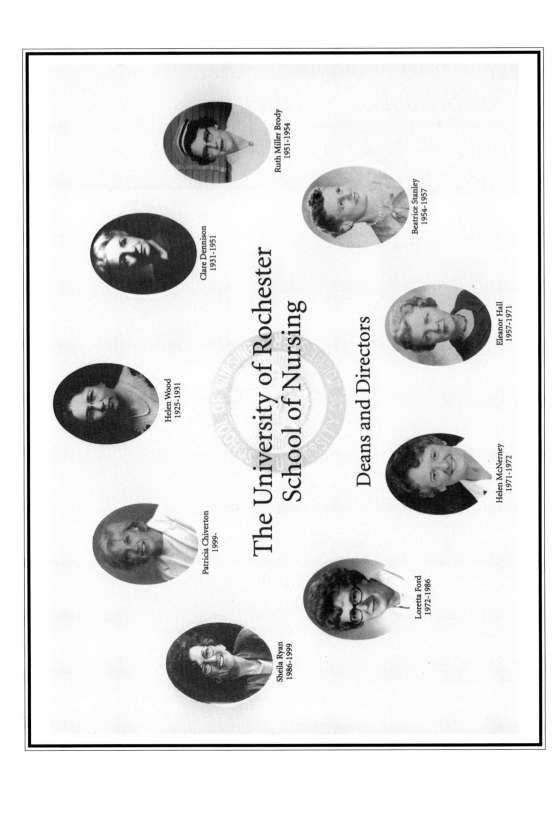

The University of Rochester
School of Nursing

Deans and Directors

Ruth Miller Brody
1951-1954

Beatrice Stanley
1954-1957

Clare Dennison
1931-1951

Eleanor Hall
1957-1971

Helen Wood
1925-1931

Helen McNerney
1971-1972

Patricia Chiverton
1999-

Loretta Ford
1972-1986

Sheila Ryan
1986-1999

scientists, prepared with Ph.D.s and post-doctoral training in nursing, are competing with the best scientists in other fields for NIH funding. These nurses are generating the knowledge necessary for the continued development of evidence-based clinical nursing practice and for nursing's future contributions to society.

Within this context, nursing at Rochester has served as a trailblazer for nursing nationally. The following can provide only a glimpse of the University of Rochester School of Nursing's rich heritage, as well as a partial account of how our future hopes and present endeavors draw strength from those who have gone before. In this chapter, we touch briefly on the formative years of the School, the post-war years, and the 1960–1971 era preceding the establishment of the independent School of Nursing (described so well and in detail by Eleanor Hall in the 1975 history, *To Each His Farthest Star*). The development of educational programs shaped by the Unification model, for which nursing at Rochester is known, along with the School's emphasis on research, innovations in practice, and regional contributions, also are discussed.

THE EARLY YEARS

Helen Wood, R.N., A.B., was appointed superintendent of nurses in 1922, but she delayed coming to Rochester until 1924 when she had com-

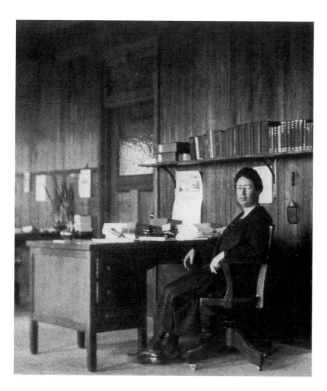

Helen Wood, R.N., A.B., *first Superintendent of Nursing, in 1925. Wood was in the forefront in setting the direction and standards for nursing education. She was involved in the influential Winslow-Goldmark Committee for the study of nursing education and the National League for Nursing Education study on grading nursing schools.*

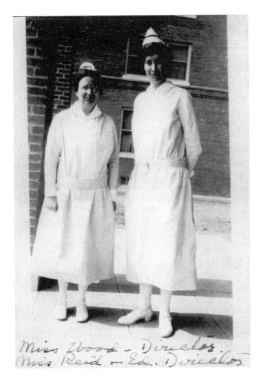

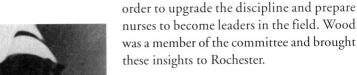

Helen Wood, R.N., A.B., *first Superintendent of Nursing, and* Grace Reid, R.N., B.S., *beloved faculty member*

pleted a master's degree at Teachers College, Columbia University. During her first year here, Wood planned the university's nursing education program. In 1925 the School of Nursing was established concurrently with Strong Memorial Hospital and the School of Medicine and Dentistry. Founding members of the faculty included Wood, Grace Reid, R.N., B.S., Leona Ivers, R.N., and Hanna Peterson, R.N.

From its earliest beginnings the nursing school was known for the quality of its graduates and the excellent patient care they provided. At the time, a university-based education for nurses was a relatively new idea. In 1925, Rochester was among a small number of colleges and universities involved in nursing education. The School of Nursing was founded in the wake of the Goldmark Report, which criticized hospital training programs and recommended university studies for nurses. (This national report, entitled *Nursing and Nursing Education in the United States,* was published in 1923 by the Committee for the Study of Nursing Education.) In order to attract adequate numbers of well-qualified students, the report recommended shortening the course of study from three years to twenty-eight months, eliminating non-educational and repetitive services. It also recommended developing and strengthening university schools of nursing in order to upgrade the discipline and prepare nurses to become leaders in the field. Wood was a member of the committee and brought these insights to Rochester.

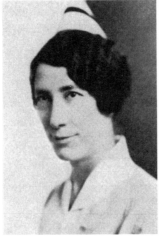

Grace L. Reid, R.N., B.S. *A founding member of the faculty, Reid served as Supervisor of Instruction from 1925 until her retirement in 1949.*

The Growth of Degree and Diploma Programs

In 1925, the School of Nursing established a five-year program leading to a Bachelor of Science degree (granted by the College of Arts and Science) with a major in Nursing (a diploma course of twenty-eight months). Three years of liberal arts study gen-

HARRIET J. KITZMAN, BETHEL A. POWERS, MADELINE H. SCHMITT

erally preceded study for the diploma in nursing, which involved two calendar years and two summers, although students could elect to complete the nursing courses first. The length of the diploma course was increased to thirty-six months in 1934; public health experience at the Visiting Nurse Association (VNA) or the Monroe County Health Department was added in 1934 and psychiatric nursing was added in 1946. By 1945, the degree program included one summer session and could be completed in four-and-a-half calendar years. Both the School of Nursing and the diploma program were administered by Strong Memorial Hospital. The liberal arts coursework that led to the baccalaureate degree was overseen by the degree-granting College of Arts and Science, with acceptance of the nursing coursework completed in the School of Nursing.

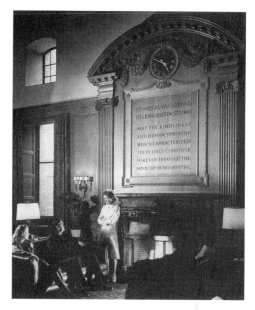

Strong Memorial Lobby, where family members waited to hear news of their loved ones

The College's Nursing Programs

The period 1941–1961 was important in the development of degree-granting programs, short courses, institutes, and workshops for registered nurses. In 1941, a Department of Nursing Education was established to provide courses for registered nurses. The first faculty member was Augusta Patton, R.N., B.S., who was succeeded in 1944 by Esther Thompson, R.N., M.A. Originally a department in the College of Arts and Science, the Department of Nursing Education was reorganized in 1951 as the Division of Nursing Education within the University School of Liberal and Applied Studies; in 1958 it became a department in the College of Education. In 1961, all nursing education was consolidated in the Department of Nursing in the School of Medicine and Dentistry.

The original courses of study focused on ward management and teaching. By 1944, however, a program for registered nurses was offered with a major in nursing education, leading to a Bachelor of Science degree. By 1947 study opportunities were available in obstetrics, operating room nursing, and public health.

In 1951 a program leading to a Master of Science degree in nursing education became available. Although focused on education and supervision, clinical experience was offered at Strong Memorial Hospital, and the program began to lay the groundwork for the clinical specialty programs that were to come.

POST-WAR PRESSURES

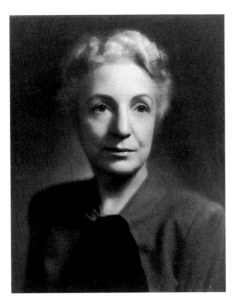

Clare Dennison, R.N., B.S., *led the School of Nursing from 1931 until 1951, first as Superintendent and then as Director of Nursing Service after the title was changed in 1947. During this time many hospitals expanded without having to acknowledge the full cost of nursing care, since most of this care was provided by nurses in training schools. Committed to Strong Memorial Hospital, Dennison attempted to constrain costs while assuring quality care.*

Clare Dennison, R.N., B.S., appointed in 1931 to succeed Helen Wood, retired in 1951, concluding her long era of leadership, both for the School of Nursing and in the development and administration of nursing services at Strong Memorial Hospital. As Director of Nursing Service (a title that replaced Superintendent in 1947), Dennison is remembered for starting one of the first recovery rooms in the nation. Ruth (Miller) Brody, R.N., M.Ed., succeeded Dennison, followed by Beatrice Stanley, R.N., M.Ed., in 1954.

Post-war changes in nursing left the University of Rochester struggling to keep pace organizationally with the national movement in nursing education. Following challenges to the school's accreditation by the National League for Nursing (NLN) in the 1950s, the university sought consultation regarding future directions for the education of nurses from NLN staff member Margaret Bridgman, R.N., Ph.D. In her assessment, Bridgman wrote: "It seems clear that the degree programs now offered by the University are not organized to use these exceptionally fine resources [within the university, Medical Center, and community] in a way consistent with the purposes, standards, and reputation of the institution and with current ideas of higher education in nursing that is well-adapted to service the needs of students and society." Thus, Bridgman brought to the university administration's full awareness the organizational changes needed in order for nursing at Rochester to retain its national leadership status, given changes in the professional discipline.

Bridgman suggested three options for organizing nursing education. The first option was to establish a true school of nursing, closely associated with all cooperating units of the university. The second was to consolidate all nursing programs in a Department of Nursing in the College of Arts and Science. The third option was to separate the degree and diploma programs, transferring the degree program to the College of Arts and Science and leaving the diploma program under the jurisdiction of the hospital.

University evaluators echoed the NLN's concerns. One recommendation made during an accreditation visit by the Middle States Association of Colleges and Secondary Schools was that "all nursing education programs be

HARRIET J. KITZMAN, BETHEL A. POWERS, MADELINE H. SCHMITT

brought together in one unit under one head and one faculty, and that this unit be given sufficient autonomy to plan and conduct such nursing programs as the University determines it requires to fulfill its objectives."

During the 1950s, nursing faculty continued to deal with functional and structural complexities. In 1956, Gertrude Stokes, R.N., B.S., instructor and supervisor of psychiatric nursing, resigned when accreditation of the School's degree program was in question; she perceived that the university had not really decided on what the fate of the program was to be. Stokes also was troubled by the complexities of her status; she served as director of the Advanced Psychiatric Nursing Program in the Department of Education of the University School, in the Department of Psychiatry, and in the School of Nursing. Responding to the resignation, the chairman of Psychiatry, John Romano, M.D., wrote the following to the dean of the School of Medicine and Dentistry, Donald Anderson: "I am writing this detailed letter to you to indicate as emphatically as I can the fundamental importance to our department, among others in the medical school, of a stable, established, collegiate nursing educational program."

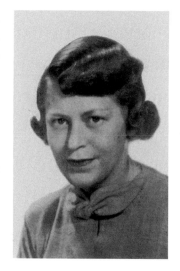

Ruth (Miller) Brody, R.N., M.Ed., *Director of the School of Nursing and Nursing Service, 1951 to 1954. Highly respected and admired for her understanding, judgment, and guidance, she served at a time when hospitals nationally were experiencing a shortage of nurses, along with increased demands for hospital services. Postwar years had brought resources to finance new hospitals and reconstruct existing hospitals. As the accrediting body placed restrictions on using student labor, the nursing shortage that had developed during the war years was intensified.*

NURSING DEPARTMENTS: SERVICE AND EDUCATION

Approval was in place in 1956 for the establishment of the Department of Nursing of the School of Medicine and Dentistry. By placing nursing education in an academic unit of the university, one of the needs identified by the NLN was fulfilled. A year later Nursing was divided into two units—nursing service and nursing education. Beatrice Stanley, R.N., M.S., directed the Department of Nursing Service at Strong Memorial Hospital until 1961. Ann Rosenberg, R.N., B.S., and Marion Nichols, R.N., served as acting directors until Claire O'Neil, R.N., M.S., arrived in 1963. In 1968, Betty Deffenbaugh, R.N., B.S., was appointed acting director and served until the appointment of Margaret Sovie, R.N., Ph.D., in 1976. The director of the nursing service was appointed to sit on the hospital's executive committee.

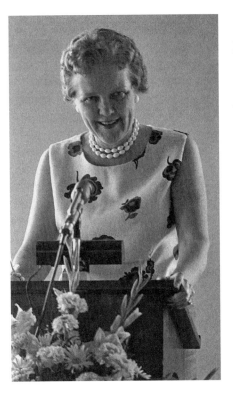

Eleanor Hall, R.N., M.A., *Chair of the Department of Nursing of the School of Medicine and Dentistry from 1957 to 1971, receiving the alumni citation to faculty from the University of Rochester in 1963. In 1975, she was granted honorary membership in the Nursing Alumni Association. Alumni remember well the strength of Hall's leadership in ensuring that nursing faculty and students were recognized and judged by the same criteria as their university colleagues.*

Eleanor Hall, R.N., M.A., was recruited in 1957 to chair the new Department of Nursing in the School of Medicine and Dentistry. She would guide the department through perilous times. NLN accreditation was lost that year (regained in 1960) and an ad hoc joint advisory committee was established by the university president to "provide assistance to the Department of Nursing in developing and strengthening the program leading to the Bachelor of Science Degree with a Major in Nursing." Major changes in program offerings enabled the School to regain accreditation and reestablish relationships within the Medical Center and the university. Hall became a member of the advisory board of the School of Medicine and Dentistry, giving nursing an inside view of policy-making in the Medical Center for the first time.

In 1960, the three-year diploma program admitted its last class; the baccalaureate program remained as the single program for entry into nursing practice. That same year, the university's board of trustees moved to consolidate the multiple nursing educational units. In 1961, the educational programs in the College of Education became part of the Department of Nursing of the School of Medicine and Dentistry. For the first time nursing education was in a single academic unit.

From a financial perspective, however, it was difficult for the educational unit to change from one in which students earned their education through the service they provided in staffing the hospital to one in which they were learners before they served. As a result, Hall needed to manage the department budget under considerable fiscal constraints. For example, in 1967–68, rising deficits were projected at 38 percent of the department's total teaching costs. Expenses for Helen Wood Hall, the building that housed Nursing, were assumed by Strong Memorial Hospital as a patient-care expense, a plan developed when nursing education was hospital-based. The endowment accounted for less than 6 percent of the department's income, and there was no direct university support for nursing education. In comparison, according to the Bates Committee Report, the comparable

Harriet J. Kitzman, Bethel A. Powers, Madeline H. Schmitt

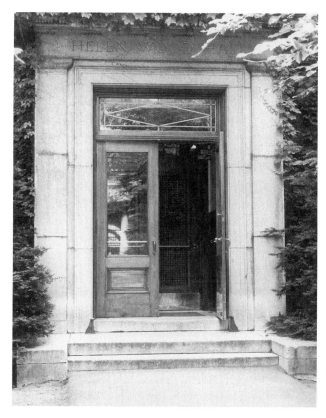

Faculty moved into Helen Wood Hall, the nursing dormitory, before it had a front door. A night watchman padlocked boards together on the outside at night and unlocked them in the morning. When the door finally was installed, Grace Reid remarked, "Never again, as long as this building stands, will these doors be locked."

endowment figure for the College of Arts and Science was 23 percent. The Bates Committee, an ad hoc committee established in 1968 by Dean Lowell Orbison to review the nursing programs, questioned the appropriateness of these arrangements at a time when hospital support of baccalaureate nursing programs typically accounted for only 5.5 percent of costs.

The realities of the pressure that resulted from contemporary educational practices—where students were to be learners rather than hospital staff—began to place constraints on the long hours of service the students were providing. These constraints were not always understood by colleagues who were less familiar with the contemporary trends in nursing education. In 1960, in an extensive memo to Dean Anderson, Hall responded to questions that were being raised about the number of clinical hours students would spend in the hospital. Hall wrote:

> As efforts are continued to improve the clinical instruction of students in order that they will learn to practice nursing effectively, we must work out satisfactory solutions to innumerable problems which prevail at present. If we believe that the major responsibility for the selection and supervision of clinical experience for the students rests with the full-time faculty, we must either increase the faculty or restrict the areas to which students are assigned. . . .

While, on the one hand, we do not favor the "over-protection" of students from the realities of the practice of nursing in hospitals, we do feel obligated to foster the concept that students are learners. As such, they need to approach each new experience thoughtfully, to learn to use the resources at their disposal to deepen their understanding of what the situation requires of them, and to reconstruct the experience with a teacher who can help them utilize it effectively in future care.

Eleanor Hall was well known for her emphasis on academic standards. In 1965, she was invited to speak on "System Barriers to Quality Nursing" at the convention of the New York State League for Nursing. Throughout her career, Hall devoted herself to the pursuit of excellence, counting as one of her highest achievements the elevation of the School of Nursing to the level of academic standards set for the university's other educational units.

Hall remained in her position until 1971, when Helen McNerney, R.N., M.S., took over as acting chair. During Hall's tenure, in countless ways—by holding fast to academic standards, encouraging faculty to develop new clinical roles, and managing the fiscal operations—she paved the way for the independent School of Nursing that was to come.

THE INDEPENDENT SCHOOL

In February 1968, the dean of the Medical School, J. Lowell Orbison, appointed an ad hoc committee to review the nursing programs and establish program goals in nursing education and nursing service. Chaired by Barbara Bates, M.D., this committee recommended strengthening the academic base in nursing, unifying nursing education and nursing service, and partnering nursing and medicine. In a sharp divergence from the direction taken by other schools of nursing, this organizational model would influence nursing nationally.

Loretta C. Ford, R.N., Ed.D., was recruited to be the first dean of the School of Nursing. In 1971, the Kellogg Foundation granted five years of funding to help form and expand this new enterprise. The money helped with the recruitment of new faculty who provided leadership in nursing practice and education, including the development of new clinical nurse specialist and nurse practitioner programs and, ultimately, the doctoral program.

At the school's inauguration, Barbara Lee, program director of the Kellogg Foundation, commented:

The extent of administrative and professional support afforded this new college by the University of Rochester, and particularly by the School of Medicine and Dentistry, must be noted. A University commitment has been made to restructure the Department of Nursing to compare organizationally with the School of Medicine in terms of autonomy, financing, and qualifications of

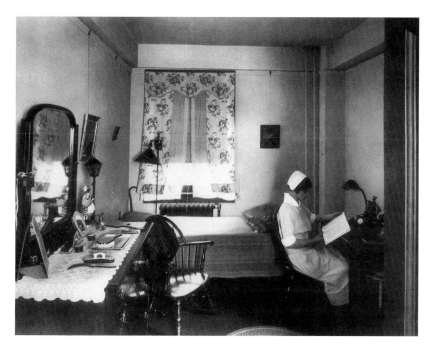

Helen Wood Hall, built to house the School of Nursing, contained the residence hall, as well as administrative offices, classrooms, laboratory, and library. It was expanded during World War II to accommodate the increased number of students in the Cadet Nurse Corps Program.

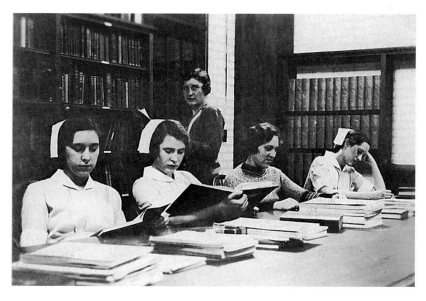

A reference library for nursing students was available in Helen Wood Hall until 1959–60 when it was integrated into the Edward G. Miner Library.

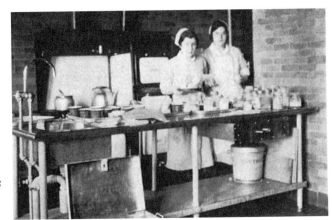

Diet kitchen in 1933

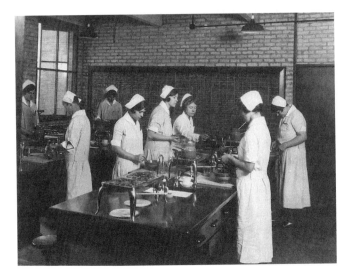

Students in a nutrition laboratory learned to prepare food for both regular and special diets in the course, Nutrition and Cookery.

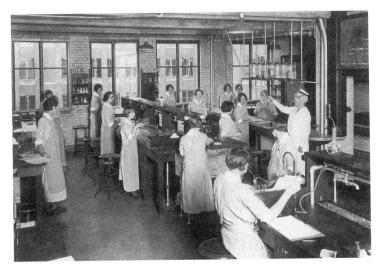

Early chemistry lab

HARRIET J. KITZMAN, BETHEL A. POWERS, MADELINE H. SCHMITT

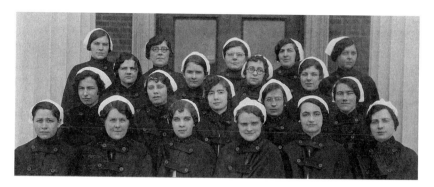

First Graduating Class, 1927

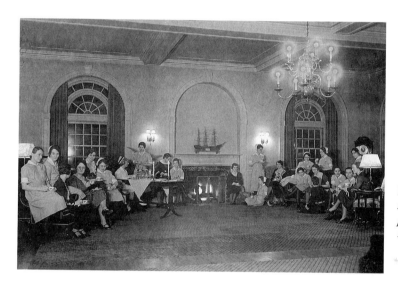

Miss Dennison *serving for a Senior tea party in Helen Wood Hall Lounge, 1932*

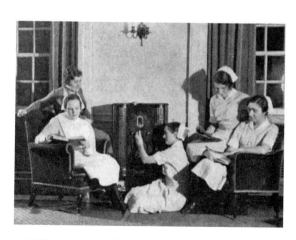

A 1933 evening around the radio in the living room, Helen Wood Hall Lounge

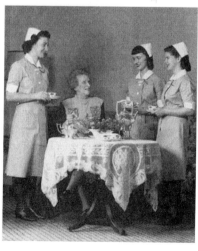

Resident supervisor, Mrs. Crosby, serves tea in 1948

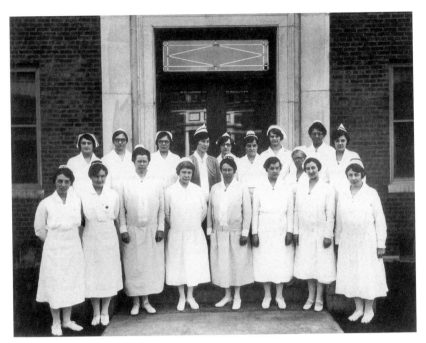

*Early
nursing
faculty*

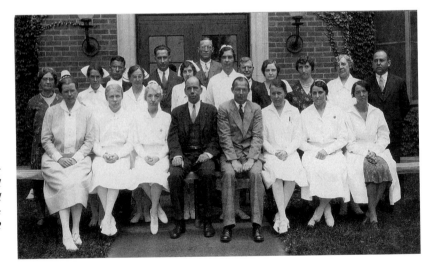

*Strong
Memorial
Hospital
administrators
in 1932*

HARRIET J. KITZMAN, BETHEL A. POWERS, MADELINE H. SCHMITT

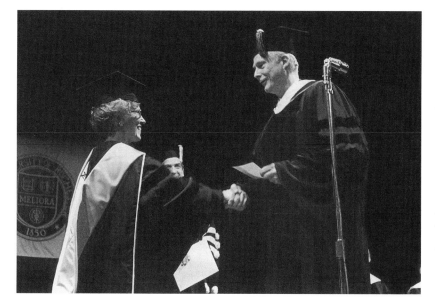

Installation of Loretta C. Ford, *at the inauguration of the School of Nursing by University Chancellor,* W. Allen Wallis, *December 8, 1972*

faculty and facilities. As this commitment becomes reality under the leadership of Dr. Ford, Rochester's School of Nursing can become a model for schools of nursing in similar settings. This alliance between medicine and nursing is as it should be, and cannot help but contribute significantly to the strength of the evolving College.

This alliance was to lay the foundation for many of the decisions that were to come, with interdisciplinary collaboration becoming a theme at the organizational, working group, and individual level.

University president W. Allen Wallis also articulated the direction of the new School of Nursing:

> A primary contribution of the School will be to provide the highly qualified teachers so sorely needed in nursing schools throughout the country. Efforts will focus on two critical problems highlighted by the National Commission for the Study of Nursing and Nursing Education established in 1967: the need for increased research in nursing and the need for new patterns of nursing education, including the education of more nurses who are qualified to teach and to engage in research.

President Wallis served as president of the National Commission for the Study of Nursing and Nursing Education, headquartered in Rochester and directed by Jerome P. Lysaught, Ed.D., professor of education in the Graduate School of Education.

Given the direction of the new school, it was no surprise that an honorary degree was conferred upon Virginia A. Henderson, R.N., M.A., during the inauguration ceremony. Henderson, a faculty member of the School of Nursing between 1929 and 1930, was described by Chancellor Wallis as hav-

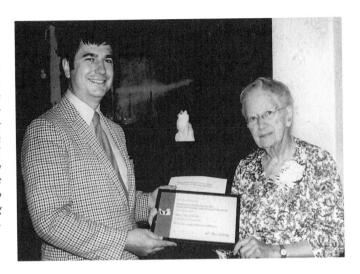

ing "had a profound and lasting effect on education, practice, and research in nursing. . . . Her rare ability to express basic principles in simple language has made her book, *The Nature of Nursing,* a landmark, and her monumental four-volume *Nursing Studies Index* ranks high among her many achievements." In accepting the honor, Henderson said: "The importance of science in undergraduate, graduate, and continuing nursing education cannot be overemphasized; nor can the importance of research as a basis for practice be overemphasized."

Dean Ford, already well established as a leader for her contribution to the development of the nurse practitioner model, brought a new vision to the

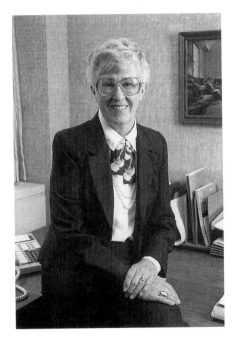

progam regarding what nurses should be doing and how they should be doing it. Her vision, consistent with the direction Rochester had set in its plans for an independent school, included the need for a highly skilled, clinically competent faculty. In addition to educating students, this faculty was to promote the development of new roles for nurses and to conduct the research needed to develop the knowledge base required for advancing the quality of patient care.

The creation of the School of Nursing as an independent school within the university provided the autonomy and authority necessary to promote major changes in nursing education, practice, and research in the context of a renowned medical center. A strong nursing system was to be implemented by nurses whose appointments reflected both academic preparation and clinical skills. This dual appointment concept was to operate at all levels, from the dean of the school, who would simultaneously be the director of nursing service in the Medical Center, to the clinical nurse specialists within the various divisions of the hospital. Designated as Clinicians I and II, these clinical nurse specialists carried academic appointments and were responsible for teaching nursing students. At the intermediate level, appropriately prepared clinical nursing chiefs directed each specialty service in all endeavors—education, service, and research. The parallelism of the clinical nursing chiefs and clinical medical chiefs facilitated the integration of nursing and medicine at the clinical department level. It also provided a mechanism for organization at higher levels. For example, the clinical nursing chiefs and clinical medical chiefs both served on the Strong Memorial Hospital Executive Committee. This organizational model remained in place until 1987.

During the 1980s, the clinical nursing chiefs experienced many competing demands, arising from the numerous responsibilities of the position. Many were new Ph.D. graduates trying to establish their research careers while managing overwhelming administrative responsibilities in practice and education. With the appointment of Sheila Ryan as dean in 1986 the organizational structure was revisited and realigned. Associate dean positions were retained but responsibilities for educational programs and research efforts were shifted from clinical chiefs to division chairs, with the clinical chiefs remaining responsible for nursing service at Strong Memorial Hospital. Responding to the national trend in nursing to enhance research efforts in university schools of nursing, three divisions were established—Health Promotion and Maintenance, Health Care Systems, and Health Restoration—based on the faculty's emerging programs of research. The divisional structure remained in place until 1995, when organizational structures in schools of nursing across the nation were flattening. A new structure then emerged, consisting of the dean and associate deans; coordinators for the Ph.D., master's, and undergraduate programs were phased in over the next three years.

In the fall of 1998, the School of Nursing was faced with a severe financial crisis related to a declining baccalaureate enrollment pattern that had al-

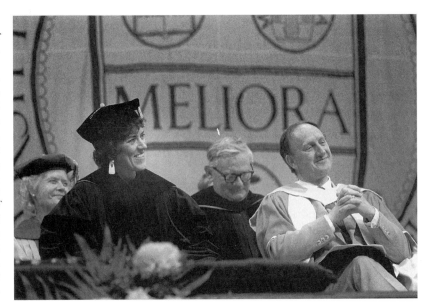

Installation of Dean Sheila A. Ryan. Shown in the picture are board member Monica McConville; Dean Ryan; Robert Joynt, *Dean of the School of Medicine and Dentistry; and* Brian Thompson, *University Provost.*

ready developed nationally and a decline in external research support. As described in that year's annual report, this crisis

> served as a catalyst for a strategic planning process that was comprehensive in its scope (over 100 School of Nursing faculty and students worked on task forces and sub-groups which covered every aspect of education, research, and practice), diverse in its participants (including School of Medicine faculty, employers, clinical staff, and senior leadership of the Medical Center), and involved a short but concentrated time frame. The outcome of that process seeks to return the School to some key aspects of past prominence—the integration of practice and education within the School of Nursing and Strong Health [the University's new health system]—and focuses research effort in a few areas of strength where cross-discipline initiatives and resources can achieve excellence.

A decision was made to phase out the generic baccalaureate program and restructure the baccalaureate program for registered nurses.

At the time of this writing, the strategic plan that emerged is in the process of being implemented. It retains a concept of unification, a nationally recognized hallmark of the School of Nursing for many years.

UNIFICATION OF EDUCATION, PRACTICE, AND RESEARCH

A harbinger of what would become a beacon for nursing at the University of Rochester throughout its seventy-five-year history is this 1924 quote by Helen Wood:

HARRIET J. KITZMAN, BETHEL A. POWERS, MADELINE H. SCHMITT

Some . . . would claim that, for the best interests of all concerned, the hospital should provide a nursing service allowing the school to supplement this service to such a degree as shall be of educational value to its students. I cannot take just this view. I should always want my position as director of a school of nursing to imply that I am by appointment also superintendent of the nursing service of the hospital. I should want to have the staff of the school given the privilege of the responsibility of the nursing services with enough funds available to employ graduates, orderlies, porters, wardmaids, or helpers, to supplement the work of the student nurse and thus maintain the efficient education of the nurse as well as the adequate care of the patient.

The joint responsibility for nursing services, nursing education, and research rested with the director of nursing from 1925 until 1957. In the late 1950s and during the 1960s, when the education and practice units were organizationally separate, tension arose between the units. Evidence suggests that the School's organizational structure was discordant with the philosophy of administrators and faculty who believed that in order to achieve the expected levels of excellence, Nursing must be recognized and governed in a manner similar to other disciplines within the university.

In the 1970s, Dean Loretta Ford strongly upheld the idea that the School of Nursing was a member of the larger Medical Center and university community. At the same time, she worked within what became known as the Unification model to reengage nursing education, practice, and research. Like Helen Wood, Ford linked education and practice through her dual appointment as dean of the nursing school and director of nursing service at Strong Memorial Hospital. Ford was widely credited for the reemergence of faculty practice in schools of nursing across the nation. She also was recognized for building relationships between medicine and nursing that would facilitate interdisciplinary education, practice, and scholarship within the integrated model.

Befitting the tenor of the times, Dorothy M. Smith, R.N., Ed.D., dean of the School of Nursing at the University of Florida, was invited to receive an honorary degree at Dean Ford's inauguration. Smith was cited by Chancellor Wallis as "having brought about fundamental improvements in health care by changes in nursing service and nursing education. She succeeded in reversing the trend toward separation of nursing service and nursing education when, as dean, she undertook the direction of nursing practice at the J. Hillis Miller Health Center, a step then controversial but now accepted." It was this leadership trend that the new School of Nursing was seeking to emulate. Smith reminded the audience: "You will see to it that nursing education does, in fact, embody research and practice, for this is what education in a university is all about."

This emphasis on research and practice was carried through in the School's Ph.D. program, established in 1978, where the focus always has been on clinical nursing research. Addressing major clinical questions through re-

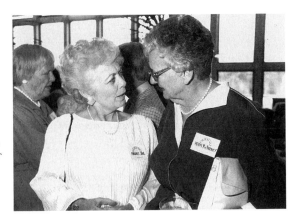

Margaret Sovie, R.N., Ph.D., *and* Helen McNerney, R.N., M.S., *enjoy a conversation at the time of the installation of Dean Sheila Ryan*

search is seen as a joint effort on the part of students and faculty advisors; matching student interests to faculty expertise depends on the support and development of faculty members' independent research programs.

At the installation of Sheila Ryan, R.N., Ph.D., in 1986 as the second dean of the independent School of Nursing, Ryan said:

> The University of Rochester School of Nursing is acclaimed for a successful model of faculty and practice collaboration called unification, which is recognized for advancing innovative nursing practices. Unification II—the next phase—is being built upon the same tenets of excellence and intellectual integration to promote the impact and efficacy of nursing through theory, practice, and research. This model, driven by scholarly productivity of nursing practice and scientific theory in education, provides multiple role opportunities, such as scientist practitioner and scientist researcher. The intellectual integration of theory, practice, and research—the intellectual adventure of disciplined inquiry—is the new goal.

As in the 1960s, nursing in the 1990s was characterized by the structural separation of Strong Memorial Hospital's Nursing Service and the School of Nursing. The concept of unification remained, however, as a template for selecting professional directions within these organizations. Since its inception, ideas about how to make the unification concept work at the level of the individual have varied widely. Because of the perceived difficulty of focusing on all three areas of excellence at any one time in one's career, nurses working within the model in the 1990s were encouraged to focus on "a dyad"—a combination of two of the model's elements (i.e., practice and education, education and research, or research and practice). This was deemed important for professional success at the individual level. It also was thought that the dyad model might bring about a beneficial effect at the organizational level as well, enhancing both nursing service and the School. History will judge how the gains achieved balance the continued striving for closer collaboration between service and education.

HARRIET J. KITZMAN, BETHEL A. POWERS, MADELINE H. SCHMITT

To some, it is a mystery how the concept of unification, which can create such tension in its application, is nonetheless revered. This respect for unification extends well beyond the University of Rochester nursing community and is a cornerstone on which the national reputation of the School has been built. The concept of unification is at its strongest when seen as a reflection of how nurses think about their profession. The inseparability of education, practice, and research, symbolized by the notion of unification, represents a gestalt for the nursing mission of service to the public, as well as for professional self-identity.

CLINICAL SPECIALIST AND NURSE PRACTITIONER PROGRAMS

Clinical Specialist Programs

From the inception of the program that led to a master's degree in nursing education in 1951, until 1968, the graduate program prepared nurses to excel in specialty areas of nursing. During these years, graduates of this and other such programs across the nation experimented with different clinical specialist roles. At Rochester, Josephine Craytor, R.N., M.S., was one of the first of these leaders. Craytor was recognized by the Oncology Nursing Society as one of a few nurses who pioneered the oncology nurse role. She developed and studied the role of the clinical specialist in cancer nursing in her interdisciplinary practice with surgeon Charles Sherman. The Rochester Regional Medical Program, described later in the chapter, brought multiple specialists in the care of the chronically ill and disabled to the faculty at Rochester. Innovations that emerged during this period laid the foundation for the master's program in medical-surgical nursing. Nurses saw new opportunities to excel in clinical practice, and the health-care community saw the contributions that advanced-practice nurses could provide in expanding and enhancing clinical services.

In 1967–68, after an intensive review, the graduate program in nursing was changed from a course of study leading to the degree of Master of Science with a major in nursing education to the degree Master of Science with a major in nursing. Virginia Brantl, R.N., Ph.D., was recruited from the University of Chicago to be associate chairman for graduate study.

A series of courses related to teaching and supervision in nursing was replaced with courses designed to support and underpin clinical practice (at that time within medical-surgical nursing). The intent was to prepare nurses for leadership roles in education, research, and practice. They were to be expert clinicians, improving patient care through use of indirect services. For example, clinical nurse specialists served as in-service educators and consultants to staff nurses, assisting with clinical problem-solving.

During the 1970s there was tremendous development in the program leading to preparation at the master's level. After the introduction in 1973 of the first program in primary care (Family Health Nurse Clinician), new clinical specialty concentrations were developed: psychiatric-mental health nursing (1974), pediatric nursing (1975), gerontological nursing (1976), and community health nursing (1976). Each specialty required four semesters of study; the medical-surgical nursing program could be completed in three semesters.

By 1984, a gero-psychiatric mental health nursing subspecialty program had been added to the gerontological and psychiatric mental health nursing programs, and psychiatric liaison nursing and adult psychiatric mental health nursing had been added to the psychiatric mental health nursing program. In addition, a women's health-care nurse practitioner program had been added.

A nursing administration program was added in 1990 and a midwifery program in 1994. The growth and breadth of program offerings followed patterns of national momentum created around identified needs. Some of the smaller programs could not be sustained as separate programs; the educational content and teaching methodologies established during their development did, however, allow these specialty preparation programs to be included in larger integrated programs. Recent records show that over 1,500 students have graduated from the combined master's programs.

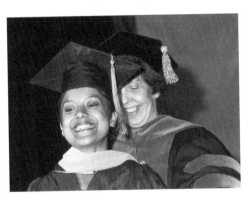

Carole Anderson, R.N., Ph.D., *Associate Dean for Graduate Studies from 1978 to 1986, adjusts the robe of master's graduate* Dahlia Rojas, *May, 1979. Anderson left Rochester in 1986 to become Dean of the Ohio State University School of Nursing.*

Pediatric Nurse Practitioner Program

In the 1960s the Department of Pediatrics, under the chairmanship of Robert J. Haggerty, M.D., was conducting research and providing leadership in the development of services for children in the community. Nursing, in the university and the community, was an important partner.

Development of the pediatric nurse practitioner program began in Rochester as early as 1966, when nurse practitioners trained at the University of Rochester began working with the pediatric resident staff in the House Officers Continuity Clinic. They provided well-child care, rehabilitative care for the ill and disabled, and acute illness screening for children of University of Rochester graduate students, as well as selected families who used the General Pediatric Clinic at Strong Memorial Hospital for primary health care. During 1967, under a Children's Bureau training project, a nurse-physician team working in the Resident Continuity Clinic of the Department of Pediatrics demonstrated that well-child care performed by the nurse member of the team was both efficacious and acceptable to the patients and professionals involved. This paved the way for a major study that was to follow.

In 1968, five nurses were prepared under a grant from the Children's Bureau research program, to work as pediatric nurse practitioners. They were trained by members of the Departments of Pediatrics and Nursing and in the offices of pediatricians' with private practices. The well-child care given by these pediatric nurse practitioner-pediatrician teams was compared to care given by the physician alone. The findings of this randomized trial, reported by Evan Charney, M.D., and Harriet Kitzman, R.N., M.S., supported the quality of care provided by the nurse practitioner-pediatrician teams. The nurses who participated in the trial (Carol Agnew, Esther Berkow, Lois Davis, Carolyn Friedlander, and Nancy Hare) continued their team practices and served as clinical preceptors for pediatric nurse practitioner students.

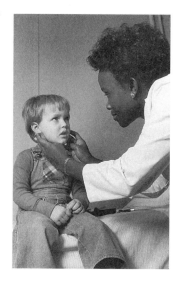

Nnenna Akwari, R.N., M.S., *a 1981 graduate of the master's program in primary care, examines a child.*

Following this study, pediatric nurse practitioners continued to be prepared in a four-month intensive program followed by a preceptorship, after which they received a certificate. Under the direction of Robert Hoekelman, M.D., and Kitzman, a three-year project was funded in 1971 to evaluate the preparation, placement, and performance of pediatric nurse practitioners. Between 1967 and 1975, eighty-seven nurses received certificates for completing the Pediatric Nurse Practitioner continuing education offering.

Medical Nurse Practitioner Program

In January 1969, a small-scale effort began by Barbara Bates, M.D., and medical outpatient department clinic nurses to change the pattern of their work. Each nurse in the clinic was freed from her usual duties to work in a team relationship with a resident physician one half day each week. The nurse-physician teams were asked to explore innovations in their roles. An informal evaluation indicated improved nurse and physician satisfaction and improved patient care; the innovative model attracted several nursing faculty members to the clinic. In May 1969, a nurse clinic was organized to enable nurses to see relatively stable chronically ill patients independently, on referral by physicians. In addition, an evening course in physical diagnosis was developed and

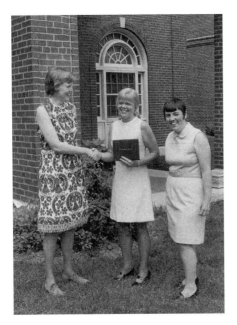

Medical Director Barbara Bates, M.D., *and Nursing Director* Joan Lynaugh, R.N., M.S., *congratulate* Carol Brink, R.N., M.P.H., *an early graduate of the Medical Nurse Practitioner Program. At Rochester, Bates and Lynaugh pioneered development of the medical nurse practitioner role.*

ten nurses from the faculty of the School of Nursing and from the staff of Strong Memorial Hospital participated as learners. Several physicians from the Department of Medicine volunteered as teachers.

By 1971, a planning grant to develop a formalized program for Medical Nurse Practitioner training was approved and funded by the U.S. Public Health Service Division of Nursing. The planning group, comprised of thirteen nurses and twelve physicians, representing a wide variety of health-care settings in the region, worked together in physician-nurse teams. Nurses in the planning group completed a five-week training program supplemented by weekly classes for an additional six months. By working through their own role realignment and practice, they helped identify problems and find solutions, giving health planners, health professionals, and the community an opportunity to see the potential of the nurse-physician team in patient care.

In July 1972, under the directorship of Dr. Bates and Joan Lynaugh, R.N., M.S., a three-year project entitled "Medical Nurse Practitioner: Nursing Education in the Care of Adult Ambulatory Patients and Implementation of Role and Practice" was approved and funded by the Division of Nursing. By 1975, ninety nurse practitioners had been prepared through the continuing education programs. Graduates of the program began working in collaborative practice settings, primarily in western New York but also across the country.

The Graduate Program in Primary Care

As a result of an ongoing study of the pediatric and medical continuing education programs, the Family Health Nurse Clinician (FHNC) Program (later referred to as Primary Care) was developed in 1972 as one component of the master's program. The other component was the Medical Surgical Program. The FHNC program was one of only six programs in the country to prepare nurse practitioners in primary care at the master's level. The program had a strong focus on health promotion and included, in addition to the core courses already in place for the master's program and the new clinical component, courses on family interaction, applied theory of small groups, and human development. The program was designed to help students under-

HARRIET J. KITZMAN, BETHEL A. POWERS, MADELINE H. SCHMITT

stand the multiple factors that affect health behavior and to support the development of interdisciplinary team skills. Clinical courses stressed the importance of always keeping the family context in mind when providing care. Nonetheless, common patterns in medical practice, affecting clinical placement of students and faculty/graduate practice, caused the older and younger tracks of the FHNC program to become synonymous with adult medical and pediatric care. The family nurse practitioner program was added later.

Enrollment climbed from six students in 1972 to forty-eight in 1980. Faculty practiced and precepted students in multiple interdisciplinary practices; indeed, the quality and quantity of preceptorships surpassed those of most programs. The program was funded originally by the Department of Health and Human Services in 1973 and was funded for expansion until 1988.

Given the strength of the commitment to interdisciplinary practice in primary care at the time, it was not surprising that the Robert Wood Johnson Foundation funded the companion proposals made by the School of Medicine and the School of Nursing for primary care education. The program was designed to prepare nurse clinicians to work with high-risk populations, to work in interdisciplinary health teams, and to work in a variety of health-care delivery systems and settings. Here were opportunities for medical and nursing school faculties to continue to work together in their education and practice. The foundation also funded, for the first time, stipends for primary care graduate students to continue their clinical practice during the summer between their first and second year, strengthening their clinical skills base.

Many graduates of the master's program in primary care have been instrumental in developing nursing and nursing education in primary care at the national level. This rigorous program, from both the theoretical and the practice perspectives, provided an excellent foundation for doctoral study in nursing, a direction pursued by many graduates.

Preparing Nursing Faculty as Nurse Practitioners in Primary Care

As nursing competencies evolved to include history taking, physical assessment, and clinical decision-making (an evolution that followed the nurse practitioner movement first conceptualized and developed by Loretta Ford and Henry Silver, M.D., at the University of Colorado), schools of nursing across the country began striving to find faculty prepared to teach these competencies. Because of the work of Rochester faculty in developing the nurse practitioner role in the late 1960s and early 1970s, the University of Rochester was in an ideal position to prepare faculty from across the country in the new methodologies. During 1973–74, the faculty developed a teaching program; by 1981, fifty-five nursing faculty from thirty-four institutions had participated. The primary care nurse practitioner faculty program involved three

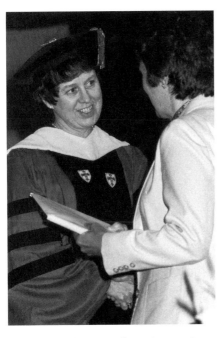

Elaine Hubbard, R.N., Ed.D., *Associate Dean for Undergraduate Studies from 1975 to 1981, presents an award at graduation. Hubbard made major contributions to the development of primary care, as a medical nurse practitioner and as Director of the Robert Wood Johnson Nurse Faculty Fellowship Program in Primary Health Care. She was architect and first director of the Community Nursing Center, serving until her retirement in 1990.*

months of intensive summer study and clinical practicum at Rochester, followed by a preceptorship at participants' home institution for the remainder of the year. The faculty returned to Rochester at the end of the academic year to share experiences, including the results of research projects, and received certificates recognizing their completion of the program.

In 1977, the School of Nursing was selected by the Robert Wood Johnson (RWJ) Foundation as one of four sites in the country to participate in a one-year fellowship program in primary care. This program was headed by Elaine Hubbard, R.N., Ed.D., a medical nurse practitioner with a long history in interdisciplinary practice and academic nursing administration. By the end of the 1981–82 academic year, fifty-one nursing faculty had completed the primary care nurse practitioner program. In addition, twenty-five RWJ fellows had completed the primary care faculty fellowship program. These efforts to instruct faculty in primary care strengthened the teaching base at Rochester and were influential in shaping the educational experiences of nursing students across the country.

The Acute Care Nurse Practitioner Program

In the late 1970s, the "acute care nurse practitioner" role (ACNP) was developed by the Surgical Nursing Service at the University of Rochester Medical Center. The first ACNP, Jill Quinn, R.N., M.S., worked with the cardiothoracic surgical team. Quinn was a graduate of the medical-surgical nursing clinical nurse specialist program and the primary care nurse-practitioner program.

The need for advanced practice nurses prepared to function in both direct and indirect patient care roles in the acute-care setting grew dramatically in the 1980s. To address this need, the medical-surgical clinical nurse specialist master's program went through a number of curriculum revisions with increasing emphasis on the knowledge necessary to deliver direct patient care at an advanced practice level. At the same time, special effort was made to maintain instruction in the knowledge and skills that nurses needed to

HARRIET J. KITZMAN, BETHEL A. POWERS, MADELINE H. SCHMITT

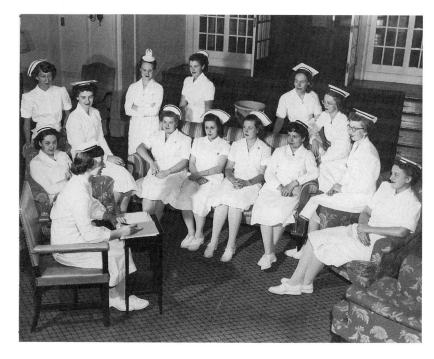

Clinical nursing leaders in conference

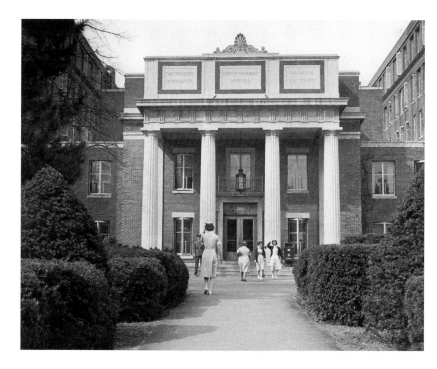

Nurses going to and from Strong Memorial Hospital

Helen Norkelunas Malarkey, R.N.,
a 1941 graduate, and her husband,
Edward, a 1941 graduate of the medical
school, both served in World War II.
Rochester was one of 1,100 schools of
nursing participating in the Cadet Nurse
Corps Program. In 1944, 243 cadet
nurses were enrolled in the School; by
1945, 79 graduates had joined the Nurse
Corps of the Army, Navy, or Air Force.

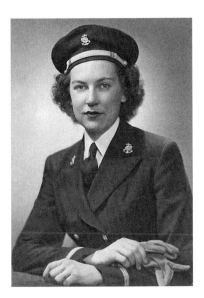

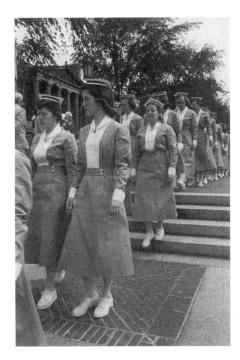

Graduating students on the Eastman
Quadrangle

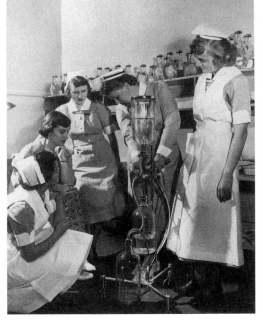

Instruction on using the Wangensteen
suction, a device that produced negative
pressure, used to suction-siphon gas and
fluid from the gastrointestinal tract

HARRIET J. KITZMAN, BETHEL A. POWERS, MADELINE H. SCHMITT

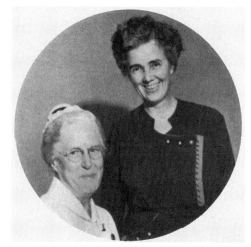

Wenona Abbott, R.N.,
B.S., *and* Helen Vickery,
R.N., B.S., *early faculty in
the School of Nursing*

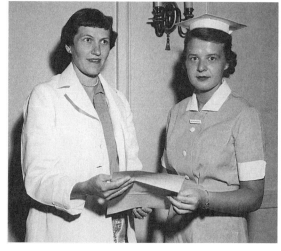

Jane Ladd Gilman, R.N., B.S., *alumnus and
Associate Director of the School of Nursing
during the early 1950s, presents the Clare
Dennison Award to* Marion Lopuszynski
Holliday, *Class of 1955.*

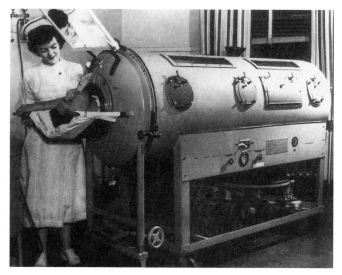

The iron lung

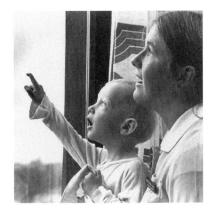

Joanne Vandevalk Clements, R.N., M.S., *in 1977, with a young patient. Clements is one of hundreds of graduates of the master's program. Many serve as administrators and advanced practice nurses at Strong Memorial Hospital.*

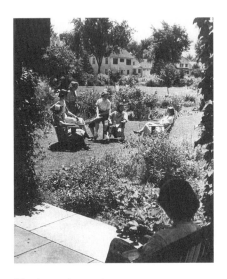

Nursing students enjoy a summer afternoon in the gardens behind Helen Wood Hall.

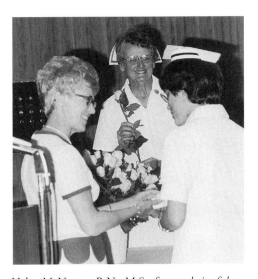

Helen McNerney, R.N., M.S., *former chair of the Department of Nursing, and* Dean Loretta Ford, *with master's graduate* Suzanne McKim, R.N., M.S., *in 1972*

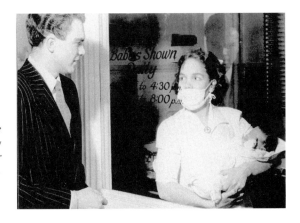

In the 1950s babies were shown through the nursery window for one-half hour twice each day.

HARRIET J. KITZMAN, BETHEL A. POWERS, MADELINE H. SCHMITT

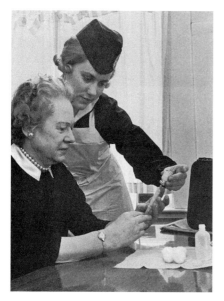

Edith Bickford, *Helen Wood Hall
residence director, poses as a patient, as a
public health nursing student teaches
preparation for an insulin injection.*

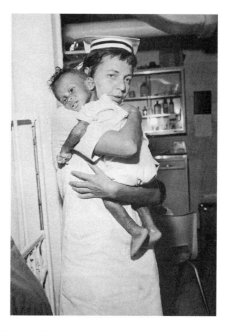

Dorothy D. Aeschliman, R.N., B.S., *Class
of 1949, aboard "Ship Hope." Aeschliman
was one of many graduates who have served in
international health.*

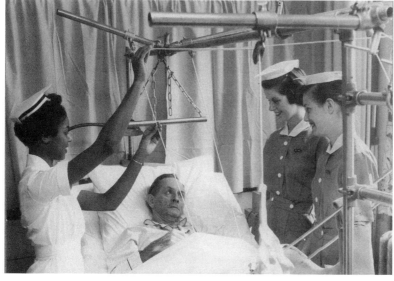

*Undergraduate
students'
instruction*

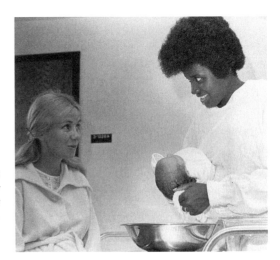

Nursing student shows a mother how best to bathe her baby, a common experience in the obstetrical unit.

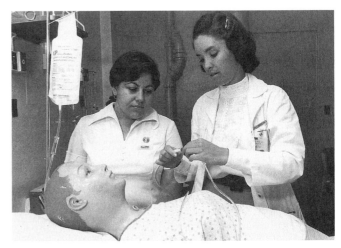

Mannequins are important aids as students learn procedures they will use with patients.

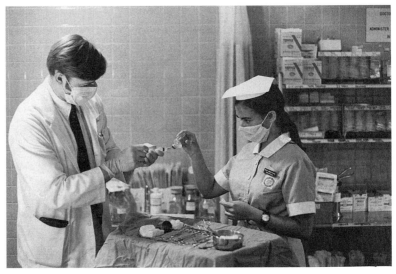

Preparing medications under sterile conditions

HARRIET J. KITZMAN, BETHEL A. POWERS, MADELINE H. SCHMITT

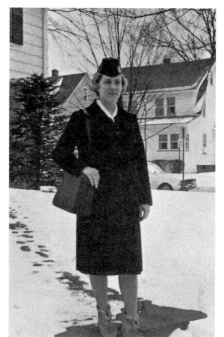

A public health nurse

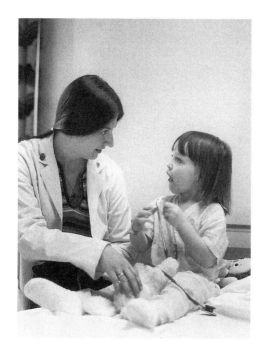

Pamela Foote, R.N., M.S., *a pediatric clinical nurse specialist, cares for a child.*

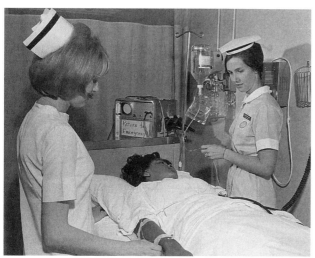

A typical clinical experience

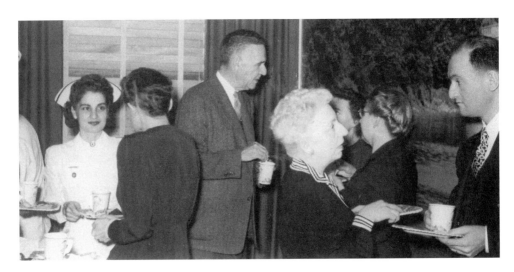

Dean George Whipple *and* Delores Orsine *(in the background) at a 1951 reception. On the right, Director of Nursing* Clare Dennison *talks with* Walter Hamburger, M.D.

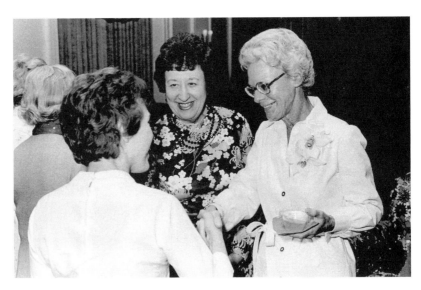

Anne Bater Young, *assistant to the dean, and* Hermine (Rusty) Anderson, *Alumni Executive Secretary for Nursing, at reception for Anderson on her retirement. Young and Anderson worked closely together fostering alumni ties. In 1965 Young, who graduated from the School of Nursing in 1941 and from the College of Arts and Science in 1952, received the University Alumni Citation for her many years of devotion and service.*

HARRIET J. KITZMAN, BETHEL A. POWERS, MADELINE H. SCHMITT

function in indirect patient care roles. By the late 1980s, it became clear that the role of the advanced practice nurse in the acute-care setting had evolved to the point that a major curriculum revision would be beneficial.

Faculty from the medical-surgical clinical nurse specialist program and the adult primary care nurse practitioner program convened to discuss the development of a formal acute-care nurse practitioner (ACNP) program. This program was designed to replace the clinical nurse specialist program and was the first formal acute-care nurse practitioner program in the United States. The educational program was designed to address three major areas: 1) master's-level core content, such as theory, ethics and public policy, and research; 2) advanced practice content, such as advanced physiology, pharmacology, and health assessment and promotion; and 3) specialty clinical content. Principles of both direct and indirect patient care were incorporated into the new curriculum, with special emphasis on collaborative practice and continuity of care. Students were admitted in 1989, and the program received approval from the New York State Department of Education. Graduates are eligible to use the title "nurse practitioner," now a legally protected title in New York State.

In some ways, the title acute-care nurse practitioner is a bit of a misnomer. Although nurses educated in the program focus their practice in a specific area of clinical expertise, their practice is not necessarily limited to the acute-care setting. For example, ACNPs in cardiovascular nursing may be responsible for the care of patients across settings, during the acute and chronic stages of disease. Even so, the title of ACNP has received national recognition.

In summary, from the 1960s evolution of nurse practitioner roles in primary care to the evolution of advanced nurse practitioner roles that is going on today, the University of Rochester School of Nursing has maintained its leading edge and plans to continue in the role of leader and national trendsetter, establishing innovative models of care and education in these areas.

PH.D. PROGRAM IN NURSING

At the inauguration of the School of Nursing, the dean of the School of Medicine and Dentistry, J. Lowell Orbison, commented:

> The inauguration today of the School of Nursing formalizes the commitment of the Medical Center and the University to this new School and to the expanded role of nursing which its inauguration implies. The School of Nursing, and through it, the Medical Center, is dedicated to a renewed emphasis on academic nursing. The continued commitment to the baccalaureate degree and expansion of the program in the master's degree, and the initiation of a program for the Ph.D. degree are all a part of these plans. From this School will

come teachers, administrators, and investigators to contribute throughout the profession to the education of future nurses and to the care of the ill and the injured.

This commitment emphasized the leadership role that the University of Rochester was to have in doctoral education in nursing. In 1969, only five universities offered doctoral programs in nursing. In addition, the number of doctoral degrees awarded to nurses nationwide was low—thirty-eight Ph.D.s and thirty Ed.D.s. By 1975 when the final proposal for the doctoral program in nursing at the University of Rochester was submitted for approval, ten schools were awarding doctoral degrees in nursing. The ten doctorally-prepared School of Nursing faculty who were to teach in the program all had degrees in fields other than nursing. Among the faculty most involved were: Carole Anderson, R.N., Ph.D., Betty Evans, R.N., Ph.D., Loretta Ford, R.N., Ed.D., Jean Johnson, R.N., Ph.D., Thomas Knapp, Ed.D., Klaus Roghmann, Ph.D., Madeline Schmitt, R.N., Ph.D., and Powhatan Woolridge, Ph.D.

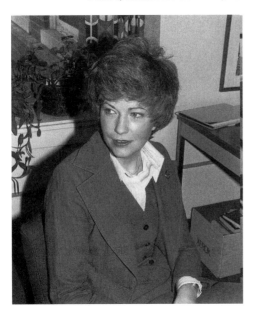

Cheryl Cox, R.N., Ph.D., *first graduate of the Ph.D. program in nursing. Cox is nationally recognized for her program of research related to health promotion.*

Debate arose among the faculty about the type of degree to be offered. The final proposal for the Ph.D. program reads:

The University of Rochester School of Nursing has chosen to pursue the development of a clinical Ph.D. Degree in Nursing. It is the belief of the faculty that a Doctor of Nursing Science Degree (professional degree program) should follow, not precede a Ph.D. in Nursing. A D.N. Sc. implies adequate nursing theory exists to be taught, whereas Ph.D. implies the need for a strong research and theory building component aimed at developing clinical nursing theory with the anticipated outcome that clinical knowledge, understanding, and skills will evolve from which a professional degree can be built. This trend appears to be the most prevalent today and the most defensible.

After approval at the university level, the proposal for a graduate program leading to the degree Doctor of Philosophy in Nursing was submitted in 1977 to the New York State Department of Education for approval. By that time fifteen universities were offering doctoral programs in nursing. The program opened in 1978, and the first students were admitted to the program in 1979, four years after the original proposal was submitted.

A decade later, twenty-nine students had been awarded the Ph.D. degree. By 1990, graduates were already having a visible impact on the profes-

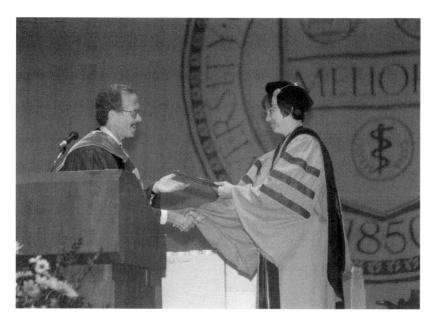

UR President Thomas Jackson *presents the University's 1993 Distinguished Alumni Medal to Ph.D. alumnus* Jacqueline Campbell, R.N., Ph.D. *Currently Anna D. Wolf Professor, Johns Hopkins School of Nursing, Campbell is internationally recognized for her policy-influencing research on family violence.*

sion, holding faculty appointments in fourteen of the major universities in the United States and Canada. Several had completed postdoctoral study and many had received prestigious awards. Rochester was rapidly gaining a reputation for producing first-rate clinical researchers who were heavily recruited as faculty. Many new programs around the country were patterned after the curriculum at Rochester.

In the 1990s, however, Rochester became only one among many universities that offered a doctoral program in nursing. At the beginning of this decade, the Ph.D. was being awarded by forty-two schools and the D.N.Sc., or other doctorate, by eleven. Nevertheless, the reputation of the University of Rochester School of Nursing's doctoral program as unique, highly focused, and rigorous, was well established. Students were highly competitive for National Research Service Award (NRSA) grants; 90 percent of the students who applied for federal funding received it. Between 1990 and 1995, the school received funding from the National Institute of Nursing Research in the form of an institutional NRSA. A total of twelve predoctoral fellows and five postdoctoral fellows received support under this award. A decade later, in 1999, there were seventy-one graduates of the Ph.D. program. About 75 percent of these graduates held faculty positions in nursing schools in the United States, Canada, Greece, and Thailand. Of those in nursing school positions, almost 70 percent had reached senior ranks. Several individuals occupied endowed chairs, dean or associate dean positions, and had been elected to the American

Academy of Nursing. Almost 25 percent of the graduates were in leadership positions in nursing practice settings or private practice. The remaining individuals were retired.

The faculty who developed or are teaching in the Ph.D. program have served as consultants to doctoral programs in many of the leading universities, nationally and internationally. The curriculum, although somewhat modified, has remained relatively consistent since its initiation and the curricula of many other programs have been influenced by it. This speaks to the strength of its original conceptualization.

ROBERT WOOD JOHNSON CLINICAL NURSE SCHOLARS PROGRAM

In the 1970s and early '80s nursing research nationally was constrained by the nearly nonexistent postdoctoral training available to nursing faculty, making it difficult for fledgling nurse investigators, most of them trained in other disciplines, to establish significant programs of clinical nursing research. In response to the need for research training, the Robert Wood Johnson Foundation (RWJF) sponsored a postdoctoral program for nurses from 1983 to 1991. The program goal was to increase the pool of nurses who had the skills to provide leadership for nursing functions in complex health agencies. In a competitive process, three sites were selected for the training of the clinical nurse scholars: University of Pennsylvania, University of Rochester, and University of California at San Francisco. The long history of interdisciplinary collaboration at Rochester, as characterized in the unification of education, research, and practice in both the School of Nursing and the School of Medicine and Dentistry, may have given Rochester a competitive edge in the selection process.

The foundation stipulated that programs would be co-directed by a nurse and a physician. Each site was provided with program planning support. Candidates for the program applied directly to the RWJF. Final selection was made by an advisory committee to the foundation. RWJF provided a stipend based on the salary that applicants were receiving from their home institutions; the maximum stipend was $40,000 a year, and the fellowship was awarded for two years.

Rochester designed a program whose unifying focus was clinical research. Participants were assisted in developing clinical research competencies that could be integrated into teaching, practice, and collaboration within a complex health agency. In addition, experiences were provided to develop skills required for successful clinical teaching and which promoted an understanding of complex political, economic, and administrative climates. The nurse program director was Jean E. Johnson, R.N., Ph.D. Three different medical directors worked with Johnson during the program's duration: Drs.

Paul Griner (1983–1986), Robert Herndon (1986–1989), and Norbert J. Roberts, Jr. (1989–1991).

Each scholar had two mentors, a nurse and a physician. These mentors provided individualized programs of study, guiding scholars in selecting learning experiences, planning a clinical research project, and conducting the pilot stage of the project. Scholars were expected to prepare a proposal for a clinical research project to be submitted to a funding agency at the end of the two-year program.

Twenty nurses received training as RWJF clinical nurse scholars at the University of Rochester. Three nurses started the two-year training program each year from 1983 to 1989. (One was unable to keep her commitment to the program.) At the program's completion, all scholars accepted positions in university-based schools of nursing. All continue to be affiliated with such schools, and most have active research programs.

RESEARCH IN THE SCHOOL OF NURSING

Throughout the lifetime of the School there has been a concern for nursing studies that has informed the quality of nursing care and the conditions that have made that care possible. Clare Dennison wrote about nursing management in emergency situations. She conducted time studies in an attempt to understand how the demands on nursing changed as a result of the increase in the number of medical students and the increasing number of untrained attendants. Faculty studied the organization of the patient care unit, specifically, the impact of the structure of medicine rooms and utility rooms on nursing activity. Esther Thompson conducted studies on the quality of nursing care in the region, eventually using students in the master's in nursing program to help gather data in the region's hospitals. During the late 1950s and 1960s some faculty began to pioneer clinical specialist roles and conduct studies related to the clinical populations for whom they provided specialty care. The fact that they saw research as part of their responsibility is a reflection of the fact that there were few doctorally-prepared nurses and so nursing research activities still rested largely with master's-prepared nurses.

After developing and studying the clinical specialist role in an oncology interdisciplinary team and becoming a cancer project nurse, Josephine Craytor, R.N., M.S., was charged with developing new educational approaches to teaching cancer care to students and nursing staff. Working collaboratively with colleagues in the College of Education, she implemented a series of educational research projects designed to develop programmed instructional materials in cancer and cancer care. These materials were tested on undergraduate nursing students in their classes. This work resulted in numerous articles and culminated in the first programmed

Josephine Craytor, R.N., M.S., *alumnus of the master's program. Craytor conducted one of the first trials of a clinical specialist role (oncology nurse specialist) in Strong Memorial Hospital in 1960. Craytor worked with an attending physician and resident physicians assigned to his service. With no administrative responsibility, Craytor moved throughout the hospital, visiting the doctor's cancer patients, identifying their needs, planning and providing patient care. She conducted one of the first studies that showed that a team approach increased patient satisfaction with physician care and enhanced the preparation for discharge. She was a member of the Bates Committee that later recommended an organizational model that integrated medicine and nursing.*

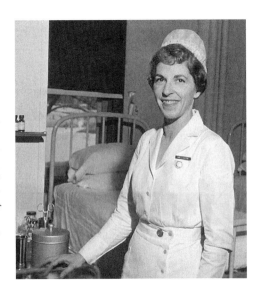

text in cancer care, *The Nurse and the Cancer Patient: A Programmed Text,* published by J. B. Lippincott in 1970. At a time when cancer still carried a social stigma, Craytor also was concerned with changing nurses' and other health-care professionals' attitudes toward cancer patients and their care. With nursing and interdisciplinary colleagues, she conducted a series of studies on the perceptions and attitudes that cancer nurses had about themselves.

Marjorie Pfaudler, R.N., M.A., who developed a specialist role in stroke/rehabilitation nursing at Rochester, also conducted studies during this period. Pfaudler's work focused on the effectiveness of various nursing interventions, such as alternating pressure mattresses to prevent decubitus ulcers from forming with bedridden patients. Mary Wemett, R.N., M.S., who taught fundamentals of nursing, was conducting research on methods to teach foundational skills to undergraduate nursing students. Working with Martha Pitel, R.N., Ph.D., Wemett also published research on the use of the gluteus medius as an intramuscular injection site; students were taught the use of this technique, based on the research findings.

The creation of the autonomous School of Nursing in 1972 resulted in the explicit

Marjorie Pfaudler, R.N., M.A., *a national expert on rehabilitation nursing, served on the faculties of the Departments of Nursing and Preventive Medicine and Community Health. Among the first clinical nurse specialists in the nation, Pfaudler was instrumental in improving the quality of care of the region's disabled.*

inclusion of research as central to the School's mission. The School's Ten Year Plan, published in 1973, stated that "the primary goal . . . is the development of nursing practice theory through research and application of the basic principles developed to the improvement of professional practice and education." The faculty voted to adopt a system of promotion and tenure, with expectations of scholarship for all faculty, that was consistent with university standards. None of the faculty had doctoral preparation to conduct research at the time of Loretta Ford's recruitment to Rochester, and recruitment of faculty qualified to conduct research became a high priority. Seven faculty, prepared at the doctoral level, were in place a year after the school was opened. One was a methodologist recruited to be a resource to the School's faculty and to support curriculum research objectives; the others were all newly graduated from doctoral programs. By 1976 ten faculty members were doctorally-prepared but retention became an issue and the number was the same five years later.

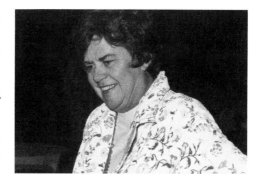

Mary Wemett, R.N., M.S., *alumnus and faculty member from 1957 to 1983, was an esteemed undergraduate teacher and loyal supporter of the university. In 1964, she and nurse-anatomist Martha Pitel, R.N., Ph.D., published research on the use of the gluteus medius as a site for intramuscular injections. Wemett developed and published self-instructional materials to teach nursing skills and was influential in the development of medical nurse practitioners and primary care practice.*

In the early 1970s several research support structures were put into place. An internal Human Subjects Review Committee was established. The nursing alumni organization created a Research Seed Fund and an Alumni Resource Directory. The Seed Fund was a source of support for pilot studies of both faculty and graduate students; it continued into the early 1990s. The resource directory identified alumni willing to assist in implementing research projects.

Research in the first few years was characterized by a large number of mini-studies. Most of these focused on promoting self-care or coping with disease; others were focused on the professional characteristics of the nurse and aspects of the care delivery system. Sustained research productivity and in-depth programs of research were, however, slow to develop, partly due to a lack of research expertise among the faculty and partly because the energies of the newly recruited, more research-oriented faculty were tied up in preparing new graduate educational programs and practice developments. Many were busy serving as clinical nursing chiefs in Strong Memorial Hospital. Under the Unification model, all faculty members were expected to fulfill responsibilities for all three parts of the School's mission: research, education and practice.

To spur the development of clinical nursing research, the School secured funding through a Clinical Research Facilitation grant from the Division of Nursing, Bureau of Health Professions. The purposes of this three-year grant were to establish an administrative support structure for research development; link doctorally-prepared investigators with clinicians to enhance the clinical emphasis of the nursing research enterprise; increase the amount of time faculty had to engage in research; assist faculty in developing, funding, and reporting their research activities; and enrich facilities, resources, and equipment for the conduct of research. Under the grant a research office was created with Madeline Schmitt, R.N., Ph.D., as its director. This position reported directly to the dean and was designed to facilitate faculty and nursing staff research efforts, rather than evaluate them.

The research office became the focal point for coordinating research support services; for expert advice and consultation related to developing research proposals and implementing research and data analysis; for disseminating faculty research money, using a format for review of proposals that followed the Federal research review process; and for programmer, methodologist, and research assistant support. A research committee was created to advise the research office staff and to advise on peer-reviewed requests for funding. (Eventually, the research committee was incorporated into the standing committee structure of the faculty organization.) Research office staff facilitated weekly Brown Bag Research Seminars, developed a research newsletter that was circulated to other schools of nursing, and acted as a conduit for information about requests for proposals, calls for papers, presentations, and the like. An annual Research Day was established, a small research library was developed, and basic research equipment (e.g., tape recorders) was made available.

Other activities during the grant period signified the further development of a research climate in the School. Faculty regulations were revised and two tracks were created, an academic-tenure track and a clinical track, in recognition of the difficulty of master's-prepared faculty to achieve university standards for scholarship. A dozen faculty members initiated doctoral study, some in the school's newly established Ph.D. program, some in other university Ph.D. programs, and some in other institutions. Student research was ongoing in the form of required master's theses, and a nursing honor society was initiated that eventually became a local chapter of Sigma Theta Tau, Epsilon Xi. Under a new associate dean for nursing practice, Margaret Sovie, R.N., Ph.D., the practice environment began to reflect staff involvement in research. A doctorally-prepared Director of Inquiry and Evaluation was sought for the practice setting. The Medical Nursing Service, under clinical chief Nancy Kent R.N., M.S., created a research committee.

At the conclusion of the Clinical Research Facilitation grant, although many research activities had been supported and projects, publications, and presentations had grown, research activities were small in scale, did not have an integrated institutional focus, and lacked further development for external funding. Many, however, were practice-based. For example, a project initiated in 1978 under Nancy Kent focused on evaluating a program to increase com-

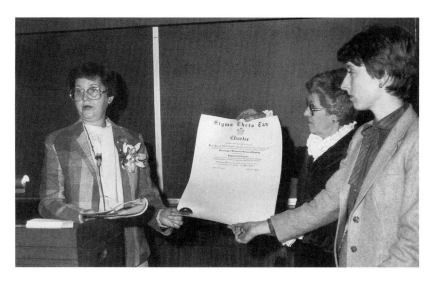

Dean Loretta Ford *and Sigma Theta Tau chapter's first president,* Maureen Friedman, *receive the group's charter from Sigma Theta Tau official,* Helene Clark. *The Epsilon Xi Chapter inducted its first members on March 22, 1979, and has remained active. The honor society sponsors and co-sponsors lecturers, awards for excellence, and provides scholarships and research grants for doctoral students and faculty. The chapter co-sponsors major research events with the school, such as the first National Research Symposium on Social Support and Health, the International Caring Conference, and the fourth Newman Health Systems International Conference. Many faculty and doctoral students have received Sigma Theta Tau International awards in support of their research activities in the 1990s. In 1999 the chapter was awarded the prestigious Research Advancement Award at the Biennial International Conference.*

munication between nurses and patients in an inpatient setting and in an ambulatory clinic. Outcomes of interest included number of broken clinic appointments, quality of patient teaching, and nurses' job satisfaction.

A report of research activity prepared by the research office in 1980 listed almost 125 active research projects. During an extension year of the grant, the research office underwent an organizational change. Between 1980 and 1986 it became a research and planning office directed by a professional health planner responsible to the associate dean for graduate/undergraduate studies. The goals were to promote research and to support the long-range planning efforts of the faculty. The activities initiated to support research under the grant were mostly continued, the network of consultants was expanded, a computing budget was negotiated, and a planning function was added. During the 1980s the office added a peer review network to help strengthen the quality of proposals being submitted for external funding. The research office also provided some instructional support, such as conducting computer classes and reviewing the human subjects approval processes for master's and doctoral students' thesis activities. The staff also conducted a series of planning studies.

In 1982 a new ten-year Long-Range Plan was published. It noted that,

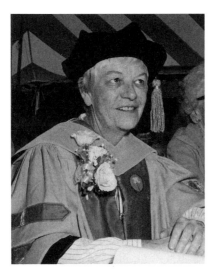

Nancy Kent, R.N., Ed.D., *served many roles during her 1971 to 1999 tenure at the university, including clinical nursing chief, head nurse of the Experimental Unit, nurse practitioner, teacher, and researcher. The nursing clinical chief role helped integrate medicine and nursing and strengthened the interdisciplinary efforts that became a prominent part of our heritage.*

although doctorally-prepared faculty had been recruited to the School, "a large proportion of faculty resources had been diverted to [the development of sound academic programs and the establishment of a model nursing practice program]. . . . The impact of the Unification Model on research productivity of faculty is unknown and needs to be determined." It was noted that a considerable expansion in the number of doctorally-prepared faculty was needed, along with increased research productivity. The goal was to have 50 percent of the faculty doctorally-prepared by 1992. A shift in the predominately junior faculty also was advocated, with a goal that at least 35 percent of the faculty be tenured and 35 percent of the faculty occupy senior ranks by 1992. In 1983–1984, a formal research committee was established. One of its first tasks was to review the research productivity of the faculty and propose strategies for enhancing that productivity.

In the final report of the Clinical Research Facilitation grant, it was noted that there was the potential for the research activities in the Cancer Center to become a research "cluster." The recruitment of Jean E. Johnson, R.N., Ph.D., as associate director for nursing in the Cancer Center, began a long and productive period of cancer-related studies that actualized the mutually beneficial investigative relationships envisioned between master's and doctorally-prepared faculty. By 1983, the work was supported by research funding from the Division of Nursing, Department of Health and Human Services, the RWJF, and the National Cancer Institute (NCI). During 1983–1984, a second cluster of studies, focused on social support processes, was funded through a Nursing Research Emphasis program grant from the Division of Nursing. Ruth Ann O'Brien, R.N., Ph.D., principal investigator, secured individual grant support from the National Institute on Aging.

Sponsored research dollars grew steadily from somewhat over $25,000, in 1977–1978, to about $425,000. In 1985–1986, the School met the external funding criteria for the receipt of a Biomedical Research Support Grant

HARRIET J. KITZMAN, BETHEL A. POWERS, MADELINE H. SCHMITT

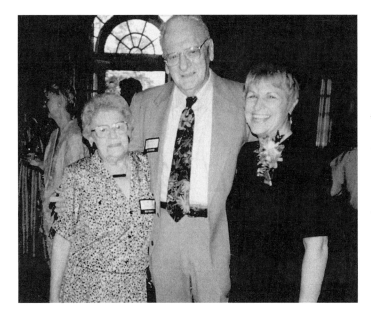

Ruth Miller Brody, R.N., M.Ed., *Director of Nursing from 1951 to 1954, and* Bernard Brody, M.D., *Rochester alumnus, welcome* Veronica Rempusheski, R.N., Ph.D., *on her appointment to the School of Nursing in 1994 as Associate Dean for Research and Director of the newly established Center for Research and Scholarly Practice*

(BRSG) for the first time. BRSG funding became an important resource for pilot research activities until the 1990s, when federal dollars for this activity were no longer available and were replaced by pilot funding internal to the School.

In early 1988, the School's faculty adopted an administrative proposal to create a Center for Nursing Science and Scholarly Practice (CNSSP). The center's director was to foster and oversee the development of a focused research program in the School, propelled by a long-range plan. Management of an array of resources, by the director, was envisioned as instrumental to the success of such a plan. Creation of the Center was delayed, however, until Veronica Rempusheski, R.N., Ph.D., was recruited as director of the CNSSP in 1994. Rempusheski, who had been responsible for nursing research activities at Boston's Beth Israel Hospital, was also appointed as the first associate dean for research.

In 1991, prior to the successful recruitment of a director for the CNSSP, Ann Marie Brooks, R.N., D.N.S., appointed Judith Baggs, R.N., Ph.D., and Nancy Wells, R.N., Ph.D., as co-directors of the Clinical Nursing Research Office. This office, housed in Helen Wood Hall, was to promote improvements in nursing and patient-care delivery via collaborative research efforts between practitioners and researchers in nursing and other disciplines.

With the recruitment of Rempusheski, the CNSSP was established in 1995, in 1,600 square feet of newly renovated space, and a five-year strategic plan for research development was created. Activities and resources that had been available in the old research office were restored and expanded, such as assistance with locating funding sources, proposal preparation, methodological and statistical consultation, regular research exchange seminars, grants management, and the like. In addition, efforts to conceptualize the focus of faculty research efforts were begun. Rempusheski actively encouraged faculty and student participation in the Eastern Nursing Research Society, the regional nursing research organization, and the School was the primary host for the tenth annual anniversary meeting of the society in 1998.

In 1999, the CNSSP was renamed by director and associate dean for research, Bernadette M. Melnyk, R.N., Ph.D., as the Center for Research and Evidence-based Practice (CREP). Renewed emphasis was placed on linking academic support for research with support for research initiatives by clinicians in the practice setting by creating the ARCC (Advancing Research and Clinical Practice through Close Collaboration) model and establishing two associate director positions, one from SMH nursing practice and one from community-centered practice, to implement the model.

Years of discussion about targeted research emphasis came to fruition in the strategic planning process in Spring, 1999. A few areas of national need were identified which coincided with Medical Center research priorities and the nationally recognized research programs of a number of the School's faculty. The identification of these areas of strength led to the establishment of the Center for High-Risk Children and Youth and the Center for Clinical Research on Aging within the CREP. A third center, the Center for Clinical Trials and Medical Device Evaluation, has recently been developed. Initiatives are underway to secure funding for the new centers, to strengthen the core of faculty resources and research efforts of the centers, and to tie the research training of Ph.D. students more closely to the centers' research programs.

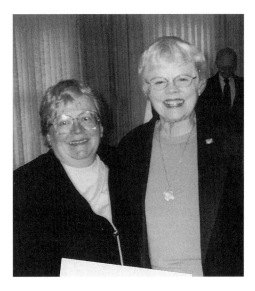

Thelma Wells, R.N., Ph.D., *and* Carol Brink, R.N., M.P.H., *experts in gerontological nursing. Highly recognized internationally for their research on urinary incontinence in older women, Wells and Brink were the first to measure pelvic muscle strength in incontinent women using a vaginal electromyography system. In 1982, they launched a full-scale program of research, using clinical trials to study interventions for urine control in older women. In 1991 they received the second Sigma Theta Tau International Baxter Episteme Award, which recognized their groundbreaking research. They are an excellent example of a researcher-clinician team, a model that Rochester has fostered.*

In summary, the development of a significant nursing research effort in the School of Nursing has been a long, slow process. Throughout its history, faculty research efforts have had a distinctive focus on clinical problems and new models of care, reflecting the strong education-research-practice links that have characterized the philosophy and organization of the School. The establishment of the autonomous School led to a significant and prolonged effort to strengthen research resources and productivity, but, especially during the School's

HARRIET J. KITZMAN, BETHEL A. POWERS, MADELINE H. SCHMITT

early years, this effort was in competition with education and practice goals. Faculty were recruited to the School to develop programs of scholarship and research, and master's-prepared faculty sought research training at the doctoral level in significant numbers. Many of these nurse scholars eventually developed significant, nationally recognized programs of research and trained a second generation of Rochester faculty researchers.

In a paper on twenty-five years of nursing research presented in 1998 to the American Academy of Nursing on its 25th anniversary, several investigators who have spent significant portions of their research careers in Rochester's Nursing School were identified by Johns Hopkins University Dean Sue Donaldson as nursing research "pathfinders." The research of these leaders has changed thinking in such areas as pain perception, female urinary incontinence, and elderly care-giving, not only within nursing but across disciplines. Thus, though the School's full research potential is yet to be realized, the way forward has been well marked by significant faculty research accomplishments.

INNOVATIONS IN PRACTICE

International Exchange Visitor Program for Nurses

Between 1959 and 1972, Strong Memorial Hospital offered an international exchange visitor program for nurses from other countries. These visiting nurses worked at Strong for one year and had the option of spending an additional six months in another hospital program. Starting with five nurses, the program grew to a maximum of fifteen visitors per year for a total of about 150. Nurses came to Rochester from all over the world, including Taiwan, India, Africa, Germany, Austria, Yugoslavia, the Scandanavian countries, and the British Isles. Rochesterians opened their homes and hearts to these visitors and friendships extend to the present.

The program's primary goal nationally was to respond to the severe shortage of nurses. The program at Strong, however, was unique. Not only did it provide clinical learning experiences for the visitors, it taught the politics of health care in the United States as well. Organized and directed by Lynn McClellan, R.N., M.S., director of staff development, the program was chosen as the exemplary program nationally and McClellan was invited to present a report on the Rochester experience at the National Council on State Boards of Nursing.

The Experimental Unit

In 1968, the Medical Center Committee on Nursing appointed a subcommittee on unit planning. A model experimental unit designed around patient needs was among the ideas developed. It was noted that: "Both nurse and physician must establish a relationship with the patient, assessing his needs, sharing appropriately, and developing a plan of care *together.*"

The goal was to demonstrate close working relationships between Nursing and Medicine. At the time that the experimental unit became operational in the early 1970s, plans were being made to build new hospital units at Strong. Thus, the goals for the multidisciplinary experimental unit, headed by Paul Griner, M.D., and Janet Mance, R.N., M.S., were expanded to include trying out new equipment, supplies, and furnishings.

Nursing wanted to try out other innovations as well. Under the guidance of Eleanor Hall, chair of the Department of Nursing, faculty member Nancy Kent, R.N., M.S., became the nursing leader on the unit and undertook the challenge of implementing a new organization of nursing care—primary nursing. Nursing nationally was being influenced by a generation of nurse theorists who were examining the importance of the nurse-patient relationship and the individuality of patient needs. Primary nursing was devised as one model that would strengthen the nurse-patient relationship, as recommended by contemporary nurse theorists. Rochester was among the leaders in the use of this organization of care.

Although some questions raised by the subcommittee were never fully answered—such as, "Is it feasible to expect [the role of the nurse] to change without change in the roles of those with whom [s]he relates?"—the unit laid the groundwork for future emphasis on primary nursing and interdisciplinary team approaches to patient care.

Strong Memorial Hospital as a Magnet Hospital

Margaret Sovie, R.N., Ph.D., was recruited to Rochester in 1976, as the first associate dean for nursing practice and associate director of nursing. An energetic, well-prepared clinician, educator, and nurse executive, Sovie was committed to quality care for patients, career opportunities for nurses, and

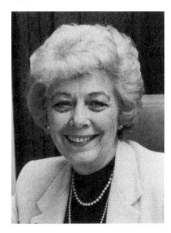

Margaret Sovie, *Associate Director for Nursing at Strong Memorial Hospital and Associate Dean for Nursing Practice from 1976 to 1987. Among Sovie's important research efforts was to "unbundle" the costs of nursing care from the costs of the room and other services. In 1985–86 she found that the cost of direct nursing care for most patients averaged only 18 to 24 percent of the room rate, a proportion far lower than assumed at the time. She is recognized as one of the nation's leading researchers on factors related to hospital nursing that affect patient outcomes.*

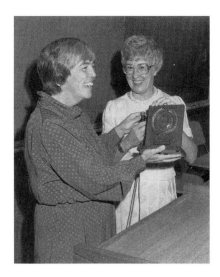

Joan Lynaugh, R.N., Ph.D., *receives the School's Distinguished Alumni Award from* Dean Loretta Ford *during the 1985 convocation. Lynaugh received her bachelor's and master's degrees here and served on the faculty from 1967 to 1975. She developed the Center for Study of the History of Nursing at the University of Pennsylvania and is widely recognized as one of the nation's most notable nurse historians.*

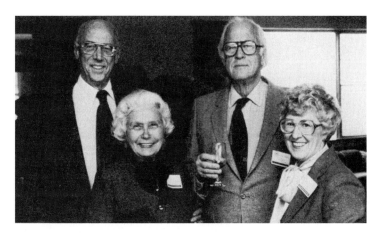

Celebrating the 10th Anniversary of the School of Nursing are honorary members of the University's Board of Trustees; (from left) J. Wallace Ely, Marie Curran Wilson *and* Edward Harris, *with Dean* Loretta Ford. *The celebration included a symposium on "The New Order of Things."*

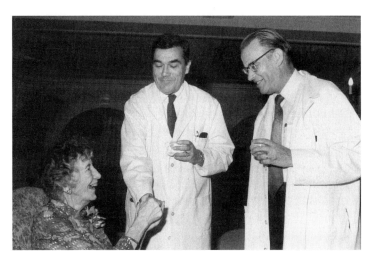

James Bartlett, M.D., *Medical Director of Strong Memorial Hospital, and* J. Lowell Orbison, *Dean of the School of Medicine and Dentistry, greet* Grace L. Reid *on the occasion of the founding of the Grace Reid Society. Reid was recognized for her high professional standards and gift as an understanding teacher.*

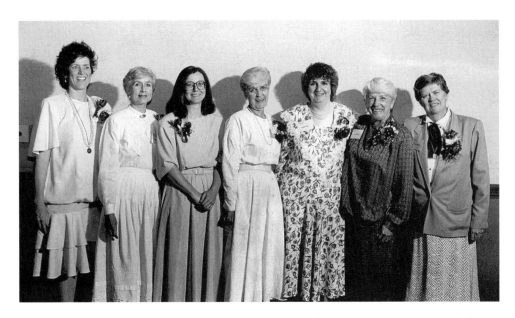

Dean Ryan *with faculty members* Cynthia Hart, R.N., Ed.D., Kathleen King, R.N., Ph.D., Jean Johnson, R.N., Ph.D., Lillian Nail, R.N., Ph.D., Josephine Craytor, R.N., M.S., *and* Mary Wemett, R.N., M.S., *at a reception of the Helen Wood Society*

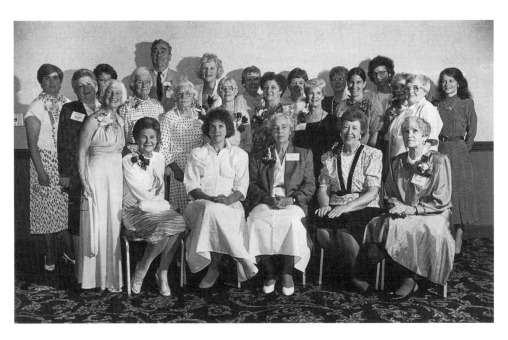

A reception of the Grace Reid Society in 1987

HARRIET J. KITZMAN, BETHEL A. POWERS, MADELINE H. SCHMITT

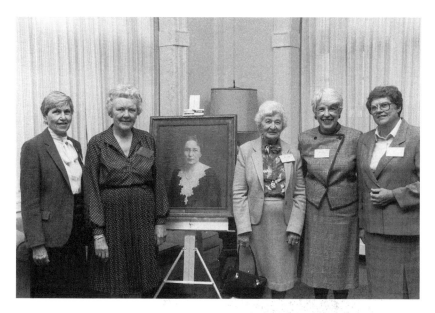

At the 1985 reunion, Helen Wood was honored and her portrait presented. From left, Jane Ladd Gilman, Eleanor Hall, *former Chair of the Department of Nursing,* S. Daphne Corbett, Josephine Craytor, *and* Mary Wemett

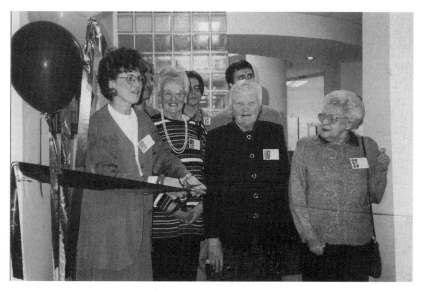

Dean Ryan, *accompanied by* Helen McNerney, Eleanor Hall, *and* Ruth Brody, *all past directors of the School of Nursing, cut the ribbon to celebrate the reopening of Helen Wood Hall on May 2, 1996. The Teaching Learning Center and classrooms were modernized and the administrative offices redesigned to make them more accessible to students. The celebration capped earlier dedication of the Jean Johnson Research Conference Room, the Miller-Brody Board Room, the Clare Dennison Student Lounge, the Jerome Lysaught Seminar Room, the Cynthia Hart Seminar Room, and the Craytor-McNerney Classroom.*

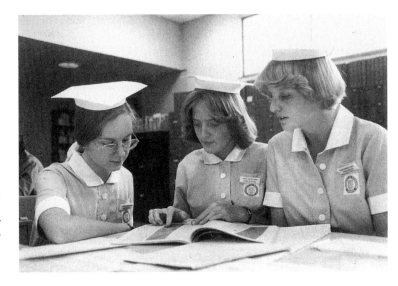

Students in Edward G. Miner Library

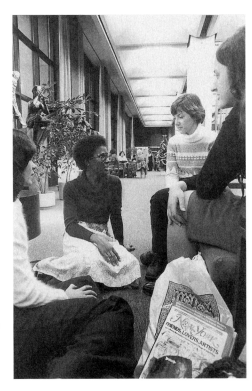

Nursing students find time for an informal discussion.

284   HARRIET J. KITZMAN, BETHEL A. POWERS, MADELINE H. SCHMITT

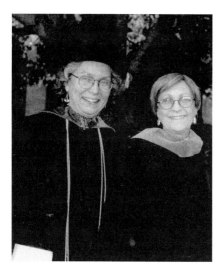

Katharine Donohoe, R.N., *Ph.D. candidate and a 1977 graduate of the master's program in nursing, advanced practice nurse, and clinical faculty member from 1977 until her death in 2000. She is congratulated by* Madeline Schmitt, R.N., Ph.D., *coordinator of the Ph.D. program, upon receiving the first doctoral student Scholarly Nurse Practitioner Award at graduation in 1999. Donohoe gained national and international recognition for her contributions to care of patients with multiple sclerosis and other neurological diseases. In 1999 she received the International Organization of MS Nurses' June Halper Award for her "leadership, innovation, and overall excellence in the field of nursing."*

research related to conditions that enhance both. Under the Unification model, implemented in 1972, Dean Ford had already established the value of having the best prepared nurses at the bedside. As a result, nurses at Strong were ready for the many innovative programs developed under Sovie's leadership. All nursing staff were to be baccalaureate-prepared R.N.s practicing in a primary care organizational model, supported by clinical nurse specialists and expert nurse managers. Conditions were right. Each clinical service was headed by an accomplished clinical chief who was responsible for the quality of patient care, education of students, and research in the specialty. High-quality clinical specialist programs provided a ready supply of graduate nurses well prepared to guide the development of services.

The resulting synergism produced an environment in which nurses could provide high-quality care. Programs that focused on opportunities for nurses included the clinical advancement system (through which nurses were recognized for clinical excellence), awards for excellence in nursing practice, and "Nurses' Week." Salaries recognized longevity and certification. Similarly, programs centered on administrative aspects included the patient classification system (with variable patient billing depending on the level of nursing care delivered) and cost centers for each nursing unit. Educational opportunities included management development, program retreats, and "think tanks." The Professional Nursing Organization and the Staff Nurse Executive Committee were developed as examples of commitment to a professional practice model.

In 1983, as the result of Sovie's leadership, Strong Memorial Hospital was selected as a Magnet Hospital by the American Academy of Nursing (AAN). The national nursing shortage in the 1980s had provided the impetus for the AAN to conduct a study to determine conditions of practice and practice environments satisfying to nurses. From 165 hospitals nominated around the nation, 41 were selected, based on high nurse satisfaction, low job turnover,

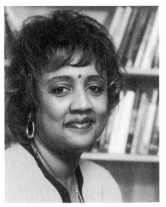

Toni Smith, R.N., Ed.D., *Associate Professor and Coordinator of Methods, Procedures, and Quality Control, Nursing Practice, like several of her contemporaries, has a career dating back to the 1970s, during which she has provided leadership in nursing practice and education at the University of Rochester. A member of the National Academies of Practice, Smith is recognized for developing systems that assure quality of nursing care and that educate students to become administrators in complex hospital environments.*

and low nurse vacancy rates in environments where other hospitals were experiencing nurse shortages. Study reports recognized Strong Memorial for its excellent nursing services. Many of its nursing innovations, including the clinical ladder, were quite different from those in other institutions. Additionally, faculty were immersed in developing and providing quality patient care through their roles as advanced practice nurses and clinical researchers, providing a rich resource for Strong Memorial Hospital.

When Sovie left to accept a position at the University of Pennsylvania in 1987, Alison VanPutte, R.N., Ed.D., acted as interim until Ann Marie Brooks, R.N., D.N.S., was recruited in 1988 as the associate dean for practice and director of nursing at Strong Memorial Hospital. Brooks refined many of the programs set in place during Sovie's tenure. Roles for advanced practice nurses continued to be developed and a position was established for a clinical researcher to support the development of hospital-based research and evaluation. Patricia Witzel, R.N., M.S., M.B.A., succeeded Brooks when she resigned in 1997 and is providing leadership to Strong Memorial nurses at present.

Nursing in the Cancer Center

Josephine Craytor, R.N., M.S., established a strong nursing presence in the University of Rochester Cancer Center. When the Cancer Center was established in 1974, Robert Cooper Jr., M.D., its first director, named Nursing as one of the core divisions and Craytor was appointed its first associate director for nursing. Under her leadership, and with support from an NIH National Cancer Institute core center grant, clinical nurse specialists developed care systems to support medical treatment and clinical trials as well as conducted their own investigations of clinical nursing problems.

After Craytor's retirement, Jean E. Johnson, R.N., Ph.D., was recruited as associate director. The former director of the Center for Research at Wayne State University's College of Nursing in Detroit, Johnson's own research fo-

HARRIET J. KITZMAN, BETHEL A. POWERS, MADELINE H. SCHMITT

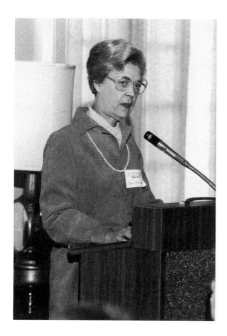

Jean Johnson, R.N., Ph.D., *faculty member from 1979 to 1995, is internationally known for her research on coping with health-care events. Early in her career she showed that people could differentiate between the physical intensity of painful stimuli and the amount of distress they experience. This finding was influential to the understanding of, the research on, and the management of pain.*

Her research on coping contributed significantly to the now accepted belief that a well-informed patient is better able to cope with the events surrounding physical illness. The research identified the specific content of the information provided to patients before a health-care event that reduced the distress they experienced and the interference the event caused in their usual activities. Dr. Johnson's research resulted in a theoretical explanation of how information that varies in content has different influences on patients' emotional and functional responses to health-care events such as undergoing surgery and treatment for cancer.

cused on the use of experimental designs to examine the effects of preparing patients for health-care procedures and surgery.

When Johnson came to the Cancer Center, there were four clinical nurse specialists and three staff nurses in the Division of Nursing. The staff nurses' salaries were covered by physicians' clinical trial research grants and they reported directly to the physicians. Johnson believed that each health-care discipline should set its own standards for practice and should evaluate members of its own discipline. If patients were to fully benefit from nursing care, nurses had to control their practice—a practice based on national standards, nursing research, and self-governance.

Over time, clinical specialists became increasingly involved with staff nurses and direct patient care. As the number of clinic patients increased, more nurses were added to the staff; staff nurse salaries and portions of clinical specialists' salaries were covered by clinical revenues. Clinical specialists and staff nurses worked together as a team, developing skills and systems needed to support a high quality of patient care. Johnson provided overall leadership, helped the nurses develop professionally, and advocated for them and for this model of care with Cancer Center administrators, Strong Memorial's nursing service, and the hospital, as well as with individual physicians. This model, of an advanced-practice nurse who was responsible for insuring the delivery of quality nursing care on each of the clinical services, continued until Johnson retired.

In a pattern consistent with the School's Unification model, Johnson and the clinical specialists held faculty appointments, taught students, and conducted research. The clinical specialists' research focused on problems such as incidence and severity of treatment side effects. Johnson conducted a series of studies to test the effects of theory-based preparatory informational interventions on patients' distress and ability to function while receiving and following radiation therapy. The purpose of the last study—conducted with radiation therapy patients—was to demonstrate the direct application of the prior research, and the theory developed from that research, to the clinical practice of nursing. Research-based preparation for radiation therapy, provided by staff nurses, was observed to be effective in decreasing patients' distress and disruption of their usual activities. Nurses continue to use this research-based knowledge when preparing patients for radiation therapy.

The Nursing Division in the Cancer Center received high marks from outside review groups. National Cancer Institute (NCI) peer review reports of applications for renewals of the center's core grant consistently contained enthusiastic ratings of the Division of Nursing. In 1992, however, Cooper, the center's director, died unexpectedly, at a time when the center was struggling to obtain renewal of its core grant from the NCI. A year later, Johnson retired from her position, and the Cancer Center, and School of Nursing were not successful in recruiting a new leader for the Division of Nursing; the Cancer Center was unable to obtain continued support for nursing from the NCI. Following the opening of the Medical Center's Ambulatory Care Center in 1998, the location of cancer clinics and the nursing structure changed. At that time the Division of Nursing in the Cancer Center was dismantled. Now, nurses caring for patients in the various clinics report to a nurse manager who in turn reports to the administrator for all of ambulatory care.

Care of the Burned Patient

Florence Jacoby, R.N., pioneered the burn nurse specialist role at Strong Memorial Hospital. After graduating from Kings County Hospital School of Nursing in 1942, Jacoby practiced as a public health nurse and private duty nurse in the Rochester area from 1943 to 1969. In 1963, as a private duty nurse, Jacoby suddenly found herself challenged to deliver high-quality nursing care to the most severely burned victim to survive an airline crash at the Monroe County airport, as well as to provide nursing leadership for the care of other burn victims of the crash. When she found little scientific literature to guide her, the care of burn patients became her professional mission. Jacoby created a partnership with her physician and nursing colleagues and, with her patients, she worked to develop burn nursing care strategies, evaluated on the basis of "what worked" for them in their long struggle toward survival and rehabilitation.

Jacoby was instrumental in designing a new burn unit at Strong that became known as one of the top ten burn centers in the nation. She also began writing about what she had learned. She worked with her physician colleagues in research to develop the scientific knowledge base for burn treat-

HARRIET J. KITZMAN, BETHEL A. POWERS, MADELINE H. SCHMITT

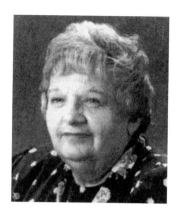

Florence Jacoby, R.N., *developed her international reputation as an expert on burn and wound care at Rochester. In 1990, she received an honorary degree from the State University of New York College at Brockport in recognition of her book,* Nursing Care of the Patient with Burns, *the bible of burn nursing.*

ments and co-published with them. She wrote the first text on burn nursing, *Nursing Care of the Patient with Burns,* published by Mosby in 1972 (translated into Japanese), with a second edition in 1976; the text became an *American Journal of Nursing* Book of the Year.

The knowledge Jacoby generated became the basis for the first national core curriculum for burn nursing care. Jacoby's work was recognized at every level—locally, regionally, nationally, and internationally. Among her numerous contributions, Jacoby served on many of the major committees of the American Burn Association. She was the first nurse appointed a member and eventually became co-chair of Nursing Training and Recruitment Committee of the International Society of Burn Injuries.

Caring for the Chronically Ill: An Interdisciplinary Study

From 1972 to 1976, an innovative practice model was designed, implemented, and evaluated at Monroe Community Hospital under the auspices of a Division of Nursing, Bureau of Health Manpower Education contract. The project, under the leadership of T. Franklin Williams, M.D., and Nancy M. Watson, R.N., M.P.H., was one of the first in the nation to gather objective outcome data on patient health status related to differing approaches to nursing care. The target population was chronically ill, diabetic, ambulatory residents in a long-term care facility.

The two approaches studied in a randomized clinical trial were the usual ambulatory nursing care model and an individualized nursing care model. A battery of outcome measures was developed covering a range of patient outcomes thought to be influenced by the quality of nursing care. Individualized nursing care was linked to a multidisciplinary planning process designed to achieve care coordination across disciplines (nursing, medicine, and dietary). Interest within the Division of Nursing in this experimental model and its relationship to outcomes led to supplementary funding and a broadening of the study goals. Madeline Schmitt, R.N., (Ph.D. candidate at the time), a School of Nursing faculty member who was the project's nursing research consultant, directed this part of the study, which included filming team meetings and studying team processes.

The Community Nursing Center

By the mid-1980s, care was beginning to shift from hospital to community, and community nursing centers were emerging across the nation. The School of Nursing had established its position as a leader in interdisciplinary primary care practice and community program development. The School's Community Nursing Center (CNC) was developed in 1988 under the direction of Elaine Hubbard, R.N., Ed.D., associate dean for community practice. The center's goal was to provide innovative services in settings that also could be used for educating students. Hubbard, a medical nurse practitioner who had been involved in a joint internal medical practice for over a decade, set about establishing "a center without walls" in the community. Unlike many centers in the nation, this one focused on existing sites for care and on the belief that the center should be economically self-sufficient through fee-for-service income. Most centers were demonstration sites supported by external funding.

Patricia Hinton Walker, R.N., Ph.D., took over the directorship on Hubbard's retirement in 1990. During Hinton Walker's tenure, the CNC became a professional corporation, contracts were established for services rendered, and its focus shifted to rural sites, in contrast to the urban settings of the earlier years.

In 1996, with Hinton Walker's departure to become dean at the University of Colorado School of Nursing, Patricia Chiverton, R.N., Ed.D., accepted the position of associate dean for nursing practice and CNC. Although CNC services are still contracted, activities are increasingly programmatic. Part of the CNC's uniqueness is its ability to offer innovative programs. For example, through Strong Health, the university's new integrated delivery system, CNC operates the travel clinic "Passport Health" for the entire health system. Although community nursing centers in other universities have closed, unable to be economically viable after external funding ended, Rochester's CNC continues to grow and flourish.

REGIONAL CONTRIBUTIONS

Supporting Quality Nursing Care in the Region

An important force in the university's nursing contribution to the community and region came with the appointment of Esther Thompson, R.N., M.A. Thompson received the first Rockefeller Foundation fellowship awarded to an American nurse. She received her master's education at Teachers College, Columbia University, and was recruited to Rochester in 1943 as director of the nursing program in the College of Arts and Science. Her charge was to provide direction for the newly established B.S. in nursing education for registered nurses, a program financed by local hospitals. In 1945, an innovative program in regional health planning was funded by the Commonwealth Fund, and Thompson seized leadership for the regional assessment and improvement of nursing care.

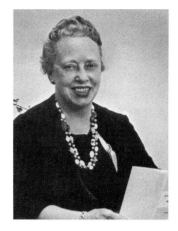

Esther Thompson, R.N., M.A., *came to Rochester in 1943 to direct the newly-established B.S. in nursing education program for registered nurses and to participate in regional health planning. Through her work at the local, regional, and state level, she became a formidable force in improving nursing care at a time when hospitals and long-term care facilities were using many untrained aides.*

Throughout the 1940s and early 1950s, Thompson's complex job responsibilities required sophistication in working with a wide range of health-care professionals—from physicians involved in the regional planning effort, to nursing faculty and students in the university setting, to staff and nursing administrators in rural as well as urban hospital settings. Few positions could have offered such a direct contrast between the realities of nursing practice and quality of nursing care at the time and her vision of what professional nursing should be.

During World War II many nurses were called away from the community, leaving the care of the sick in hospitals to poorly trained aides and those nurses who remained. An anticipated post-war surplus of nurses did not materialize. Madeline Schmitt interviewed Thompson in her retirement and wrote:

> Miss Thompson was "appalled" by the nursing care she observed in her travels about the region. Aides and nurses alike were poorly prepared for their jobs, with much overlap in what various categories of personnel were actually doing. She gathered systematic data on nursing attitudes, activities, and the quality of nursing care, completing numerous regional studies in the 1940s and 1950s. Miss Thompson noted, in a personal interview, that these should have been published, but "we were finding out too much about poor nursing, poor safety practices. Administrators wanted the results squelched."

Thompson served on many local advisory boards, including the local School of Practical Nursing, sponsored by the Board of Education. She stimulated a collaborative agreement to have practical nurses prepared in two hospitals where professional nurses were trained, the first such program in the country, according to Thompson. By the later 1940s, a time when team nursing was common, she initiated and facilitated the incorporation of the practical nurse in a team relationship with the professional nurse.

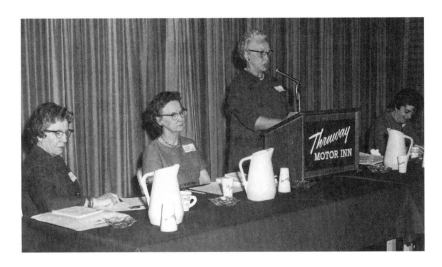

Esther Thompson *speaks to the New York State Nurses Association Workshop on Education.*
She is presenting the Blueprint for the Education of Nurses in New York State, *the*
historic document that recommended professional nursing preparation be set at the
baccalaureate level. With her are Lucille Notter, Katherine Disosway, *and* Veronica
Driscoll. *(Photo courtesy of NYSNA Collection, Foundation of NYSNA Archives.)*

Replacement of untrained aides with better prepared personnel was
Thompson's goal. In the early 1950s, as chair of a study to improve care by
aides, she obtained support from the state health department and the state
hospital association to develop a vocational program for teachers of hospital
aides. While some of Thompson's activities seemed, even to her, contrary to
her commitment to prepare nurses at the baccalaureate level, she was a prag-
matist. She did what she had to do to bring immediate improvement in the
quality of nursing care in the region.

For many years, Thompson conducted continuing education workshops
on a variety of topics for nurse representatives from hospitals in the region.
She had an unusual ability to network and bring together nurses with dispar-
ate agendas, such as directors of nursing services, around a common goal. She
also started the Interagency Inservice Education Committee in 1964, first
chaired by Lynn McClellan, R.N., M.S. This innovative committee was organized under the hospitals in the Rochester Regional Hospital Council, for
which Thompson was the nurse coordinator.

In the early 1950s, Thompson accepted the first in a series of positions
with the New York State Nurses Association (NYSNA) an organization with
which she had a long history, serving as vice president and president, as well as
chair of multiple committees. Under a directive from the NYSNA board in
1966, the Committee on Education, chaired by Thompson, wrote and published *The Blueprint for Nursing Education in New York State.* This became an
important statement that generated extensive debate within the nursing community nationwide. NYSNA recommended that preparation for professional

HARRIET J. KITZMAN, BETHEL A. POWERS, MADELINE H. SCHMITT

nursing be in baccalaureate programs, preparation for technical nursing be in associate degree programs, that diploma nursing schools be phased out by 1972, and that no new practical nursing programs be started.

Thompson's efforts to clarify levels of practice in nursing and to move nursing in New York State toward the goal of baccalaureate education for professional practice were central to her work. Her knowledge of nursing practice, based on her intensive studies, enabled her to articulate a complex understanding of how nursing education was linked to various practice domains. She retired from the university in 1968, leaving a long legacy of support for the development of quality nursing care in the region. Although efforts by the university to retain the regional focus continued for several years, it never reached the level of commitment it had under Thompson's leadership.

The Rochester Regional Medical Program

Edith Olson, R.N., M.S., was recruited by Eleanor Hall in the 1960s to be the nursing director for the Rochester Regional Medical Program (RRMP); Ralph Parker, Jr., M.D., was medical director. Hall had become acquainted with Olson, a national expert on rehabilitation, when they taught together at Yale. Olson subsequently recruited a strong team of nurse specialists to provide nursing leadership in the region.

The RRMP, federally enacted and funded in 1965, was designed to close the gap between existing knowledge about the treatment of heart disease, cancer, and stroke and its application in clinical practice. Later, these diagnoses were expanded to include diabetes, renal disease, and blood dyscrasias.

The University of Rochester School of Medicine was designated as the leader

Edith Olson, R.N., M.S., *was nursing director of the Rochester Regional Medical Program. Recruited from Yale, Olson developed one of the most effective nursing teams in the country, helping to develop care for those with chronic illness in the Finger Lakes region.*

for developing and conducting the RRMP program (largely consisting of continuing education and consultation) in its ten-county region. This region had had a successful decade offering similar activities under the auspices of the Rochester Regional Hospital Council; these activities would be expanded in scope and direction under the RRMP. RRMP was unlike all other such programs in the nation, in recognizing and respecting an interdisciplinary and collegial approach to learning and problem-solving.

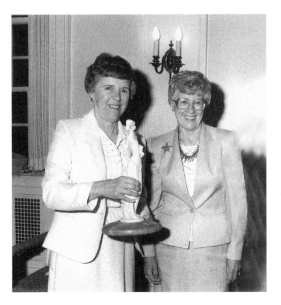

Rose Pinneo, R.N., M.S., *and Dean* Loretta Ford *at the time of Pinneo's retirement. Pinneo was among the first coronary care clinical nurse specialists in the nation. As a faculty member in the Rochester Regional Medical Program, Pinneo contributed to coronary care in the region through continuing education and consultation.*

According to Olson: "When professional persons learn together and stay focused on the patient and his/her needs, there is no need to compete for identity or one-upsmanship."

Rose Pinneo, R.N., M.S., a nurse who helped establish one of the country's first coronary care units in Philadelphia, was recruited to Rochester. Noted cardiologist Paul Yu, M.D., and Pinneo wrote the first coronary care text for nurses. As part of the RRMP, Pineo recruited nurses from all the region's hospitals to come to Rochester for an intense three-week continuing education program; she then helped these nurses set up coronary care units in their own hospitals. Other nurses in the RRMP were Josephine Craytor, R.N., M.S. (cancer), Marjorie Pfaudler, R.N., M.A., and Janet Long, R.N., M.S. (stroke/rehabilitation), Maria Smith, R.N., M.S. (diabetes), Virginia Hanson, R.N., M.S. (renal disease), and Nancy Clark, R.N., M.S. (cardiac disease). The program for each of these disease categories was similar to that designed for coronary care, requiring intensive continuing education and on-site consultation. Monographs were prepared by each group to help people in the region develop the services.

Continuing Education

Nationally, the continuing education movement in nursing started with the first conference in Williamsburg, Virginia, in 1968. Lynn McClellan, R.N., M.S., (who directed staff development in the hospital) was on the national meeting planning committee. The ANA sponsored continuing education groups, which helped establish standards for continuing education. Between 1978–1981, the School of Nursing had a federal Health and Human Services grant to study "A Regional Approach to Continuing Education" for thirteen counties, which included Rochester and New York State's Southern Tier. This project involved convening two northeastern regional meetings and conducting needs assessment; over 20,000 nurses were surveyed. Despite initial grant support, further funding to develop an infrastructure for ongoing regional continuing education could not be secured, and nursing's regional focus was fractured.

Although continuing education programs are still offered by the nursing service of Strong Memorial Hospital and by the School of Nursing, systematic needs assessments have not been done, nor have programs in any area been offered consistently. This in no way has reduced the School's involvement in developing health services in the region. As earlier described, the School's programs have infused the region with advanced practice nurses. Support for quality nursing care in the region has changed only in the means used to achieve this end.

Community Health Nurse Connections

A close connection developed between nursing at the University of Rochester and nursing at the Visiting Nurse Service (VNS) and the Monroe County Health Department. Both were to become among the most progressive community health nurse agencies in the nation. For example, the first "meals on wheels" service of VNS was developed in Rochester under the leadership of its director, Elizabeth Phillips, R.N., M.S. Similarly, the nursing division of the Monroe County Health Department, under the leadership of Katherine Neill, R.N., M.S., initiated the development of many innovative nursing services that were to gain national recognition.

Katherine Neill, an early graduate of the master's program at the University of Rochester, taught a course on community aspects of nursing in the mid-1940s and served as a senior associate on the faculty of the School of Nursing until her retirement in 1982. An innovator and researcher, she is credited with pioneering many programs that have become standard care.

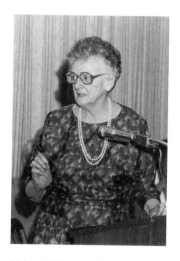

Helen McNerney, *alumnus of the early master's program, esteemed teacher and able administrator. McNerney served in multiple roles, always bridging to the community. As the first Nursing Director of the Rochester Neighborhood Health Center, she paved the way for new nursing services in the urban area. From 1975 to 1981 she served as Executive Director of the Visiting Nursing Service of Rochester and Monroe County and was a member of more than twenty community boards and advisory committees.*

Undergraduate students at the University of Rochester received their public health/community nursing experiences at VNS and at the county health department. In 1975, Helen McNerney, R.N., M.S., past interim chair of the Department of Nursing, became the director of the VNS, where she served until 1981. In 1999, the VNS became part of Strong Health, the university's integrated health delivery system.

The Rochester Neighborhood Health Center

The Rochester Neighborhood Health Center was developed during the 1960s under the leadership of Evan Charney, M.D., associate professor of pediatrics, and Helen McNerney. Emphasis was placed on team care, with both physicians and nurses assuming responsibility. The first center, established in the inner city, was funded by the Office of Economic Opportunity and originally administered by the university through the aegis of the local anti-poverty agency, Action For A Better Community. Kenneth Woodward, M.D., an alumnus and assistant professor of preventive medicine and community health at the medical school, was its first medical director and McNerney was its first nursing director. By 1972, the center was offering comprehensive family-based health care to its 15,000 registered patients, including preventive and therapeutic services.

Innovative community programs were not new to nurses in Rochester. They were involved in what was to be the forerunner of the Community Mental Health Center (CMHC). Under the leadership of the Department of Psychiatry, public health nurses employed by the county health department were assigned by nursing director Katherine Neill to work in teams with psychiatry residents and social workers, delivering mental health services to inner-city families where one family member had been diagnosed with a serious mental health problem. Several features made the Neighborhood Health Center noteworthy from a nursing perspective. First, planning was an interdisciplinary collaborative effort, with faculty members from Medicine and Nursing and members of the community participating. Second, the first six nurses were full-time employees of the county health department; Neill assigned nurses to cover public health nursing needs at the center. Third, the nurses were prepared as nurse practitioners through programs at the School of Nursing, enabling them to enhance their contributions to the health-care team.

THE COMMONWEALTH EXECUTIVE NURSE FELLOWSHIP PROGRAM

In the early 1980s, directors of the Commonwealth Fund recognized that nursing leaders needed to "adopt a comprehensive view of health-care institutions and their social contexts or wholes, and the mission they undertake." With the help of Dean Loretta C. Ford, the Commonwealth Fund supported the development of a national cadre of outstanding nurse executives who would have the potential to improve the delivery of health care in the United States. The Commonwealth Executive Nurse Fellowship Program

HARRIET J. KITZMAN, BETHEL A. POWERS, MADELINE H. SCHMITT

began in 1983, and Ford was named national program director. Dean Sheila A. Ryan later accepted the directorship when Ford retired. Although the program was modified over its twelve years of operation, its primary emphasis was to support nurses with advanced degrees in clinical nursing during their M.B.A. studies. Thus, it acknowledged the need to combine clinical expertise and management in health care.

Between 1986 and 1993, 147 fellowships were awarded to nurses in the Executive Nurse Fellowship Program of the Commonwealth Fund. This important national program, headquartered at the University of Rochester, has been influential in preparing a large number of nurses for hospital executive and management positions.

SUMMATION

Themes emanate from the history of the School of Nursing. One is an ongoing commitment to unification and the belief that high-quality care is best accomplished when education, clinical practice, and research occur in close proximity. Educational and research programs have emphasized the need for rigor in science, the need to understand the art of practice, and the importance of human values that underpin the care of people. Research programs have focused on developing the science necessary to address important challenges and perplexing problems encountered in clinical practice.

Another theme is commitment to developing and providing quality nursing care for the institution and the region, along with a commitment to interdisciplinary collaboration. There has been a persistent underlying belief that the highest quality nursing care comes from joint efforts with other disciplines to prepare care providers, to plan, deliver, and evaluate services, and to form the discourse that drives health policy. Many organizational and programmatic decisions have reflected this belief. The result of these commitments is a rich and uncommon history of concern for the quality of nursing care in the region.

Nursing at the University of Rochester has faced many challenges. Although Helen Wood in the early 1920s envisioned a school that offered postgraduate as well as basic nursing instruction, postgraduate instruction did not become a reality until 1941. The years 1941–1972 were times of struggle, growth, and change, as Nursing was administered in multiple divisions within the university. Faculty worked across departments and services in order to provide diploma, baccalaureate, postgraduate certificate, master's, and continuing education programs. During this period, the educational activities of the School of Nursing, originally administered by Strong Memorial Hospital, were gradually acknowledged within the academic framework of the university.

Although Rochester may have been behind the times in establishing an independent school of nursing (autonomy only came in 1972), nursing at the University of Rochester, from its beginning to the present, has been ahead of the times in conducting research, developing new models of nursing care, and preparing generations of nurses as master clinicians, scholars, and leaders. The School of Nursing's current vision and strategic plan chart a bold forward course, no less challenging than what has gone before and grounded in values and commitments that have inspired important innovations in practice and advances in research and education throughout its history.

HARRIET J. KITZMAN, BETHEL A. POWERS, MADELINE H. SCHMITT

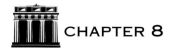

CHAPTER 8

Eastman Dental Center: Its History and Relationship to the Medical Center

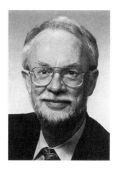

RONALD J. BILLINGS,
D.D.S., M.S.D.

In 1915, a unique institution was founded in upstate New York to provide dental care for children. The Rochester Dental Dispensary was George Eastman's gift to the city of Rochester and its children, but more than one man's vision has shaped the institution. Over the years, the Eastman Dental Center (as the dispensary was renamed after the philanthropist's death) has been a major force in dentistry worldwide, educating generations of dental leaders and providing new levels of oral health care through research, education, and patient care.

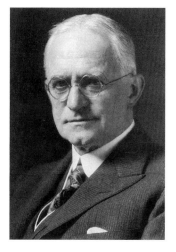

George Eastman

Now a division of the University of Rochester Medical Center, the center's diverse programs have been nurtured and expanded by some extraordinary individuals during the past eighty-five years. Rochester had enlightened leadership in the early part of the 20th century, not only from George Eastman but from Captain Henry

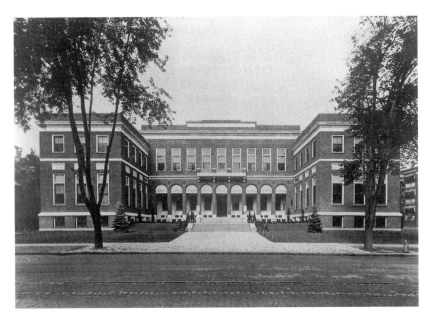

Lomb and William Bausch, as well. These two industrialists persuaded Eastman to donate funds to build and equip the dispensary and added their own donations to the funds. They convinced the city of Rochester to budget annual funds to help cover the costs of caring for children who had little or no access to dental care.

Eastman viewed his gift to create the dispensary as one of his wisest philanthropic investments. By the time he died in 1932, he had donated about $3 million to the dispensary. He also made its charter sufficiently broad to ensure that his original intention of providing care for Rochester's underserved children would be preserved; he gave those who came after him the latitude to

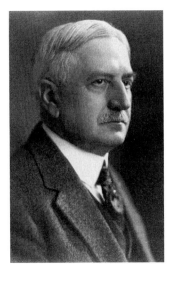

*Harvey J.
Burkhart,
D.D.S.,
1916–1946*

develop the dispensary in ways that would be responsive to the times. The dental dispensary was a favorite interest of Eastman's during the first two decades of its existence. Later he became interested in extending his concept of dental health care to other countries. During the 1930s, he donated the money to build and equip dental clinics in Stockholm, Brussels, Paris, London, and Rome. Although each evolved differently, all but one are still active.

Harvey J. Burkhart, D.D.S., a nationally and internationally prominent dentist and civic leader from Batavia, New York, was named the dispensary's first director in 1916. At the same time, the first licensed school for

RONALD J. BILLINGS

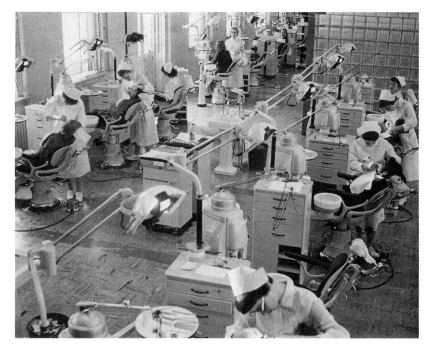

The Rochester Dental Dispensary's School for Dental Hygienists was the first institution of its kind to be recognized by the Board of Regents of the State of New York. (Photo c. 1945)

dental hygienists in New York State was established at the dispensary, with Burkhart as its director. Under his leadership, the dispensary became a model for patient care. Several pioneering concepts took root here, including dental research, the education of children and their parents on the importance of dental care, and the training of dentists in children's dentistry. During his lifetime, Burkhart oversaw the creation of the Eastman European Dental Clinics and presided at their dedication. He received many awards and is one of the namesakes for the New York State Dental Society's highest honor, the Jarvie-Burkhart Award.

Following Eastman's death in 1932, the Rochester Dental Dispensary was renamed the Eastman Dental Dispensary. His generous gift has been carefully managed and today the nearly $50 million endowment provides support for the Dental Center, the Eastman Department of Dentistry, and the Center for Oral Biology.

In 1947, following Burkhart's death, Basil Bibby, B.D.S., Ph.D., dean of the Tufts Dental School, was appointed as the dispensary's second director. Bibby received

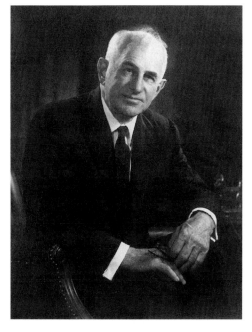

Basil G. Bibby, D.D.S., Ph.D., *1947–1970*

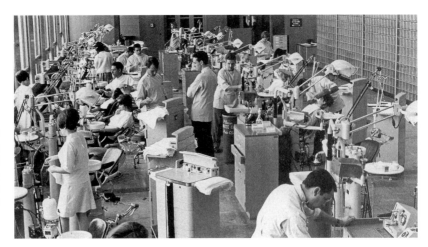

A busy day in Eastman Dental Center's main clinic (photo c. 1967)

a dental degree from Otago University of the University of New Zealand, a Ph.D. in bacteriology from the University of Rochester, and later a D.M.D. from Tufts. He was one of the first dentists accepted into the Dental Fellows program at the University of Rochester. The fellows program was created following the abandonment of the D.D.S. program and was intended to provide advanced education for academic and research-oriented dentists.

During Bibby's tenure as director of the Dental Center, research was incorporated into the fabric of the institution and formal specialty education programs were developed. Adults as well as children were accepted for treatment, and the institution's national and international reputation grew. Studies by center researchers, including Bibby, Michael Buonocore, and Helmut Zander, altered the path of dental history. Among the most noteworthy discoveries was the observation by Bibby that fluoride applied directly to the teeth would prevent dental caries. He also is credited with advancing knowledge about the cariogenicity of foods and the role of oral bacteria in the formation of dental caries. For his outstanding achievement in dental research, he received the second Gold Medal Award for Excellence in 1988 from the American Dental Association.

Michael Buonocore discovered that etching the enamel surface of the tooth with a weak acid would enhance the adhesion of plastic fillings to the teeth, revolutionizing the fields of restorative and esthetic dentistry. His studies also advanced the prevention of dental caries through the development of dental sealants. Buonocore is recognized as the father of the dental bonding process.

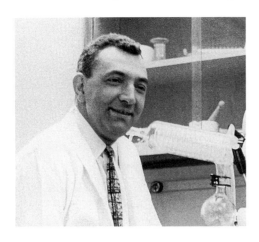

Michael Buonocore, D.D.S., M.S., *father of the dental bonding process*

RONALD J. BILLINGS

In the same way, Helmut Zander is widely regarded as the father of modern periodontology. Zander established much of the underlying scientific basis of periodontology and he is one of the most influential periodontal scientists of the 20th century. Many of the academically-oriented dentists who studied under these and other Eastman or University of Rochester faculty have become leaders in dental research and dental education. In 1964, the Eastman Dental Dispensary became Eastman Dental Center, a name chosen to reflect the diversity of its academic, research, and patient care activities. Bibby retired as director in 1970 but contin-

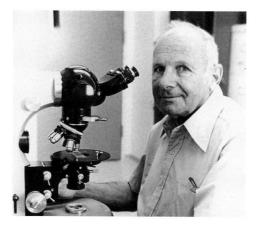

Helmut A. Zander, D.D.S., M.S., *father of modern periodontology*

ued his research as senior scientist emeritus, almost to the time of his death in 1998.

William McHugh, D.D.S., was named Eastman Dental Center's third director in 1970. McHugh, like Burkhart and Bibby, became a prominent dental leader and served as president of the American and international associations for dental research. Like his predecessors, he received several awards during his illustrious career and his contributions to the development of the center were numerous. Most notable was his role in guiding the center's 1978 move from the original building on East Main Street to its new location on the University of Rochester Medical Center campus.

Under McHugh's leadership, the center was rededicated to its traditional mission of providing patient care and community service, to its academic mission of offering the best possible post-doctoral clinical training to dentists, and of conducting field-advancing research. The location on the campus of another great research, educational, and clinical institution was designed to nurture and enhance interaction between the Medical Center and the Dental Center. This formal affiliation with the University of Rochester was further strengthened with McHugh's additional appointment as associate dean for dental affairs. McHugh served the center and the university in this dual capacity until his retirement in 1993.

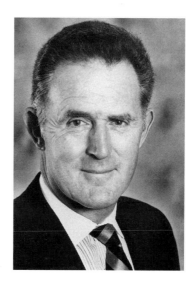

William D. McHugh, D.D.S., *1970–1993*

Ronald Billings, D.D.S., M.S.D., was appointed the fourth director in the spring of 1994. He led the center through

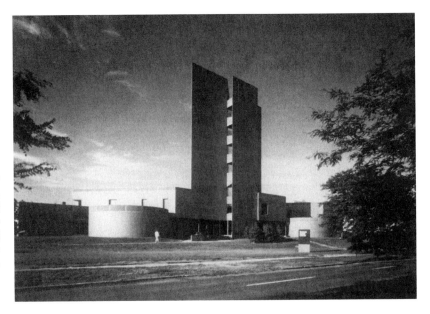

*The "new"
Eastman
Dental
Center on the
Medical
Center
campus*

a period of a significant change and was instrumental in the merger of the
center with the Medical Center. That merger, formalized on July 1, 1997,
joined all the resources and energies of each organization into one organization dedicated to becoming the foremost institution worldwide for oral health

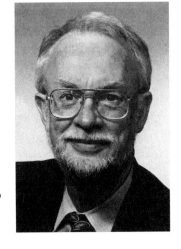

*Ronald J.
Billings,
D.D.S.,
M.S.D.,
1994–1999*

care, dental post-graduate education, and
dental research. Eastman Dental Center
joined the Medical Center as a peer organization alongside Strong Memorial Hospital,
the School of Medicine and Dentistry, the
School of Nursing, and the Medical Faculty
Practice Group. Eastman Dental Center now
serves as the Medical Center's oral health clinical arm.

On January 1, 1998, dental faculty
from Eastman Dental Center and the School
of Medicine and Dentistry's departments of
Clinical Dentistry and Dental Research
were integrated into a new department, the
Eastman Department of Dentistry. Cyril
Meyerowitz, D.D.S., M.S., was appointed
chair of this new department. At the same time, the Center for Oral Biology
(COB) was formed to pursue basic research in oral health under the direction
of Lawrence Tabak, D.D.S., Ph.D. COB was the first of the basic science
research centers formed in the Aab Institute of Biomedical Research. Tabak
also serves as senior associate dean for research in the School of Medicine
and Dentistry. Billings was named director emeritus in 1999.

Cyril Meyerowitz succeeded Billings as the fifth director of Eastman Dental Center in January 1999. His years of experience as an educator, researcher, and clinician make him unusually well qualified for his dual position. This coalescence of leadership provides a unique opportunity for academic dentistry to flourish in the ways envisioned by so many for so long.

The University of Rochester dental enterprise provides training at the postdoctoral level in general dentistry, oral surgery, orthodontics, pediatric dentistry, periodontology, and prosthodontics to dentists from around the world. Academic and research-oriented dentists pursue graduate degrees at the master's level, mainly in the Department of Community and Preventive Medicine and in the COB, while students at the doctoral level are concentrated primarily in basic science departments. NIH-funded training grants support nearly all students working toward an advanced academic degree.

Cutting-edge research in both clinical and basic science is extensive and varied. Basic science studies are conducted under the auspices of COB, while clinical and translational studies are performed in the Eastman Department of Dentistry. Most research is supported by a blend of government and corporate grants or contracts.

The commitment to Eastman's vision of making dental care accessible to those most in need has been preserved and extended. More than 30,000 adults and children receive their oral health care from faculty and resident clinics located in Eastman Dental Center, Strong Memorial Hospital, Highland Hospital, Monroe Community Hospital, and in the community. Eastman Dental Center's community outreach program treats an additional 10,000 underserved children who would otherwise not receive care, in mobile, and in school- or community-based clinics

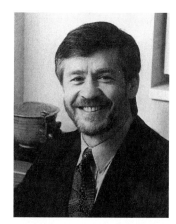

Cyril Meyerowitz, D.D.S., M.S., *1999–present*

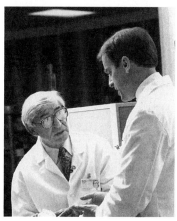

J. Daniel Subtelny, D.D.S., M.S., *one of EDC's great teachers*

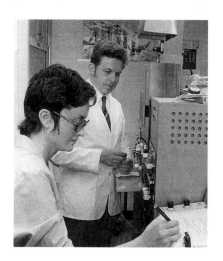

Martin Curzon, D.D.S., *directs student researcher in the use of the mass spectrometer*

located throughout the Rochester metropolitan area and western New York.

Specialty clinics provide oral health care for adults and children with complex oral/facial diseases or disorders and Eastman Dental Center is among the largest providers of dental care for the developmentally disabled in New York State. In addition to these latter efforts, a unique program to provide basic oral health care for the homeless was recently established in downtown Rochester and is overseen by the Eastman Dental Center's community outreach program.

No longer separate and independent, but now united and interdependent, the two organizations are one, fulfilling Eastman's wish of the center to be "part of a great project for a higher grade of dental education." As a combined organization, the resources and potential are there to set new standards of excellence in the years ahead. The words of Dr. McHugh, written for the 50th anniversary of the School of Medicine and Dentistry, still resonate today:

> While what develops will depend greatly on the will and abilities of individuals, the opportunities are immense. The essential and important role of dentistry in health care has been recognized, and the value of scientific research in dentistry has been demonstrated. Rochester has a proud tradition of educating leaders in dental education and research. I am confident that the future will add luster to that heritage.

Bringing Dental Care to Rochester's Schools

Eastman Dental Center faculty are joining their medical and nursing colleagues in providing health care and preventive services at family-oriented "wellness centers" in more than thirty schools in the Rochester metropolitan area. School-based preventive dental care disappeared during the latter years of the century with the advent of fluoride dentifrices, and as city and county funding was redirected to address the acute problems of drug use, AIDS, and teen-pregnancy.

In the 1990s, the Dental Center, in collaboration with school districts, county health and social service departments, New York State Bureau of Dental Health, and the Rochester Primary Care Network, launched a major collaborative school-based outreach dental program in Rochester's inner city and neighboring rural communities. The program focuses on providing preventive and primary dental care to economically disadvantaged children who otherwise would not receive care.

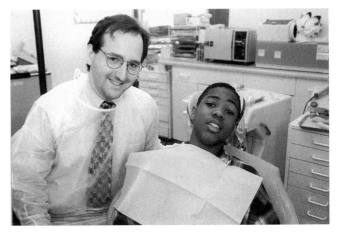

RONALD J. BILLINGS

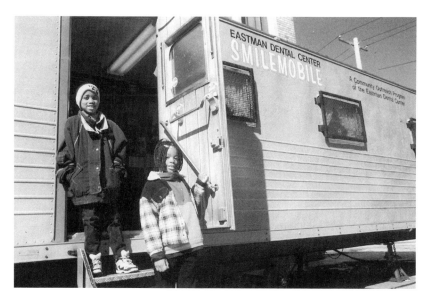

Dentistry with a Smile

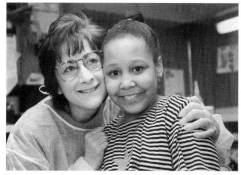

Two mobile Smilemobiles *now bring preventive dental care to more than 2,200 schoolchildren throughout the Greater Rochester region. Each* Smilemobile *is a traveling dentist's office that visits eleven schools for periods of from six to eight weeks each. Within this comfortable, child-centered environment, EDC dental hygienists clean teeth and apply fluoride and sealants, while faculty from the Dental Center fill cavities and provide other basic dental services. Children with problems beyond the scope of the* Smilemobile *program are referred to the Dental Center for care.*

The Smilemobile *service was begun in 1970 as a cooperative effort by the Monroe County Dental Society and Eastman Dental Center. Today, the program is run entirely by EDC's Division of Community Dentistry. A third* Smilemobile, *made possible by a grant from the Daisy Marquis Jones Foundation, will be placed in service during 2000.*

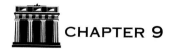

CHAPTER 9

Strong Memorial Hospital of the University of Rochester: A History

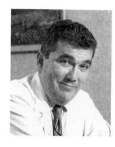

JAMES W. BARTLETT, M.D.

The sign at 601 Elmwood Avenue, near the University of Rochester's River Campus, reads "Strong Health, Strong Memorial Hospital, University of Rochester Medical Center." The sign is simple, the building it announces is massive and complex. Within these walls, more than a half million men, women, and children rely on Strong for some or all of their medical needs. Most come because they are ill or injured and they know they will find skilled diagnosis and treatment. Others come for psychological and emotional support and guidance. Some come here from far off places, seeking specialty care from physicians who have national and international reputations.

The visitor to Strong Memorial Hospital may arrive first at the handsome new Elmwood Avenue entrance, where the Wolk Pavilion joins the main hospital building, with its inpatient beds, to the ambulatory care building and a multi-tiered parking garage. Other entrances on Crittenden Boulevard direct patients and visitors to the Gannett Emergency Center, the Cancer Center, the Musculoskeletal Unit, and the University Health Service. Farther down Crittenden Boulevard, a sign over the entrance to the Department of Psychiatry announces "Strong Behavioral Services." Circling back toward Elmwood Avenue are new entrances to the Medical Center's educa-

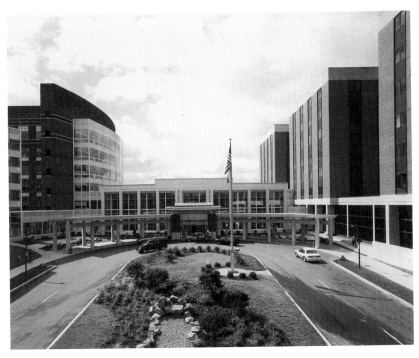

In 1999, the hospital's operating budget was $450 million, a significant portion of the entire budget of the University of Rochester. Two-thirds of the hospital's revenues come from inpatient services, one-third from outpatient care. Forty percent of the revenue comes from patients living outside of Monroe County who come to Strong Memorial for treatment and care.

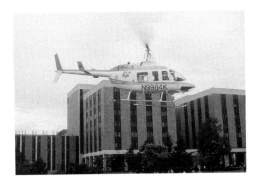

Medical helicopter approaching original landing pad at Strong Memorial Hospital. Designated as a Level I trauma center, Strong Memorial Hospital is served by a Mercy Flight helicopter that transports seriously ill and injured people from throughout a twelve-county region.

tional and research facilities. A new Emergency Department is rising on the north side of the complex, while the Eastman Dental Center (now part of the School of Medicine and Dentistry) rises nearby, looking, some say, rather like a healthy molar.

This impressive complex is the shell within which comprehensive health care is delivered 24 hours a day to the residents of the 12-county Finger Lakes region. Strong Memorial Hospital, with its 750 beds, extensive outpatient facilities, and dozens of diagnostic and treatment facilities last year counted 42,737 admissions to its inpatient service and more than 580,000 outpatient visits.

In recent years, the University of Rochester has consolidated and extended its clinical operations, as the organization of medical care in Monroe County has changed and as educational and research activities have grown. Strong Memorial Hospital, for years a distinct entity within the university system, is now part of Strong Health, a University of

JAMES W. BARTLETT

Rochester health-care organization that includes Highland Hospital, two nursing homes, a senior living center, and the Visiting Nurse Service.

More than 900 physicians are part of the Strong Health system, including the University of Rochester Medical Faculty Group; more than 700 of these are employed by the University of Rochester. Last year, Strong Health's total annual budget, including Strong Memorial Hospital, was $650 million.

1926: 260 CRITTENDEN BOULEVARD

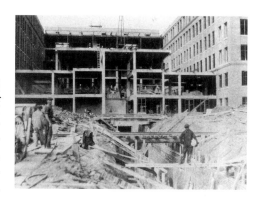

"In an era dominated by infectious and nutritional diseases, the accomplishments of scientific medicine were astonishing—and achieved at relatively low cost. The predominance of acute diseases made the hospital a logical center of medical care should a serious illness or surgical emergency strike. Requirements for ongoing office care were much less in an era when chronic diseases and conditions associated with aging were not as frequent. The relatively modest level of hospital

The original Strong Memorial Hospital entrance under construction (note tunnel connecting to Helen Wood Hall)

costs led to few complaints about underwriting the expense of clinical education through hospital charges. Moreover, the long duration of hospital stays (average stay in 1900—two to three weeks), lack of life-sustaining technologic equipment, and strong reliance on bedside observations in managing

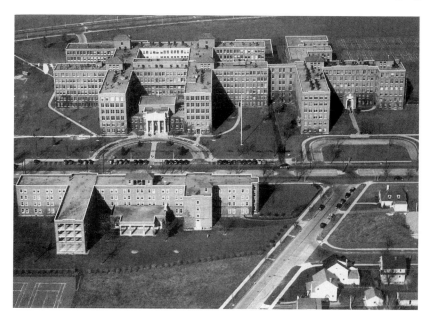

1925

patients, resulted in an outstanding opportunity for students. They could follow the natural history of disease, learn principles of therapy, develop personal relationships with patients and families, and make real contributions to patient care. The educational system was well suited to the medical practice of the era, and provided students a nearly ideal introduction to the life of a physician."[1]

—From *Time to Heal*, by Kenneth M. Ludmerer

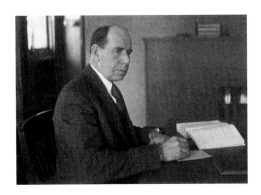

Nathaniel W. Faxon, M.D., *founding director of Strong Memorial Hospital*

Seventy-five years is a long time, and Strong has come a long way since January 4, 1926, when Nathaniel W. Faxon, M.D., first unlocked the door of Strong Memorial Hospital, proclaimed it open, and walked back up the seventeen steps of the main entrance to await patients. The first classes of medical and nursing students had been admitted in September 1925. Now, with the advent of clinical services, the proverbial three-legged stool had all its supports in place: education, research, and patient care.

Strong Memorial Hospital looked very different then than it does now. There were only three entrances: the classic door that Faxon had unlocked, with its four columns and the words above that read "University of Rochester—Strong Memorial Hospital—Medicine—Dentistry"; the entrance to the Emergency Department, just

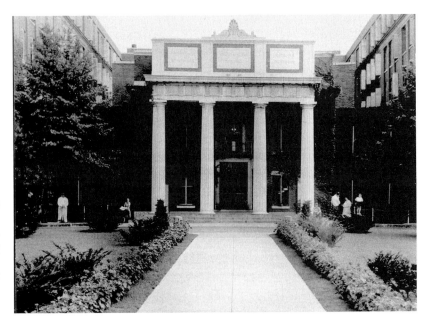

Original entrance to Strong Memorial Hospital, 1926

JAMES W. BARTLETT

east of the main entrance; and, further east, a more modest portal that served as the entrance to Rochester Municipal Hospital.

The presence of the Municipal Hospital was solid evidence of Strong's commitment to the health of the community and, conversely, of the city's firm support of the new School of Medicine and Dentistry and School of Nursing. The original Municipal Hospital, established in 1868, grew out of a smallpox epidemic; it eventually became a dilapidated pest house that served the city (but barely) through several severe epidemics. In 1902 a new Municipal Hospital on Waring Road focused on infectious diseases; it too became woefully inadequate.

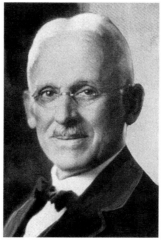

George W. Goler, M.D.

In 1922, George W. Goler, M.D., the innovative health officer of the city of Rochester, and the staff of the city's health bureau were preparing plans for a new hospital to be erected on the Waring Road site. Goler took the initiative in suggesting to the University of Rochester that the Municipal Hospital become a geographic and architectural part of the new university hospital, then being planned. This was a daring idea, modeled on the arrangement forged between the University of Cincinnati and that city's municipal hospital. A fifteen year contract between the university and the city of Rochester was drawn up, stipulating that Strong would provide all the health-care services for the Municipal Hospital. Rochester's Bureau of Municipal Research had determined, through a study done in February 1921, that 500 additional beds were needed in the community. Thus Strong Memorial and Rochester Municipal Hospitals were built to that number.

All but twenty-six of Strong's beds were designated as semi-private, four-bed units, with three single rooms on each wing reserved for gravely ill patients. A unique feature in Strong was a provision to set aside ten beds to be designated by the hospital director for the study and care of patients whose diagnoses were of research interest to the full-time clinical faculty. These beds, which could be designated any place in the hospital, were used for example by William S. McCann, M.D., first chair of the Department of Medicine, in his early metabolic studies. They may be seen as a precursor to the development of a special metabolic unit, and, even later, the Clinical Research Center.

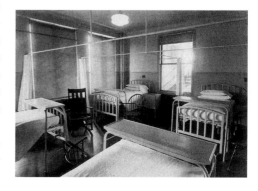

Semi-private facilities in the original Strong Memorial Hospital

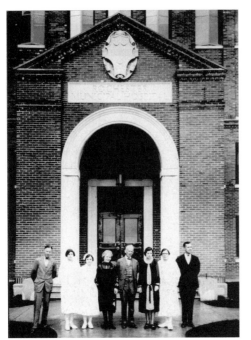

George W. Goler, M.D., *and staff at the entrance of Rochester Municipal Hospital, 1926. The new Municipal Hospital opened on July 28, 1926, with the transfer of patients from an older facility on Waring Road. Designed to be linked architecturally with the new university hospital then being planned, the Municipal Hospital's wards were 8- to 12-bed units, except for the infectious disease floor that had isolation facilities. A new feature was a psychiatric floor, the first effort to provide inpatient care for psychiatric patients outside of the Rochester State Hospital. The city paid Strong for the care of Municipal's patients, all of whom were medically indigent.*

Patients in the Municipal Hospital and semi-private patients at Strong paid no professional fees for their care. The few private patients at Strong were cared for exclusively by the full-time salaried faculty and their fees were credited to the hospital. Medical and surgical floors were segregated by sex, and patients were grouped according to their economic status.

Another important link between the new hospitals and the community was the on-site presence of the Rochester Health Bureau Laboratories. Physically and professionally part of the medical school's Department of Bacteriology, the laboratories also served as the microbiology laboratory for the two hospitals.

While it would take decades to integrate the hospital's operations into the community, the links that Goler forged were an important bond between the new facilities and the community they served.

The city of Rochester, of manageable size and with a fairly stable economy, provided fertile ground in which the seed for a university hospital could be planted. Innovative practices had been put in place, many of them suggested and financed by Eastman. For example, the city had its own health department bureau and a bureau of

---

The founding of the University of Rochester's medical school and associated hospital in the 1920s was brought about by Rush Rhees, president of the university; George Eastman, local industrialist and philanthropist; and Abraham Flexner, secretary of the General Education Board of the Rockefeller Foundation. Flexner's 1910 report on the need to reform American medical education emphasized the direct involvement of faculty and students in the laboratory and at the bedside, as well as rigorous standards for student admission and testing. While his proposals to integrate medical education—especially the basic sciences—into the university are often emphasized, he also stressed the concept that the hospital should play an integral part in medical students' education. With the backing of the General Education Board, Flexner's ideas for establishing university-run hospitals were being put in place at private universities such as Duke, the University of Chicago, and Rochester.

That once rare phenomenon—a hospital owned and operated by a university—was becoming more common. George Eastman, the Rockefeller Foundation, and a major gift from the family of Eastman's business associate Henry A. Strong made it possible for the University of Rochester to be in the vanguard of this national movement.

JAMES W. BARTLETT

municipal research. At the private level, well-organized agencies were established and functioning, such as the Chamber of Commerce and the Council of Social Agencies; the latter directed an integrated Community Chest program that supported health-care agencies. Five private hospitals were in operation: St. Mary's, Rochester General, Genesee, Highland, and Park Avenue. If the new enterprise could put down roots in this environment, then the capacity for growth and change was considerable.

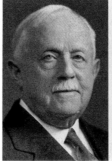 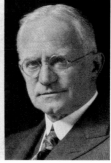

President Rush Rhees   George Eastman

THE FIRST DECADE: 1926–1936

The first ten years of the combined hospitals' history were exciting and challenging. Patient care grew significantly; the number of admissions rose from 3,632 in 1926 to 12,072 in 1934. The outpatient department, organizationally a part of Strong Memorial Hospital, grew from six patients on opening day to an average of over 400 per day ten years later. A reasonably large population lived on site, including student nurses, resident physicians, and several administrators; there were 226 rooms in the nurses' dormitory and 88 rooms in the staff house. As the size of the student bodies increased, so did educational activities, especially in the area

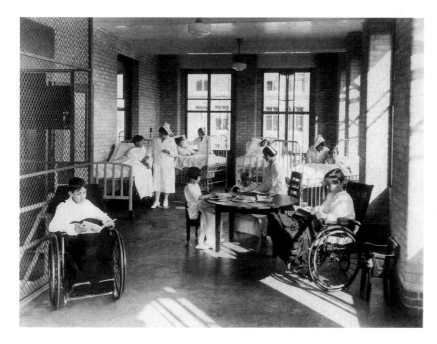

Pediatric patients and nurses on a solarium porch in the original hospital facility

of graduate medical education, where interns and residents proliferated almost exponentially.

The founding faculty in the clinical departments was entirely full-time and salaried, and provided exclusive care for the hospital's patients. As the outpatient department grew, some local practitioners with special skills were appointed as consultants. Most clinics (surgical, medical, pediatric) were general rather than specialized, with consultants such as cardiologists and allergists appointed from the community to provide particular services. Subspecialty divisions began to develop first in the Department of Surgery, with skilled specialists being recruited (mostly from outside Rochester) and given authority to develop the patient care, education, and research activities. These specialists had the benefit of hospital resources but they received no salary and supported themselves with fees from their own practices.

Community practitioners began to play an increasingly significant role in the hospital. As early house staff completed their residencies, a few were appointed full-time faculty, while others established their own practices and were given clinical (part-time) appointments and admitting privileges to the hospital. (Then, as now, a faculty appointment in the School of Medicine and Dentistry was required for a clinician to have practice privileges at Strong Memorial Hospital.)

The first few years were difficult. Strong Memorial was somewhat isolated from the rest of the medical community. Some practitioners viewed it as an unnecessary intrusion into an already well-established and competent medical community. Why, they wondered, hadn't the university used already available community resources in establishing its School of Medicine and Dentistry? Although a few physicians applauded the new teaching hospital, others were vocal in expressing what they viewed as the potentially negative impact of teaching and research on patient care.

Only three years after the opening of the hospital, the Great Depression swept over the country, compromising the community's ability to support medical care and welfare—and the medical profession's ability to support itself. Many adjustments were called for; one of these was the faculty compensation plan. Abraham Flexner's model of a full-time, fixed-salaried faculty with no outside professional income—a plan most notably attempted at the Johns Hopkins School of Medicine—proved not to be sustainable in Rochester, nor in Baltimore, or elsewhere. As universities competed for severely shrinking clinical dollars and for ways to attract patients, the faculty salary system was changed. Full-time clinical faculty were paid a base salary and permitted to earn up to a fixed amount above that base; any overage reverted to the medical school.

This model was adopted at the University of Rochester in the early 1930s, and with it came the practice of charging professional fees for semi-private patient services at Strong Memorial Hospital. Full-time faculty now had a direct incentive to engage in patient care; part-time faculty who brought their patients to Strong Memorial Hospital also charged for the services they provided.

Reviewing these first ten years, we see a growing Strong Memorial Hospital, an expanding faculty, and an increasing number of physicians entering the Rochester community after graduation from the medical school and the hospital residency programs. Volunteer organizations were formed for the hospital, supported by faculty spouses and women from the community. Especially noteworthy was the founding of the patients' library at Strong and the establishment of "the surgical dressing group" which brought people from the community into the hospital to support the professional staff.

During its first decade, the hospital began to attract attention in professional and scientific organizations within the state and nationally. In 1934 Faxon served as president of the American Hospital Association; even before this appointment he had often written on the establishment of and innovations at the new Strong Memorial Hospital.

A new idea began to be circulated in the early 1930s—the founding of a not-for-profit voluntary hospital insurance program. The idea for the program that eventually became known as Blue Cross was generated first in Houston, Texas, and soon spread to other parts of the country. Faxon took the lead in establishing the program locally, and Rochester's Blue Cross opened its doors on June 4, 1935.

By that time Faxon had left Rochester to become the director of the Massachusetts General Hospital in Boston. His departure from Strong in 1935 was followed soon after by the arrival of Basil MacLean, M.D., from New Orleans to take over the hospital's directorship. The roots of Strong Memorial Hospital had been securely planted. In the next decade more visible growth would be seen.

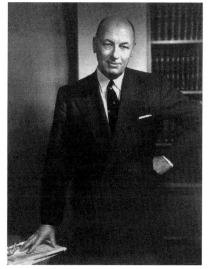

1936–1950

Many changes occurred over the next fourteen years, in the hospital, the university, and the community. At Strong, all the numbers increased. If we compare statistics for

Basil MacLean, M.D., *second director of Strong Memorial Hospital*

1936/37 with those of 1948/49, we see the number of inpatient admissions and patient days increasing by a third, while clinic visits decreased by the same percentage. The apparent decrease was probably at least partly due to increasing faculty office practice not recorded in clinic statistics. These trends were reinforced by the rapid spread of Blue Cross hospital insurance, an improved economy, and the presence of more practitioners in Rochester, both those with faculty appointments and those without.

By 1937, Strong Memorial was a founding member of the University Hospital Executive Council (UHEC), a group that included the hospitals associated with the University of Minnesota, the University of Wisconsin, the University of Iowa, the University of Chicago, the University of Indiana, the University of Michigan, and Lakeside Hospital in Cleveland. The group met twice a year at one of the member hospitals, and directors often were accompanied by senior staff. Each institution would submit questions that were addressed over a two-day period. The UHEC provided a forum where leaders of hospital departments (such as Nursing, Pharmacy, Personnel, and Social Work) could draw on the experiences of others. Confidential data such as salaries and other costs were also shared.

Later in the 1940s, after Strong's assistant director, Albert Snoke, M.D., had left to become director of the Yale–New Haven Hospital, a second group was formed—the Council of Teaching Hospitals (CTH). This group included Massachusetts General Hospital, Yale–New Haven Hospital, New York Hospital, Presbyterian Hospital of New York City, the Hospital of the University of Pennsylvania, Johns Hopkins Hospital, Lakeside Hospital in Cleveland, and Strong Memorial Hospital. CTH members met once a year in a format similar to UHEC except that the medical school deans often joined the hospital directors. (The Council of Teaching Hospitals (COTH) of the Association of American Medical Colleges, which represents all the major teaching hospitals in the United States, was formed considerably later.)

By 1950 approximately half the physicians practicing in Monroe County had strong ties to the University of Rochester, having received either their medical degrees there or their specialty residency training at Strong Memorial Hospital, or both.

Even while the integration of Strong into the medical community progressed, pockets of suspicion and distrust continued. In 1938, when the university's contract with the Municipal Hospital was up for renewal, a powerful push came from a part of the medical community to have the tax-supported institution give staff privileges to all licensed physicians in the city. This would radically change a pattern in which all the hospital's services were provided by the university. It was a bitter battle. Although ultimately unsuccessful for the insurgents, the struggle showed the continuing resistance to a teaching hospital with its firm commitment to education.

By the late 1930s the city of Rochester had made considerable progress in planning and financing community services. Although George Eastman had died in 1932, two new leaders were on the scene. Marion Folsom, a statistician from the Harvard Business School and Eastman's special assistant at Kodak, became a dominant force in organizing the city's planning efforts. Folsom was helped considerably by Luther Fry, the newly arrived chair of the university's Department of Sociology, an expert at identifying and measuring social trends and needs.

Based on the insights of Folsom and Fry, Rochester was able to view itself as an interrelated social system, where each individual part—such as unemployment, health care, education, and welfare—was affected by all the others. The community moved toward integrating services, and structures were developed to support the effort. The Rochester Hospital Council was formed in the late 1930s; the Council of Social Agencies established a Health Planning Committee and brought in Walter Wenkert from Yale to spearhead its efforts.

Up to this point, Strong Memorial was predominantly a ward and semi-private room hospital, with few private rooms. This pattern changed dramatically when a new wing with several floors of private rooms was opened in May 1941. Now faculty had the facilities to attract and care for patients of all socioeconomic levels, a distinct teaching advantage for medical and nursing students, as well as residents. The numbers of faculty grew considerably, both full-time and part-time, and many subspecialties were developed in the now large clinical departments of Medicine, Surgery, Pediatrics, and Obstetrics/Gynecology. By the time World War II started in December 1941, the size of the house staff had doubled, as it would again by the end of the 1940s.

World War II was a difficult time for all Rochester hospitals, and Strong was no exception. The number of employees decreased, and some of the medical staff were called to duty in the armed forces. After the war, however, Rochester had in place the structure and talent to enable it to move forward rapidly in regional planning, including health care. Planners viewed the region as a single system and realized that certain controls were in order. Two examples may be cited. In 1946, with help from a Commonwealth Foundation grant, the Rochester Hospital Council was transformed into the Rochester Regional Hospital Council. About the same time, the Health Planning Council took firm control in determining the number of hospital beds needed; random expansion by individual hospitals was not permitted, and strict standards of need and cost were established.

Two new additions were added to Strong Memorial Hospital after the war. The Edith Hartwell Clinic in LeRoy, New York, was given to the university and became a children's long-term rehabilitation facility, staffed by the orthopaedic faculty and physical therapists. (In many ways this was the beginning of the hospital's involvement in long-term care and rehabilitation medicine.) In 1948, the Department of Psychiatry opened the new R-wing, endowed by Helen Woodward Rivas, which provided an inpatient unit and outpatient facilities.

There was suspicion in some parts of the community about the research and experimentation carried on at the university hospital, a concern that patient welfare did not always come first. Early on, the anti-vivisectionists had

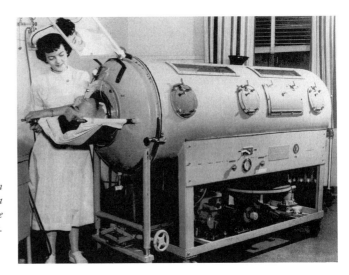

Caring for a patient in the iron lung: Poliomyelitis was a recurrent epidemic until the late 1950s.

protested Whipple's research on anemia in dogs, work that led to the successful treatment of pernicious anemia and a Nobel Prize. In fact, many medical discoveries and treatments have come from Rochester through the careful, systematic, and thorough care of patients, especially in hematology, heart disease, surgery, and pediatric infectious disease.

Research at the Medical Center and elsewhere in Rochester has led to better patient care and better outcomes of medical treatment. Over the years increasing safeguards have been developed to insure fully informed and documented consent and high standards of safety through human subject review boards and ethics committees whose membership includes representatives from the community and other professions in addition to Medicine and Nursing.

During the early years, medical educational opportunities in the community were scarce, although a few students and house officers may have accompanied faculty consultants to other hospitals, especially in pediatrics. Formal affiliations involving residents and students amongst the Rochester hospitals were developed starting in 1945 with the Genesee Hospital. In 1947, some Strong Memorial residents did begin to broaden their experience by rotating to some of the outlying hospitals. This was done at the urging of the

---

"The Monica Story": A Classic Case Study

A good example of research in Rochester is the famous study of "Monica" by George Engel, M.D., and Franz Reichsman, M.D. Monica was born in 1953 in New York's Southern Tier without a complete esophagus. The first months of the infant's life were spent in the hospital where she was fed through a hole created in her stomach. In a "first" for Rochester, surgeon Charles Sherman was able to replace the child's incomplete esophagus with a part of her intestine, after which she was able to eat and swallow. Monica's development and the impact of these early difficulties were recorded and studied by Engel and his collaborators for many decades, years during which she grew, married, and became a mother. Many generations of medical students came to know Monica through Engel's lectures and the remarkable films made of her progress.

JAMES W. BARTLETT

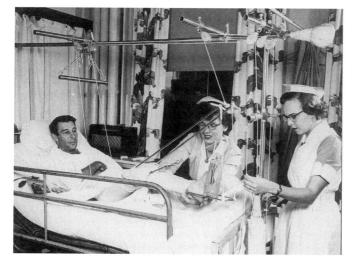

Nursing care and education at the bedside: instructor Marjorie Pfaudler *and a student with a patient in traction*

Rochester Regional Hospital Council, in the expectation that the presence of residents, and the need to teach, would stimulate greater attention to quality and evenness of care. As psychiatric facilities increased, student nurses from the Genesee Hospital began to come to Strong Memorial for their psychiatric experience.

As we can see, the years from 1935 to 1950 saw a considerable expansion of Strong Memorial Hospital—in patient care, education, research, and community affairs.

1950–1965

The fifteen years between 1950 and 1965 saw major changes occurring at Strong Memorial Hospital, the university, and in the regional environment.

In 1953, at the age of 75, George Whipple retired as dean of the School of Medicine and Dentistry. Donald G. Anderson, M.D., an internist who had been dean of the Boston University School of Medicine and then secretary of the American Medical Association's Council on Medical Education, was appointed as Whipple's replacement.

The comfortable relationship that had existed for so many years between the medical school and the hospital (with the hospital acting as a rather independent department within the school's administrative structure) was now stressed, as Anderson energetically and aggressively pursued Medical Center-wide planning. MacLean left as the hospital's director to become Commissioner of Hospitals in New York City and later the head of that city's Blue Cross. A professionally educated administrator, J. Milo Anderson, was recruited from Ohio State University Hospital to take over the stewardship of Strong.

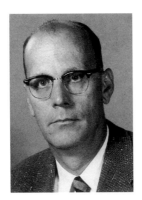

J. Milo
Anderson,
Administrator,
Strong
Memorial
Hospital

The problem of how best to integrate the medical school, nursing school, and hospital continued to be a vexing one. In 1960 Milo Anderson left—somewhat precipitously—to become administrator of Presbyterian Hospital in San Francisco. Robert Berg, M.D., recently recruited from Massachusetts General Hospital to chair the new Department of Preventive Medicine and Community Health, agreed to act as interim administrator while Dean Anderson and senior faculty redefined the hospital position and recruited a new director. Recognizing that education and patient care were interwoven, the Dean's committee recommended that the next director should have a background in medical education, as well as administrative skills,

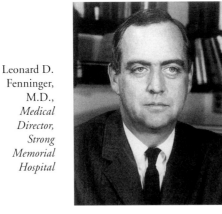

Leonard D.
Fenninger,
M.D.,
Medical
Director,
Strong
Memorial
Hospital

and that he also should serve as an associate dean in the School of Medicine and Dentistry. After a nationwide search, Leonard D. Fenninger, M.D., an associate dean in the School of Medicine and Dentistry, was appointed medical director of Strong Memorial, a position he held until late in 1965.

By 1950, all functions of the Medical Center were cramped for space. Except for the private and psychiatric wings and the annex built across Elmwood Avenue for the Atomic Energy Project, not much new space had been added to the complex. Increasing specialization in patient care, research, and education made it difficult for the center to adapt to these new needs. New departments and divisions were being formed—such as Psychiatry, Radiology, Preventive Medicine, and Rehabilitation, to name a few—all of which had highly differentiated requirements. Some surgical divisions, most notably Orthopaedics, required discrete units with specially trained staff. Although clinical studies were being carried out in all parts of the hospital, a special metabolic research unit of four beds was converted into a clinical research center. Often interim solutions were found; for example, to meet an increasing demand for intensive care beds, part of C5 was renovated into a medical / surgical intensive care unit.

Each year more space was needed. Many plans for conversion were considered, such as filling in the courtyard spaces or building a replacement hospital to the west of the Medical Center (on the then sacrosanct baseball field). During the late 1950s and early 1960s, the contractual relationship between Strong Memorial and the Rochester Municipal Hospital once again became

JAMES W. BARTLETT

tenuous. At this time of rising hospital costs and shrinking tax base, the city decided it could no longer afford to be in the hospital business. In 1962, Municipal Hospital was sold to the university for a modest sum; with it came sixteen acres of land that the university had originally lent to the city. Here was a major opportunity. A decision was made to rebuild Strong Memorial Hospital (except for the psychiatry service) on that property.

While change was sweeping the Medical Center, the community also was undertaking major advances in planning and financing. One of these resulted in the Rochester Hospital Fund Drive of 1960. Since the city's hospitals received support from the Community Chest, all plans for separate fund-raising activities had to be registered with the Chest. Just at this time Marion Folsom returned to Rochester, having completed his tenure as Secretary of Health, Education, and Welfare in the Eisenhower Administration, and he resumed a leadership role in health planning. It was decided that a joint fund drive would be mounted in support of all the hospitals.

By this time, almost the entire community was covered by health insurance, with Blue Cross covering 80 percent of the population; Blue Shield was gradually offering more benefits while the Rochester Municipal Hospital was the safety net for the city's medically indigent. The Health Planning Committee, led by Walter Wenkert working with Blue Cross, the Monroe County Medical Society, and the university, had undertaken a community-wide review of hospital utilization. The committee discovered that the chronically ill were occupying 16 percent of the acute hospital beds. Clearly better and more cost-effective care could be provided for these patients at a different kind of facility. These findings energized the fund drive and helped ensure its success.

A similar cooperative approach was taken in 1964, when the issue fo-

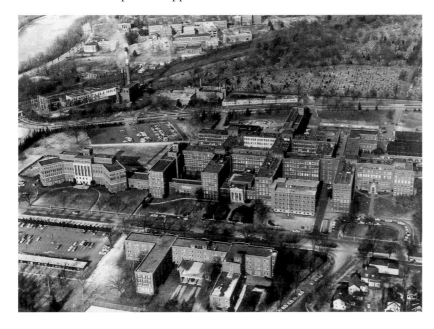

1962

cused on consolidating pediatric beds scattered throughout the community hospitals. Once again the university, the hospitals, and the industrial community researched the problem together, and made difficult decisions designed to preserve and improve the quality of patient care, education, and funding.

In 1962 the U Wing of Strong Memorial Hospital was completed, adding space for an inpatient rehabilitation floor, physical therapy, industrial and vocational medicine, faculty practice, and the Combined Clinic. The latter was an interdisciplinary continuity-of-care effort where fourth-year students followed their patients throughout the final year of medical school. Funding for the new wing came from the Hill-Burton Act, grants from the Commonwealth and Ford Foundations, and the Hartwell family. Approval by the Folsom committee for this addition was contingent on the willingness of the university to take responsibility for medical services to the Monroe County Home and Infirmary (later renamed Monroe County Hospital).

During the same period, state and national resources, as well as new regulations, were coming into effect. Passage of the Hill-Burton Act, providing monies for hospitals (especially in rural areas), brought an opportunity that was seized by the Rochester community and used to define a regional system. In New York State, the Metcalf-McCloskey Act established a state review system for health-care facilities that further enhanced planning efforts in the Genesee region.

In 1965, several important events occurred at Strong Memorial Hospital. Dean Anderson took a sabbatical leave; several months later, after talks with university president W. Allen Wallis, he relinquished the deanship. Fenninger, Strong's medical director, left to go to the Bureau of Health Manpower at the National Institutes of Health. At the national level, President Lyndon Johnson signed the Medicare/Medicaid Act into law.

1965–1975

In 1965 J. Lowell Orbison, M.D., chair of the Department of Pathology, was appointed dean of the School of Medicine and Dentistry. After consulting with the clinical chairs, Orbison asked James Bartlett, M.D., to serve as acting medical director for Strong Memorial Hospital; the following year, Bartlett accepted the post on a permanent basis. Realizing that hospital management had become a complex job, Clarence Wynd, retired head of Kodak Park and chair of the University Trustees Visiting Committee to the Medical Center, and Bartlett invited Allan C. Anderson, then administrator of Highland Hospital, to become the executive director of Strong Memorial.

In 1972, bids were received for the remaining structures, bids that exceeded the funds available. Several design changes were made (for example in the heating and air-conditioning systems) and the completion of the new Emergency Department was postponed. Thanks to a generous grant from the

The design and construction of the new hospital facility to the east of the Medical Center occupied most of the decade between 1965 and 1975. Ellerbe Architects of St. Paul, Minnesota, worked closely with the faculty to design a first-rate facility. As soon as plans for the foundation were completed, bids for that portion of the work were received and digging got underway.

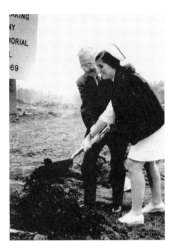

Dr. Whipple *with staff nurse, ground breaking ceremony for the new Strong Memorial Hospital*

Eli Lilly Foundation, it became possible to add a connecting wing that joined the new hospital to the old at all floor levels, as well as to establish a separate Clinical Research Center. A revised contract, within budget, was awarded to Huber, Hunt and Nichols of Indianapolis.

The new building rose slowly over the next several years. It consisted of modern hospital space and housed all ancillary services, teaching and conference space, but had almost no faculty offices; these remained in the old building. The 900,000-plus square-foot project was budgeted at $66 million, a far cry from the million-dollar gift by the Strong family for the original hospital.

The principal source of funds for the new hospital was a $44 million tax-exempt bond issue levied by the New York State Dormitory Authority. The bonds were secured by the university, which deposited an appropriate portion of its endowment portfolio in the Lincoln First Bank; there it remained as income-producing property for the university, while ensuring creditors that the bonds were solidly backed. An additional $10 million grant from

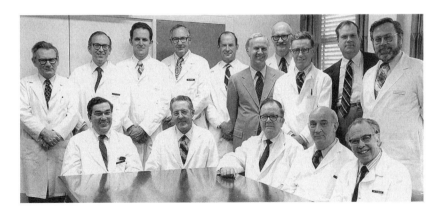

Clinical chiefs Wednesday lunch group, early 1970s

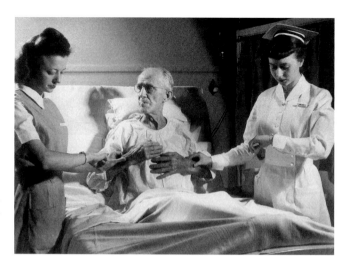

*Caring for
the patient*

the National Institutes of Health was based on the expanded educational manpower associated with the new hospital. The fund drive for the community's hospitals, mentioned earlier, raised four million more dollars for Strong; the remaining monies came from gifts, grants, and other university resources. When finally completed, the project came in several hundred thousand dollars under budget.

Exciting changes were contemplated in nursing. Two committees, one chaired by Robert France, the university's vice-president for finance, and the other by Barbara Bates, M.D., of the Department of Medicine, explored how best to integrate nursing into patient care, education, and research functions at the Medical Center. Nursing education and hospital nursing care had drifted apart, even as the nursing faculty worked hard to improve standards of teaching and scholarship. The plan agreed upon was to reintegrate these activities with a new School of Nursing and a revised Medical Center administrative structure. The concept was approved and implemented through a five-year grant from the Kellogg Foundation. Loretta Ford, R.N., Ed.D., was recruited from Colorado to be the founding dean. She would also serve as director of Nursing in Strong Memorial Hospital, delegating some of those responsibilities to an associate director who would also be an associate dean in the nursing school. Nursing chiefs were appointed in each of the major clinical departments to work closely with the physician chiefs in providing quality clinical care and education. Other nursing faculty were expected to develop special areas of clinical competence.

The plan was ambitious and not easy to implement, but its successes were impressive. At the bedside, the concepts of team nursing were largely replaced by primary nursing. Each nurse had a roster of assigned patients and took responsibility for organizing all their nursing care (even that delivered by other nurses and nursing consultants) and integrating that care with the medical services. The system at its best delivered much more informed,

JAMES W. BARTLETT

coordinated, and personal care. Because of the case management format, patient care often was delivered more economically. As a result of the changes, Nursing became a major integrating force in managing the institution.

How best to set up work patterns in the new hospital was determined by creating an experimental in-patient unit within the old Municipal Hospital. Although the study could not model the physical configuration of the new patient units, the functional duties of the staff could be examined closely. This project was headed by Paul Griner, M.D., and Janet Mance, R.N., with major support from Betty Deffenbaugh, R.N., acting director of Nursing. By this time, many categories of workers were required to staff the hospital, including dietary aides, housekeeping assistants, registered nurses, licensed practical nurses, nursing assistants, secretaries, orderlies, etc. The work of the experimental unit helped simplify and consolidate roles. By moving day, there were many fewer categories of employees, all working much more closely together. Primary nursing and ward management fit well into the new scheme.

The opportunity to build the new hospital also led to the development of better technical resources. For example, the new building was equipped with an automated transportation system, with its own tracks and lifts, for moving basic supplies such as laundry, pharmacy, and food to the clinical units. This innovation kept traffic out of the corridors and elevators used by patients and staff. Each floor could provide hot meals (previously prepared and then reheated) at flexible times, as needed by a patient who may have missed a regular mealtime.

The late 1960s and early 1970s were times of rapid unionization in the hospital and health-care fields. A union election was held at Strong early in 1966. The hospital's dietary, housekeeping, and floor secretaries voted against joining a national union, while the engineering and maintenance department decided to establish its own local and independent union. Over the next several years, two other elections were held; the third time around, hospital service workers did accept national union representation. With help from the university's Personnel department, the Medical Center learned the principles of labor relations well. The union did not object to the changing roles that accompanied the expansion to the new hospital. Later, nurses voted to decline unionization.

When the new hospital building was finally complete, tested, and ready to go (a few months behind schedule), a detailed plan for the move was developed. For many reasons it was not practical to shut down the hospital, so patients and staff were moved in a single day—February 25, 1975. Three-hundred-eighty patients were transported by staff and special teams in a scheduled and orderly fashion. (Among the patients moved was George Whipple, the school's founding dean.) An emergency resuscitation team directed by Frank Colgan, M.D., was set up halfway between the old and new hospitals; fortunately their services were not required. Howard Spindler, M.D., delivered the final patient in the old obstetrical unit, then walked over to the new

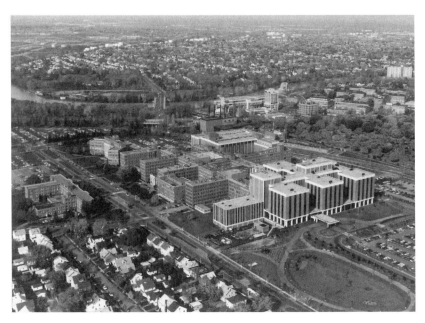

1975

facility and delivered the first baby born there. The move had been expected to take six hours, but was completed in less than four. Staff and patients were thrilled with the colorful new facility. But as staff turned back to look at the empty and barren floors where they had labored long and hard, many were overcome by an unexpected wave of nostalgia and sadness.

The Medicare/Medicaid law, implemented in 1966, resulted in major changes in hospital financing and reimbursement. While the law was a boon to facilitating hospital care for the elderly, it imposed strict reporting and accountability standards that were often procrustean and not always helpful. The differences between Part A (hospital charges) and Part B (professional fees) set different standards, facilitated unbundling of fees, and became an opening wedge in the efforts to move away from community rating in health insurance. Community rating, coupled with the high penetration of Blue Cross/Blue Shield in Rochester, was the cement with which the Monroe County health-care system had been constructed.

To implement the new Medicaid programs, certain standards were required for federal financial participation, while eligibility requirements for medical indigency were set by the states. Gov. Nelson Rockefeller pushed through one of the first state Medicaid programs in the country, a program generous in benefits and broadly inclusive, with about 25 percent of the total population of New York qualifying for medical assistance. The immediate result was a great rush for hospital care, at a cost that the state could not bear, even with federal assistance. The legislature and the governor then gave the State Health Department authority to regulate Medicaid hospital rates statewide. The resulting complex system, which grouped hospitals, required uniform financial reporting, and then established rates designed to save Medicaid

JAMES W. BARTLETT

dollars was the first answer. Rate regulation later was expanded to include Blue Cross hospital per diem rates. The results, which did not take geographic regions and their differences into account, were difficult for several of the Rochester hospitals, including Strong.

At the time the Medicare/Medicaid Act was implemented, the state had a certificate-of-need policy requiring that all new hospital facilities have prior approval on both programmatic and financial grounds, with depreciation recognized and funded. The state then approved bond issues that would be repaid through depreciation funding. At a later date the state should set a reimbursement rate at a level that allowed the institution to meet the funding and operation of the already approved facilities.

As Strong moved into the new hospital building, a new rate was necessary to cover expanded programs and depreciation. The NYS Health Department balked, and a cumbersome appeal process moved at a snail's pace. A crisis arose over Strong's continued ability to participate in Blue Cross, then a voluntary agreement between the hospital and the Blue Cross Association, and considerable local tension was generated. The issue was finally resolved one Sunday afternoon when James Wilmot, a university trustee, called Governor Carey at his Shelter Island home, and said to the governor, "You've got to do something for Strong." The governor did. The health department promptly reviewed its prior approvals and established a somewhat spartan rate for the new hospital, but one that allowed it to move forward.

The university's Trustees Visiting Committee to the Medical Center, headed by Clarence Wynd, became more active in the early 1970s. Rochester General Hospital, Genesee, St. Mary's, and Highland all had requested and developed major affiliations with the Medical Center, and full-time faculty, students, and residents from the university were well established in all the hospitals. Community planning and state regulations required a considerable level of board and executive participation in these affiliations.

It had also become evident that for educational and patient-care activities to prosper, Strong must be even more oriented toward the community, while the community needed a more thorough understanding of the university's mission. The fiftieth anniversary of the Medical Center in 1975 and the concurrent opening of the new hospital building offered a good opportunity to address these goals. A Board of Overseers for Strong Memorial Hospital was established, initially chaired by Wynd and consisting of five other university trustees, as well as representatives from throughout the community.

During this decade, increasing specialization and subspecialization developed in all the Rochester hospitals, and especially at Strong. Private, semi-private, and Medicaid patients were all grouped according to their medical requirements in single or double rooms within units devoted to specialty care—surgical intensive care, coronary care, medical intensive care, orthopaedics, urology, neurosurgery, etc. Patients now were completely integrated as to economic status and sex. A single standard of care within the hospital was finally achieved and supported by the Rochester region.

Within the community (and outside the hospital), other forces affecting the organization and delivery of medical care were stirring. The early 1970s saw the establishment of three managed-care organizations, including a Kaiser Permanent–style HMO established by Blue Cross in a wooded grove near Rochester General Hospital. The Monroe County Medical Society required Blue Cross to sponsor Health Watch, a more open, less restrictive delivery system. The Office of Economic Opportunity encouraged and financed the development of several neighborhood health centers, known collectively as the Rochester Health Network. While Strong Memorial had no direct involvement in establishing these organizations, several faculty members played prominent roles in advising and facilitating their establishment. In spite of these advances in health-care delivery, many chronically ill patients (especially those on Medicaid) whose home care had collapsed were spending weeks in the Emergency department while social workers struggled to find long-term care beds for them.

1976–1989

These were crucial years for Strong Memorial Hospital—and for the Rochester community. The flexibility of the new hospital facilitated the development of specialized services, which created new opportunities to improve patient care and to advance clinical research and clinical education. For example, a revised pediatric intensive-care unit, a bone-marrow transplant unit, and a long-term care unit all were introduced.

The space designated for the Emergency department in the new hospital had been left empty because of lack of funds and a desire to redesign its plan. With the generous help of Caroline Gannett and the Gannett Foundation, the new plan was accomplished in the late 1970s. When the old hospital building, fully depreciated, reverted to the university, its 350,000 square feet of vacated space became available for renovation into research and office space, as well as room for additional clinical care services. The Musculoskeletal Unit, for example, was built on the ground floor in the old Emergency department

---

The Malpractice Crisis

During the 1970s, a medical malpractice crisis developed. As claims increased in number and size, insurers withdrew from the market, leaving hospitals and physicians with inadequate coverage. A particular problem for hospitals—and for some physicians—was the lack of sufficient coverage through reinsurance. The University of Rochester joined with Columbia, Cornell, Johns Hopkins, and later Yale, to form an off-shore insurance corporation in Bermuda. The new insurer covered all the university's liability including their hospitals and full-time medical faculty; reinsurance could then be obtained through Lloyds of London.

JAMES W. BARTLETT

area; the unit provided a focused and accessible outpatient and treatment facility for orthopaedics and (for several years) neurology. A Cancer Center was built as an addition to the new hospital. Located at what had been the entrance to the old Municipal Hospital, the new center provided integrated outpatient facilities, radiation therapy, chemotherapy, and certain surgical procedures.

Strong continued to be very busy, as many of the old barriers of suspicion and distrust between the community and the university were removed. Classes expanded in the medical and nursing schools, and there was a considerable increase in resident staff and fellowship programs, an effort well supported by the affiliated hospitals and the faculty located there. Two thousand of the 3,000 acute-care beds in Monroe County (including Strong's 750 beds) were available for educating medical students and residents. Continuing medical education for physicians and health-care professionals also grew considerably during the decade.

A number of administrative changes occurred at the Medical Center during these thirteen years. In 1978, Lowell Orbison retired as dean of the School of Medicine and Dentistry and director of the Medical Center. In 1979, Frank E. Young, M.D., Ph.D., chair of the Department of Microbiology, was appointed dean, director, and vice president; he served in that position until 1984 when he left to become commissioner of the Food and Drug Administration.

When Allan Anderson left in 1979 to be president of Lennox Hill Hospital in New York City, Gennaro J. Vasile, Ph.D., replaced him as Strong's executive director. Vasile left in 1984 and, shortly thereafter, Paul Griner, professor of medicine, became general director of Strong Memorial; Leo Brideau was named chief operating officer. In 1984, Dennis O'Brien succeeded Robert Sproull as president of the University of Rochester; he appointed Robert J. Joynt, M.D., Ph.D., professor and chair of the Department of Neurology, as dean of the School of Medicine and Dentistry, and later vice president.

These were interesting, trying, and demanding years, years which required the whole community to work as a team in forging responsible leadership, especially in the health-care field. Many regulatory agencies—federal, state, regional, and local—were eager to guide the health-care community in improving access, maintaining and advancing quality, and containing costs. The Finger Lakes Health System Agency, which covered the Rochester region from Lake Ontario to the Pennsylvania border, had staff and citizens' committees that reviewed all new programs. New York State continued its mandatory certificate-of-need process and extended its control of hospital per diem rates to Blue Cross, as well as to Medicaid. In Rochester, where 80 percent of the insured population had been covered by Blue Cross, that meant rigid control of almost all hospital reimbursement by Albany. Reimbursement rates were determined by a number of factors, none of them regional in nature; thus Rochester, with its long history of controlling the number of hospital beds, was at a serious disadvantage.

In the late 1970s, Rochester's hospitals found their revenues inadequate to sustain existing programs. In a remarkable display of community ingenuity and cooperation, the hospital boards, industrial leaders, the university, and the Rochester Hospital Council worked together to form a new organization, the Rochester Area Hospital Corporation (RAHC). In 1979 RAHC designed an innovative program in which Blue Cross, Medicare, and Medicaid agreed to provide an annually adjusted sum to be divided among the hospitals in a prospective manner. Under the terms of the Hospital Experimental Payment Program, the hospitals submitted their budgets to RAHC in a common format. Part of the monies allocated was set aside for unexpected contingencies and new programs, while so-called "volume corridors" were established to handle unexpected fluctuations in hospital usage. These contingency funds might be tapped for capital projects, if the projects were approved by the RAHC board and its medical advisory committee. Funds were also set aside for charity care and medical education costs.

In what was becoming elsewhere a morass of contradictory reimbursement policies, Rochester became an area of relative calm, where planning, budgeting, and implementation were accomplished in a responsible and accountable manner. The story of RAHC has been well told elsewhere;[2,3] it is important to point out, however, that many university leaders were involved in the effort, particularly Laroy Thompson, vice president and treasurer, and Robert Joynt, then dean of the School of Medicine and Dentistry, as well as the Strong Memorial Hospital administrative staff.

In summary, throughout the 1980s and early 1990s Rochester hospitals were able to contain costs, at a time when they were rising rapidly throughout the state and nation. At the same time, they were able to maintain quality and initiate appropriate innovations (although occasionally belatedly) without the disruption and competition that was occurring elsewhere. Critical to the success of the effort were waivers granted to the Rochester region by the federal government's Health Care Financing Agency and by the State of New York. Managed cooperation was the hallmark of these "Camelot years" for the Rochester health-care system, a system now to be tested by the unleashed dragons of competition.

1990–2000

The pace of change quickened during the last decade of the century. The Medical Center completed several large building projects at the Elmwood Avenue site. The first of these was the hospital's Ambulatory Care facility, with its seven floors, totalling 285,000 square-feet of new space; next to it rose a large parking garage, on land formerly occupied by the Municipal Hospital.

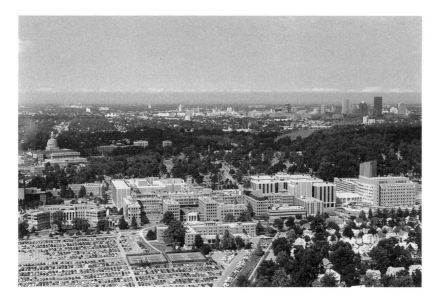

1995

These major construction projects were accomplished with little disruption of clinical activities; a shuttle service transported patients and visitors to and from a nearby parking lot until the new facilities were completed. With its expanded, improved, and more differentiated clinical services, the addition of the ambulatory care building enabled Strong Memorial to accommodate to an increasing emphasis on out-of-hospital care.

The most recent major building project was the construction in 1998–1999 of the Arthur C. Kornberg Medical Research Building at the west end of the Medical Center, and the development of the Aab Institute for

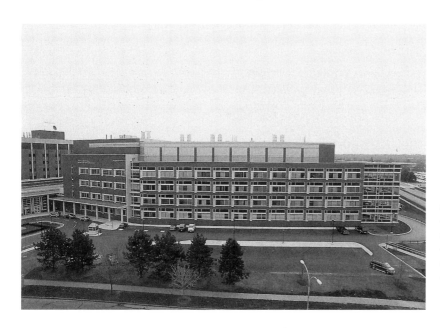

Arthur Kornberg Medical Research Building, 1999

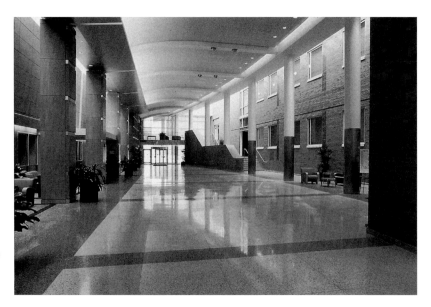

Biological Sciences. The new research center is the centerpiece of a plan to invest $550 million over ten years to build new research facilities and to recruit 100 scientists—the largest recruitment effort since the medical school was founded in 1924.

Reorganization within the Medical Center and the university, as well as within the region's health-care leadership, also marks the end of the century. Paul Griner left his position as general director of Strong Memorial to become senior vice president of the Association of American Medical Colleges, while Leo Brideau, the hospital's second in command, became its CEO.

With the appointment of Jay H. Stein, M.D., as senior vice president

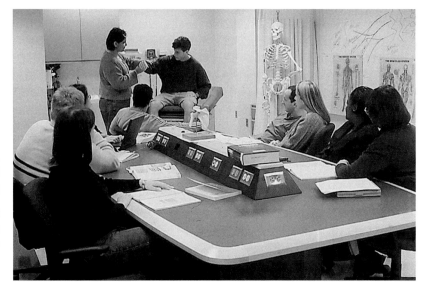

JAMES W. BARTLETT

and vice provost for Health Affairs, a single individual was identified with executive decision-making authority for the entire Medical Center. Stein is also the chief executive officer of Strong Health, the university's integrated health-care system.

This health-care system includes two acute care hospitals, Highland and Strong Memorial; two skilled nursing facilities, The Highland Living Center and The Highlands at Brighton; a home care group, including the Visiting Nurse Service and Community Care of Rochester; a senior living facility, the Highlands at Pittsford; the medical faculty group; a network of community-based physicians and scores of outreach clinics located throughout Monroe County and fourteen other counties of upstate New York.

Stein reorganized the health-care system along functional lines. Leo Brideau is vice president for the regional health system; Steven Goldstein, former president of Rochester General Hospital, is vice president for acute care at both Highland and Strong Memorial Hospitals; Sally Leiter, president of the Visiting Nurse Service, is vice president for home care; Raymond Mayewski, M.D., is the vice president responsible for the medical faculty group; and Michael Weidner, former president of Highland Hospital, is vice president for primary care and long-term care services.

Realignments have occurred recently among the other Rochester hospitals. Rochester General and Genesee have merged to form Via Health Care, while St. Mary's and Park Ridge hospitals joined to form Unity Health. At this time, for-profit corporations have not yet invaded New York State. They are discouraged by law from doing so, as well as by the fact that the capacity for profit to be gained by reducing unnecessary and unprofitable programs is not as great in the Rochester region as in other parts of the nation.

As the year 2000 begins, the predominance of a single regional insurer with community-rated premiums has seriously eroded. At one time, Blue Cross ensured 80 percent of the population and a single premium rate applied to all, young and old; the dominant role played by Eastman Kodak in the local economy helped facilitate this state of affairs. Differing rates began to be introduced with the coming of Medicare. Experience rating (i.e., basing premiums on the actual health-care costs expended on a designated group of people, such as corporate employees) has become widespread as health-care costs escalate.

Although health-care costs in Rochester rose at a considerably slower pace than elsewhere in the nation, largely because of community wide controls on hospitals, the clamor for experience rating increased as local companies downsized and as other insurers expanded their position in the Rochester market. The Hospital Experimental Payment Program that had flourished in the 1980s and that had made Rochester a model for health-care cost containment fell apart as different insurers offered different reimbursements with different rates. When it began to appear that one or two hospitals might do better outside the RAHC reimbursement system, the plan collapsed, and the era of cooperation continued its decline.

The events that unfolded on Memorial Day weekend in 1993 provide a good illustration. From Friday to Tuesday, leaders of the Preferred Care Medical Group and Eastman Kodak Company were able to design and price a plan for Kodak's senior and retired employees that would exclude any use of Strong Memorial Hospital or St. Mary's Hospital. Patients requiring complicated services available locally only at Strong would be referred to out-of-town specialists. After much turmoil, the plan eventually was withdrawn; there was considerable doubt about its long-term economy and it failed to offer open competitive bidding by rival providers. This sounded the funeral dirge of community rating, and it heightened an era of direct competition among Rochester's health-care providers.

The economic forces that were reshaping Rochester's reimbursement patterns had a very considerable impact on medical and nursing education. The Rochester medical community had opened almost all of its facilities for the education of medical students and residents and for the continuing education of practicing physicians. Significant numbers of full-time faculty were at work at Rochester General, Genesee, Highland, and St. Mary's; the university also contracted to provide medical services at Monroe Community Hospital, a long-term care facility. The fact that medical education was taking place in clinical-care settings had been viewed as a strong force in improving the quality of health care, advantageous to all. Now, efforts to squeeze out associated costs have led to considerable distress, as residency programs have been consolidated and their size and locations reduced. The pinch has often been painful for education and patient care, when trying to meet financial needs and national accrediting requirements.

On the other hand, out-of-hospital programs in offices and clinics are now better integrated and have become valuable sites for medical education, especially since the brief hospital stays that are today's norm leave little time for interviewing, discussion, and follow-up. If continuity of care is further interrupted, radical shifts in the educational effort will be required. Nursing education has also felt the effects of cost reductions, especially in hospitals. Nursing education programs that developed in hospitals and universities have been taken over by colleges (especially community colleges) that cannot exercise sufficient pedagogic control over the facilities where their students receive clinical experience.

2000 AND ON

The story of Strong Memorial Hospital begins in 1926 with a description of a rather isolated institution. At the turn of the millenium, that institution has become closely intertwined with its community and is now a valuable

JAMES W. BARTLETT

asset for the whole region. What was once a single teaching hospital has been transformed into a teaching community. Generations of physicians, nurses, and other caregivers have been educated here, and the community has benefited from their high level of skill and dedication, as well as from the progress made by medical researchers here and elsewhere.

George Eastman's goal was to have Rochester become "one of the healthiest communities in the world."[4] Thanks to the community and the Medical Center he helped shape so significantly, a very good start has been made toward reaching that goal.

In the original lobby of the old Strong Memorial Hospital (now part of the Reading Room of the Miner Medical Library) an inscription reads:

> HENRY ALVAH STRONG
> HELEN GRIFFIN STRONG
>
> MAY THE KINDLINESS
> AND HUMAN SYMPATHY
> WHICH CHARACTERIZED
> THEIR LIVES CONTINUE
> FOREVER THROUGH THE
> MINISTRY OF THIS HOSPITAL

May that legacy long continue.

REFERENCES

1. Ludmerer, K.M. Time to Heal. Oxford University Press, New York. 1999.
2. Block, J.A., Regenstreif, P.I., Griner, P.F. A Community Hospital Payment Experiment Outperforms National Experience. JAMA: 257:193–197, 1987.
3. Hall, W.J., Griner, P.F. Cost-Effective Health Care: The Rochester Experience. Health Affairs. 58–59, spring 1993.
4. Brayer, E. George Eastman: A biography, p. 429. The Johns Hopkins University Press, Baltimore. 1996.

POSTSCRIPT

A healthy institution, like a healthy organism, is one that can respond and adapt successfully to challenges, while preserving its traditional strengths and values. This volume documents the ways in which the men and women working within the several components that comprise the University of Rochester Medical Center have met the challenges that have arisen—decade by decade—over the past three-quarters of a century.

Approaches to medical and nursing education, scientific concepts, and the approaches to patient care that were state-of-the-art in 1925 often seem relatively primitive now. Innovative educational approaches, the ability of researchers to look into every aspect of the human organism at the molecular and genetic level, and an extraordinary array of new diagnostic and treatment modalities have presented us with both challenges and opportunities. This institution is now poised to respond with its characteristic attention to excellence and capacity for innovation, but with a commitment to preserving its traditional values.

It would be a mistake, however, to see this proud continuum as a closed circuit. Every advance in education, medical science, and patient care raises a new challenge. At the University of Rochester, new teams of physicians, scientists, nurses, medical and dental educators, ethicists, and technologists are building on the work of their talented predecessors.

And still the questions multiply. How can we make life healthier and more secure for the growing millions of our elderly? How can we teach young people the importance of healthy living, of rejecting the lure of high-risk behaviors? How can we ensure that our babies are born healthy, their parents nurturing, their homes safe and non-violent? How can we better provide for those of us living with diseases that once were fatal, but that now require complex, life-long treatment? How can we afford to provide the kind of care we are called on to provide? How can we afford to fund the research needed to answer these compelling questions?

As a new century begins, the University of Rochester Medical Center is taking bold steps to meet these challenges. We are proceeding along a path made straight and secure by those who came before us. In this year 2000, the "farthest star" that has lighted our way for so many years continues to shine brightly, leading us into a future that holds great promise.

Meliora!

—The Editors